T0211571

Lecture Notes in Artificial Intelligence 9794

Subseries of Lecture Notes in Computer Science

More information about this series at http://www.springer.com/series/1244

Huiping Cao · Jinyan Li · Ruili Wang (Eds.)

Trends and Applications in Knowledge Discovery and Data Mining

PAKDD 2016 Workshops, BDM, MLSDA, PACC, WDMBF
Auckland, New Zealand, April 19, 2016
Revised Selected Papers

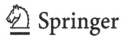 Springer

Editors
Huiping Cao
New Mexico State University
Las Cruces, NM
USA

Jinyan Li
University of Technology
Sydney, NSW
Australia

Ruili Wang
Massey University
Auckland
New Zealand

ISSN 0302-9743   ISSN 1611-3349 (electronic)
Lecture Notes in Artificial Intelligence
ISBN 978-3-319-42995-3   ISBN 978-3-319-42996-0 (eBook)
DOI 10.1007/978-3-319-42996-0

Library of Congress Control Number: 2016944916

LNCS Sublibrary: SL7 – Artificial Intelligence

Printed on acid-free paper

This Springer imprint is published by Springer Nature
The registered company is Springer International Publishing AG Switzerland

Preface

This edited volume contains selected papers from the four workshops that were held on April 19, 2016, in Auckland, New Zealand. These workshops were run in conjunction with the 20th Pacific-Asia Conference on Knowledge Discovery and Data Mining (PAKDD 2016), a leading international conference in the areas of data mining and knowledge discovery. The four workshops are: Workshop on Biologically Inspired Data Mining Techniques (BDM), Workshop on Machine Learning for Sensory Data Analysis (MLSDA), Workshop on Predictive Analytics for Critical Care (PACC), and Workshop on Data Mining in Business and Finance (WDMBF). The aim of these workshops was to provide forums for discussing research topics related to emerging data mining theories and real-life applications, where knowledge discovery was found to be necessary and/or useful.

The PAKDD 2016 workshops received a total of 38 full-length paper submissions. Each submitted paper was rigorously reviewed by at least two Program Committee members. Although many papers were worthy of publication, only 23 regular papers could be accepted for presentation at the workshops and publication in this volume.

The general quality of submissions was high and the competition was tough. We would like to thank all the authors who submitted their papers on many exciting and important research topics to the PAKDD workshops. We thank the workshop organizers for their tremendous effort and valuable time to make the workshops possible. We also thank all the workshop participants and presenters for attending these workshops. It is our hope that the workshops will provide a lasting platform for disseminating the latest research results and practice of data-mining approaches and applications.

These workshops would not have been possible without the help of many colleagues. We would like to thank the Program Committee members for their invaluable review time and comments. Given the extremely tight review schedule, their effort to complete the review reports before the deadline was greatly appreciated. In addition, we found some reviewers' comments were truly excellent, as good as what is usually found in a survey paper—critical, constructive, and comprehensive. These comments were very helpful for us in selecting the papers.

Thank you all and may the papers collected in the volume inspire your thoughts and research.

May 2016

Huiping Cao
Jinyan Li
Ruili Wang

Organization

Workshop Co-chairs

Huiping Cao   New Mexico State University, USA
Jinyan Li   University of Technology Sydney, Australia

BDM Workshop (The 5th PAKDD Workshop on Biologically Inspired Data Mining Techniques)

Workshop Organizers

Shafiq Alam Burki   University of Auckland, New Zealand
Gillian Dobbie   University of Auckland, New Zealand

Program Committee

Patricia Riddle   University of Auckland, New Zealand
Kamran Shafi   DSARC, UNSW, Australia
Stephen Chen   York University, Canada
Kouroush Neshatian   University of Canterbury, Christchurch, New Zealand
Ganesh Kumar   Missouri University of Science and Technology, USA
   Venayagamoorthy
Yanjun Yan   Western Carolina University, USA
Ming Li   Nanjing University, China
Ismail Khalil   Johannes Kepler University, Austria
David Taniar   Monash University, Australia
Redda Alhaj   University of Calgary, Canada
Lean Yu   Chinese Academy of Sciences (CAS), China
Fatos Xhafa   Universitat Politecnica de Catalunya, Spain
Xiao-Zhi Gao   Aalto University, Finland
Emilio Corchado   University of Burgas, Bulgaria
Michela Antonelli   University of Pisa, Italy
Khalid Saeed   AGH Krakow, Poland
Richi Nayek   QUT, Australia
Saeed u Rehman   Unitec, Institute of Technology Auckland,
                               New Zealand
Zawar Shah   Whitireia Comunity Polytechnic, New Zealand

MLSDA Workshop (Machine Learning for Sensory Data Analysis)

Workshop Organizers

Ashfaqur Rahman	CISRO Australia
Bernhard Pfahringer	The University of Waikato, New Zealand
Jiuyong Li	The University of South Australia
Jeremiah D. Deng	University of Otago, New Zealand

Program Committee

Adnan Al-Anbuky	AUT, New Zealand
Weidong Cai	Sydney, Australia
Rachael Cardell-Oliver	UWA, Australia
Paulo De Souza	CSIRO, Australia
Jeremiah Deng	Otago, New Zealand
Alberto Elfes	CSIRO, Australia
Clinton Fookes	QUT, Australia
Jia Hu	Hope, UK
Yuan Jiang	Nanjing, China
Eamonn Keogh	UCR, USA
Irena Koprinska	Sydney, Australia
Daniel Lai	Victoria, Australia
Ickjai Lee	James Cook, Australia
Ivan Lee	South Australia, Australia
Christopher Leckie	Melbourne, Australia
Jiuyong Li	South Australia, Australia
Craig Lindley	CSIRO, Australia
Ann Nowé	VUB, Belgium
Mariusz Nowostawski	Gjøvik University College, Norway
Paul Pang	Unitec, New Zealand
Matthew Parry	Otago, New Zealand
Yonghong Peng	Bradford, UK
Bernhard Pfahringer	Waikato, New Zealand
Martin Purvis	Otago, New Zealand
Ashfaqur Rahman	CISRO, Australia
Daniel Smith	Data61, CSIRO, Australia
James S.C. Tan	(UniSIM), Singapore
Duc A. Tran	Massachusetts, USA
Zhiyong Wang	Sydney, Australia
Brendon Woodford	Otago, New Zealand
Haibo Zhang	Otago, New Zealand
Jun Zhang	Sun Yat-sen, China
Zhi-hua Zhou	Nanjing, China
Xingquan Zhu	UTS, Australia

PACC Workshop (The First International Workshop on Predictive Analytics for Critical Care)

Workshop Organizers

Vaibhav Rajan	Xerox Research Centre, India
Geetha Manjunath	Xerox Research Centre, India

Program Committee

Chiranjib Bhattacharyya	Indian Institute of Science (IISc), India
Sakyajit Bhattacharya	Xerox Research Centre India (XRCI), India
Inderjit Dhillon	University of Texas, Austin, USA
Shuai Huang	University of Washington, USA
Gang Luo	University of Utah, USA
Sriganesh Madhvanath	Palo Alto Research Centre (PARC), USA
Chandan Reddy	Wayne State University, USA
S. Sadagopan	IIIT-Bangalore, India
Jing Zhou	Palo Alto Research Centre (PARC), USA

WDMBF Workshop (Workshop on Data Mining in Business and Finance)

Workshop Organizers

Ling Liu	Southwestern University of Finance and Economics, China
Qing Li	Southwestern University of Finance and Economics, China
Yuanzhu Chen	Memorial University of Newfoundland, Canada
Weidong Huo	Southwestern University of Finance and Economics, China

Program Committee

Ting Hu	Memorial University of Newfoundland, Canada
Sung Hyon Myaeng	KAIST, Korea
Keng Siau	Missouri University of Science and Technology, USA
Sa-kwang Song	KISTI, Korea
Shengyan Sun	IBM, China
Zhangxi Lin	Texas Tech University, USA
Juchen Yang	Tianjin Tech University, China
Weiwei Yuan	Harbin Engineering University, China

Contents

Predictive Analytics for Critical Care (PACC)

Data Mining in Business and Finance (WDMBF)

Biologically Inspired Data Mining Techniques (BDM)

Towards a New Evolutionary Subsampling Technique for Heuristic Optimisation of Load Disaggregators

Michael Mayo[✉] and Sara Omranian

Department of Computer Science, University of Waikato, Hamilton, New Zealand
mmayo@waikato.ac.nz, sara.omranian@gmail.com

Abstract. In this paper we present some preliminary work towards the development of a new evolutionary subsampling technique for solving the non-intrusive load monitoring (NILM) problem. The NILM problem concerns using predictive algorithms to analyse whole-house energy usage measurements, so that individual appliance energy usages can be disaggregated. The motivation is to educate home owners about their energy usage. However, by their very nature, the datasets used in this research are massively imbalanced in their target value distributions. Consequently standard machine learning techniques, which often rely on optimising for root mean squared error (RMSE), typically fail. We therefore propose the target-weighted RMSE (TW-RMSE) metric as an alternative fitness function for optimising load disaggregators, and show in a simple initial study in which random search is utilised that TW-RMSE is a metric that can be optimised, and therefore has the potential to be included in a larger evolutionary subsampling-based solution to this problem.

Keywords: Non-intrusive load monitoring · Disaggregation · Imbalanced regression · Fitness function · Evolutionary undersampling

1 Introduction

A significant problem facing modern society is ensuring the efficient use of energy resources. One area where energy efficiency improvements can be made is in the domestic arena. If householders understand their own individual energy usages, down to the level of detail of individual appliances, then they are more likely to change their behaviour in way that conserves energy [11]. However, the main problem with this is that a household typically has tens of appliances and power outlets, and for accurate monitoring and reporting to householders, sub-meters must be physically installed at each outlet.

Non-intrusive load monitoring (NILM) is an alternative to this that attempts to replace sub-meters with machine learning algorithms. The algorithms are used to train models that predict individual appliance/power outlet energy usage from the stream of whole-house energy usage that is provided by a typical smart meter.

© Springer International Publishing Switzerland 2016
H. Cao et al. (Eds.): PAKDD 2016 Workshops, LNAI 9794, pp. 3–14, 2016.
DOI: 10.1007/978-3-319-42996-0_1

Although this field has been a focus of research for many years (ever since Hart's seminal 1992 paper [5]), it has developed dramatically with the much more recent advent of smart meters capable of measuring household energy consumption at high frequency. New and massive datasets have been captured and are currently being analysed in research contexts.

To put the disaggregation problem into a more formal context, let us assume that there are n appliances and/or power outlets (hereafter simply referred to as an appliance), labelled $A^{(1)}, A^{(2)}, \ldots A^{(n)}$ and that ith appliance's energy usage at time t is $A_t^{(i)}$. The values of $A_t^{(i)}$ are unknown (except in the training data) and to be predicted for each appliance. The only values that are known are the stream of whole house energy use measurements $Z_1, Z_2, \ldots Z_{t-2}, Z_{t-1}, Z_t$ leading up to the current time (t).

We note that the unit of measurement can be any acceptable measure of energy usage. In this work, we adopt *current*, measured in amperes (A), as the stream to measure and predict. This follows Makonin et al.'s [7] analysis showing that current is the most reliable measure for data analysis because it fluctuates to a much lesser degree than other measures such as real power (which is frequently used in other research works in this field).

The remainder of this paper is organised as follows. In Sect. 2 a brief background provided. In Sect. 3 a new metric named target-weighted RMSE (TW-RMSE) is introduced to address the problem of imbalance that occurs in the of regression target variables in most disaggregation datasets. Then, in Sect. 4, a random search–based algorithm is presented to select a regression model that optimizes TW-RMSE. Section 5 evaluates the presented approaches on the AMPds dataset [7] and makes a complete comparison between RMSE and TW-RMSE. Lastly, Sect. 6 concludes the paper.

2 Background

2.1 Load Disaggregation

Non-intrusive load monitoring/disaggregation research goes back many years. One of the first researchers who proposed a disaggregation method was Hart [5], who stated that in order to decompose the total load into its components, models of individual appliances and their combinations were needed. He was also the first to observe that the power consumed by appliances was additive, i.e. if the loads of all appliances in a household are known, then at any time t the following equality holds: $Z_t = \sum_i A_t^{(i)}$.

With the introduction of more powerful computers and significantly more memory and processing power, disaggregation research took a large step forward. Zeifman and Roth [12], for example, proposed an algorithm that uses stepwise power changes, power surges, and time-on and time-off durations as features. His approach used historical data for initial training of a disaggregation model. The main aspect of his algorithm was the use of approximate semi-Markov models which could make robust computationally-efficient predictions. The downside of his algorithm was that it only worked with on/off appliances and not general appliances which may be in multiple discrete states, or transition continuously between states.

2.2 AMPds v2 Dataset

The Almanac of Minutely Power dataset ("AMPds") was introduced by Makonin et al. [7] in 2013, and a revision (version 2) released sometime afterwards. This dataset is a record of one house containing both total and submetered power data from 25 submeters at one minute intervals for two years (from 1 April 2012 until 31 March 2014). The dataset comprises 1,051,200 records and includes, besides the meter readings, additional data about water usage and climate. As Fig. 1 depicts, the measurements of current draw which are the focus of our predictive experiments are highly imbalanced. The figure shows the log frequencies of current draws for a washing machine for one year's worth of data.

As mentioned in the Introduction, a major finding of the authors of the AMPds dataset and its associated paper was the fact that current provides better quality predictions than real power. Another new idea in this paper was the introduction of a novel method for discretising current draws, to fit the notion of appliances being like finite state machines (i.e. many appliances operate in discrete states, such as ON/OFF or LOW/MEDIUM/HIGH).

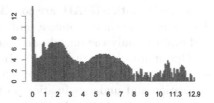

Fig. 1. Log frequencies of washing machine current draws. Shown are current draw (x) vs. the log frequency (in seconds) when that level of current usage was metered (y).

While a classification approach to solving this problem is reasonable, we focus in this paper instead on regression and attempt to predict appliance current draw directly. If a good regression-based solution to the problem is found, the approach can be adapted to the classification setting by discretising current using the approach described by Makonin et al. [7]. Another reason for adopting a regression-based approach to the problem is that the finite state machine abstraction is not true for all appliances: some devices clearly vary continuously in their energy usage, and even for appliances that do appear to operate in discrete states, the number of and boundaries between each state are not always clear (as Fig. 1 attests).

2.3 Evolutionary Machine Learning for Massive Imbalanced Regression Problems

To date, few prior works exist on the problem of regression using imbalanced datasets [1]. This is because most of the classical imbalanced dataset research in machine learning concerns classification rather than regression. Furthermore, the authors are unaware of any prior evolutionary machine learning works on the imbalanced regression problem, let along any works considering the problem in the context of load disaggregation. This is a potentially rewarding area for research, therefore. Given the paucity of evolutionary approaches to this problem, some of the few non-evolutionary approaches will be briefly mentioned.

The earliest work on regression with imbalanced data is the paper by Torgo and Ribeiro [10] in which the standard SMOTE algorithm [3] was adapted to a regression setting. Essentially, the modified SMOTE algorithm under-sampled examples with target values that occur more frequently in the data. They also considered the two different ways of creating a balanced sample: under-sampling and over-sampling. They believed over-sampling was generally better than under-sampling, especially when small samples were involved. This made sense to the authors, since by using under-sampling full use of the available data was not made.

Beyond that, further works concerning imbalanced regression have only been published very recently. A common approach is to define new metrics for the problem As justification, Branco et al. [1] argue that performance measures commonly used in regression, such as Mean Squared Error (MSE) and Mean Absolute Deviation (MAD) are not adequate for imbalanced regression problems. This is because they assume a uniform relevance of the target variable domain and evaluate only the magnitude (and not the direction) of the error.

One approach was presented by Hernández-Orallo [6], which introduced ROC space for regression (RROC). RROC space is defined by plotting total over-estimation and under-estimation on the x and y axes respectively. The author also proposed area over the RROC curve (AOC) as a metric, but the drawback of his approach was it only accounted for under-predictions. Another metric proposed by Ribeiro [9] and Torgo and Ribeiro [10] is based on the concept of utility-based regression for precision/recall metrics. Utility-based regression uses the notion of non-uniform relevance of the target variable values across the domain of the target to define a metric. For example, certain parts of the target variable domain may be more critical than others; therefore the utility is higher. This notion of utility led to the proposal of metrics such as the Mean Utility and the Normalized Mean Utility by Riberio [9], and then to a utility-based regression algorithm based on regression rule ensembles called ubaRules [9].

3   Target-Weighted RMSE Metric

To address the problem of massive imbalance that occurs in the AMPds dataset we propose a modification to the standard RMSE metric for evaluating regressors. We name the new metric target-weighted RMSE (TW-RMSE).

The basic idea is related to the notion of macroaveraged accuracy [8] in information retrieval. Macroaveraged accuracy is a alternative metric for evaluating classification models in which individual classes are weighted equally in the accuracy calculation, as opposed to the weighting being on individual examples (which is the case for normal or "micro"-averaged accuracy). As Manning et al. state, common classification metrics such as the F1 measure fail when the imbalance is overwhelming. And this is largely because the F1 metric is a micro-averaging approach. Macroaveraging, on the other hand, is an attempt to eliminate the problem of massive class imbalance.

Since our problem domain is regression, however, we do not have readily available class labels to make use of. Therefore we define proxy class labels for each example by dividing the range of the predictive target variable into equal-width bins, and we treat an example's bin as its class label for the purposes of balancing, resampling, and computing performance metrics.

Furthermore, we allow the user to specify (i) the number of bins and (ii) an individual weight for each bin. The weights serve a similar purpose to utility in utility-based regression, in that they allow the user to focus the metric on particular ranges of current draw. For example, if the user is only interested in particular states that an appliance may be in, then the weights for the corresponding ranges of current usage can be increased when the metric is calculated.

Once the ranges and weights are set, an RMSE value is calculated for test example predictions in each range. The TW-RMSE is the weighted average of these individual RMSE values. Algorithm 1 shows pseudocode for performing this calculation.

Input: $\mathbf{Y} = \{(y_1, y_1^*), (y_2, y_2^*) \ldots (y_n, y_n^*)\}$, a vector of predicted (y_i) and actual (y_i^*) values for n training or test examples; m, number of bins; $\mathbf{w} = \{w_1, w_2 \ldots w_m\}$, a vector of weights for the bins

begin

$\quad$ $l \leftarrow min(y_1^*, y_2^* \ldots y_n^*)$;
$\quad$ $u \leftarrow max(y_1^*, y_2^* \ldots y_n^*)$;
$\quad$ Divide the range $(u - l)$ into m equal-width bins $\mathbf{B} = \{b_1, b_2 \ldots b_m\}$;
$\quad$ Assign each $(y_i, y_i^*) \in \mathbf{Y}$ to the appropriate bin in $\mathbf{B}$ (using the y_i^* value);
$\quad$ Delete any empty bins from $\mathbf{B}$;
$\quad$ Compute the RMSE $r(b_j)$ for the predictions in each $b_j \in \mathbf{B}$;
$\quad$ $t \leftarrow \sum_{b_j \in \mathbf{B}} w_j r(b_j)$ where $w_j \in \mathbf{w}$ is bin b_j's weight;

end

Output: t, the TW-RMSE metric

$\quad$ **Algorithm 1.** Algorithm to compute the TW-RMSE metric.

Effectively, this approach should give an unbiased error estimate if the dataset is imbalanced. As the number of bins is reduced, however, the TW-RMSE metric becomes an approximation of the RMSE metric: therefore the user must ensure that the number of bins is set correctly.

4 Random Search-Based Algorithm to Optimise TW-RMSE

To demonstrate the potential utility of the TW-RMSE metric for appliance energy usage modelling, we propose a simple random resampling-based algorithm that uses TW-RMSE to select an optimal training sample for a regressor.

The approach can be divided into two parts. Firstly, Algorithm 2 depicts a method for creating a balanced resample from the original, highly imbalanced, training dataset. The approach taken is similar to the algorithm for computing TW-RMSE, except that instead of binning predictions, this time the examples in the training set are iteratively resampled into bins that are the same size. A parameter s governs the overall size of the sample.

Input: $\mathbf{X} = \{(\mathbf{x_1}, y_1^*), (\mathbf{x_2}, y_2^*) \ldots (\mathbf{x_n}, y_n^*)\}$, a training dataset of examples $(\mathbf{x_i})$ and targets (y_i^*); m, number of bins; s, desired sample size $(s << n)$;

begin

    $l \leftarrow min(y_1^*, y_2^* \ldots y_n^*)$;

    $u \leftarrow max(y_1^*, y_2^* \ldots y_n^*)$;

    Divide the range $(u - l)$ into m equal-width bins $\mathbf{B} = \{b_1, b_2 \ldots b_m\}$;

    Assign each example $(\mathbf{x_i}, y_i^*) \in \mathbf{X}$ to the appropriate bin in $\mathbf{B}$ (using the y_i^* value);

    Delete any empty bins from $\mathbf{B}$;

    $\mathbf{S} \leftarrow \emptyset$;

    repeat

        foreach $b \in \mathbf{B}$ **do**

            if $|\mathbf{S}| < s$ **then**

                | Randomly resample one example from b into $\mathbf{S}$

            end

        end

    until $|\mathbf{S}| \geq s$;

end

Output: $\mathbf{S}$, a balanced resampling of the dataset

Algorithm 2. Algorithm to create a balanced resample of examples.

The second part of the algorithm is a simple random search procedure, pseudocode of which Algorithm 3 depicts. The algorithm essentially repeatedly resamples the entire training dataset, creating a small balanced resample with each iteration. A regressor is then trained on each sample, and the TW-RMSE metric computed for the sample. The regressor with the smallest TW-RMSE is returned after a fixed number of iterations.

In the next section, it will be shown that this approach results in a significant decrease in TW-RMSE for most appliances, but that RMSE on the whole is unchanged (thus validating our rationale for TW-RMSE).

5   Evaluation

In order to evaluate the effectiveness of TW-RMSE as a metric for evaluating and selecting regression models in the presence of imbalance, we performed an extensive set of experiments on portions of the AMPds v2 dataset [7]. The dataset itself contains energy usage data (including current, real power and voltage) for a large number of sub-metered appliances.

Input: $\mathbf{X} = \{(\mathbf{x_1}, y_1^*), (\mathbf{x_2}, y_2^*) \dots (\mathbf{x_n}, y_n^*)\}$, a training dataset of examples $(\mathbf{x_i})$ and targets (y_i^*); m, number of bins; s, desired sample size $(s << n)$; i, number of iterations

begin

    $\mathbf{S}_{best} \leftarrow$ a subset of the training data $\mathbf{X}$ selected using Algorithm 2;

    $R \leftarrow$ a regressor trained on $\mathbf{S}_{best}$;

    $t_{best} \leftarrow$ TW-RMSE of R_{best} evaluated against $\mathbf{S}_{best}$ calculated using Algorithm 1;

    for $iteration \leftarrow 2 \dots i$ **do**

        $\mathbf{S} \leftarrow$ a subset of the training data $\mathbf{X}$ selected using Algorithm 2;

        $R \leftarrow$ a regressor trained on $\mathbf{S}$;

        $t \leftarrow$ TW-RMSE of R evaluated against $\mathbf{S}$ calculated using Algorithm 1;

        if $t < t_{best}$ **then**

           | $R_{best} \leftarrow R$

        end

    end

end

Output: R_{best}, the best regressor obtained.

Algorithm 3. Training algorithm based on random search and model selection.

We selected nine sub-meters to analyse, specifically the same sub-meters as previously analysed in a classification setting by Makonin et al. [7]: the basement plugs and lights (BME), the clothes dryer (CDE), the clothes washer (CWE), the dishwasher (DWE), the kitchen fridge (FGE), the HVAC/furnace (FRE), the heat pump (HPE), the entertainment unit (TVE) and finally the wall oven (WOE). In each case, we extracted and built predictive models for the current (A) time series only. These formed our (unknown) $A_t^{(i)}$ values for the evaluation. We also extracted from the dataset the whole-house (WHE) current draw, which were our (known) Z_t values. As mentioned previously, the total length of each time series, covering two years worth of data sampled once per second in each case, is 1,051,201 samples.

A sliding window approach was used to generate a dataset suitable for learning regression models. Essentially, this approach generates examples by "sliding" a fixed-size window along the WHE series, creating one each example for each position that the window can occupy. Since the window size we chose was fixed at 60, each example's features therefore correspond to whole-house energy usage for the past 60 s.

Unlike standard time series prediction, however, the prediction target for each example is not the next WHE value. Instead it is the corresponding sub-meter reading. Notation-wise, the features are $Z_{t-59}, Z_{t-58} \dots Z_{t-1}, Z_t$ and the prediction target is $A_t^{(i)}$ where i is the sub-meter index and t is the current time in seconds.

This procedure produced a dataset with $(1,051,201 - 60 =)\,1,051,141$ examples. Since the examples are ordered in time (and therefore the i.i.d. assumption does not hold), we further divided these examples into two subsequences: the

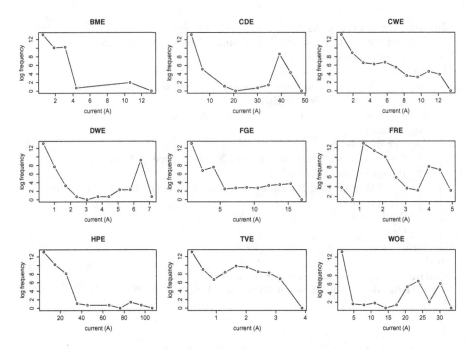

Fig. 2. Distribution of target (i.e. appliance current) values in the test sets. Note that the y axis shows the *log* frequencies rather than the raw frequencies.

first 50 % of examples (a year's worth of data) were used for training, and the second 50 % (a second year's worth of data) for testing. A total of nine datasets for the nine sub-metered appliances were created in this way.

Figure 2 shows distributions of current in the test data by appliance, which reinforces seriously imbalanced nature of problem.

We used the standard random forest classifier adapted for regression for our experiments [2]. The number of random trees in the forest is set to 100, and the number of random features selected per tree was $\lfloor log_2(60) + 1 \rfloor = 7$.

In our first experiment, we trained a random forest regressor on each *entire* training set (i.e. we ignored Algorithms 2 and 3), and then we evaluated its performance on the corresponding test sets.

Figure 3 shows the distribution of RMSE by bin across the test data for this first experiment. This figure illustrates nicely how error generally increases with current draw. Increased current draw usually corresponds to smaller frequencies in the datasets.

Table 1 gives values for both RMSE and TW-RMSE (using $m = 10$ bins and uniform $w_i = \frac{1}{m}$ weights) computed on the test datasets. These values are useful for determining the effects of Algorithms 2 and 3 in our next experiments.

Next, we trained the random forests model on a single resample of the training data (obtained using Algorithm 2) and tested it against the entire test dataset.

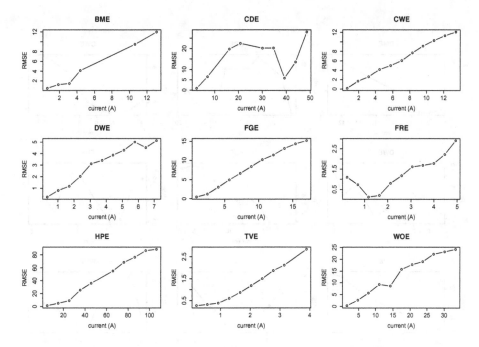

Fig. 3. RMSE values calculated for each bin in the test sets, using regressor trained on full training sets.

Table 1. Test results after training a random forest classifier on the entire training dataset.

Appliance	RMSE	TW-RMSE
BME	0.62	4.78
CDE	1.09	15.26
CWE	0.43	6.37
DWE	0.66	3.05
FGE	0.54	8.06
FRE	0.29	1.30
HPE	1.82	45.04
TVE	0.43	1.20
WOE	1.13	13.49

The number of bins m and the weights w_i are the same as in the previous experiment, and we set the sample size $s = 10,000$. Figure 4 and Table 2 depict the results.

Two observations can be made from these results. Firstly, TW-RMSE is reduced by a significant amount when the regressor is trained on the small resampled training dataset compared to being trained on the entire training dataset.

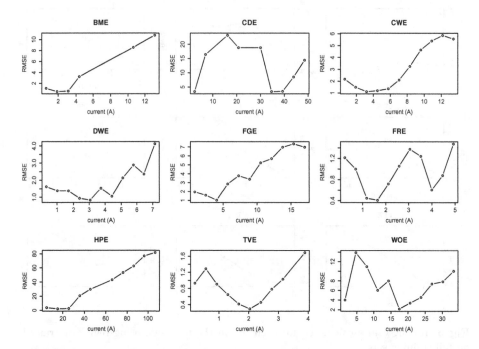

Fig. 4. RMSE values calculated for each bin in the test sets, using regressor trained on a balanced resample of the training set selected using Algorithm 2.

Table 2. Test results after training a random forest classifier on a balanced resample of the training dataset selected using Algorithm 2. Results marked [a]indicate an improvement compared to training on the entire training dataset. Results marked [b]indicate that the improvement is more than 10 %.

Appliance	RMSE	TW-RMSE
BME	1.07	4.13[b]
CDE	3.47	12.29[b]
CWE	2.16	3.10[b]
DWE	1.63	1.84[b]
FGE	1.95	4.26[b]
FRE	0.46	0.95[b]
HPE	3.74	37.63[b]
TVE	0.91	0.85[b]
WOE	4.03	7.11[b]

Table 3. Test results after training a random forest classifier using Algorithm 3. Results marked [a]indicate an improvement compared to training on only a single balanced sample. Results marked [b]indicate that the improvement is more than 10 %.

Appliance	RMSE	TW-RMSE
BME	1.07	3.40[b]
CDE	3.34[a]	12.02[a]
CWE	2.18	3.13
DWE	1.57[a]	1.78[a]
FGE	1.94[a]	4.27
FRE	0.46	0.67[b]
HPE	3.84	32.08[b]
TVE	0.90[a]	0.45[b]
WOE	4.31	7.24

This is clearly evident graphically when Figs. 3 and 4 are compared: for many appliances, e.g. the wall oven (WOE), the error curve no long approximately increases with increasing current draw. This graphical difference is reflected in changes in the TW-RMSE metric which in all cases is more that 10 % and sometimes 50 % reduced in magnitude (comparing Tables 1 and 2).

In contrast, comparison between the tables also shows that the RMSE metric does not decrease at all. In fact, the more balanced subsampling results in an overall increase of RMSE because of the much greater emphasis given to the majority of examples in which the appliance is in an off or low energy state.

Finally, we ran Algorithm 3 for $i = 100$ iterations, and the results are shown in Table 3. Comparing to Table 2, there is a further marked decrease in TW-RMSE for seven of the sub-meters as a consequence of the random search. The only appliances that did not show improvement when Algorithm 3 was applied with 100 as opposed to 1 iteration were the clothes washer (CWE), the kitchen fridge (FGE) and the wall oven (WOE). However, on the whole, most of the sub-meter predictions further improve compared to Table 2. This show that the TW-RMSE metric, when computed on a training set, is a good indicator of generalisation performance.

6   Conclusion

This work represents our first step towards the development of an evolutionary subsampling technique for solving the NILM problem. The main contribution of interest here is a new fitness metric, namely TW-RMSE, which can counter the effect of massive imbalance that occurs in typical NILM datasets. A further lesser contribution is an algorithm inspired by TW-RMSE for generating balanced random under-samples of examples.

The results here are promising and demonstrate that TW-RMSE has potential to be a useful fitness metric. Our next steps will be (i) to investigate the potential sensitivity of the metric to its key parameters, such as the number of bins; and (ii) to couple TW-RMSE with a more state-of-the-art evolutionary subsampling algorithm (e.g. a method reviewed by Derrac et al. [4]) in order to more properly evaluate its potential.

References

1. Branco, P., Torgo, L., Ribeiro, R.: A survey of predictive modelling under imbalanced distributions (2015). arXiv:1505.01658v2
2. Breiman, L.: Random forests. Mach. Learn. **45**(1), 5–32 (2001)
3. Chawla, N.V., Bowyer, K.W., Hall, L.O., Kegelmeyer, W.P.: SMOTE: synthetic minority over-sampling technique. J. Artif. Intell. Res. **16**(1), 321–357 (2002)
4. Derrac, J., Garcia, S., Herrera, F.: A survey of evolutionary instance selection and generation. Int. J. Appl. Metaheuristic Comput. **1**(1), 60–92 (2010)
5. Hart, G.W.: Nonintrusive appliance load monitoring. Proc. IEEE **80**(12), 1870–1891 (1992)
6. Hernández-Orallo, J.: ROC curves for regression. Pattern Recogn. **46**(12), 3395–3411 (2013)
7. Makonin, S., Popowich, F., Bartram, L., Gill, B., Bajic, I.: AMPds: a public dataset for load disaggregation and eco-feedback research. In: 2013 IEEE Electrical Power Energy Conference (EPEC), pp. 1–6 (2013)
8. Manning, C.D., Raghavan, P., Schütze, H.: Introduction to Information Retrieval. Cambridge University Press, Cambridge (2008)
9. Ribeiro, R.: Utility-based regression. Ph.D. thesis, Department of Computer Science, Faculty of Sciences, University of Porto (2011)
10. Torgo, L., Ribeiro, R.: Utility-based regression. In: Kok, J.N., Koronacki, J., Lopez de Mantaras, R., Matwin, S., Mladenič, D., Skowron, A. (eds.) PKDD 2007. LNCS (LNAI), vol. 4702, pp. 597–604. Springer, Heidelberg (2007)
11. Vine, D., Buys, L., Morris, P.: The effectiveness of energy feedback for conservation and peak demand: a literature review. Open J. Energy Effic. **2**, 7–15 (2013)
12. Zeifman, M., Roth, K.: Nonintrusive appliance load monitoring: review and outlook. IEEE Trans. Consum. Electron. **57**, 76–84 (2011)

Neural Choice by Elimination
via Highway Networks

Truyen Tran$^{(\boxtimes)}$, Dinh Phung, and Svetha Venkatesh

Centre for Pattern Recognition and Data Analytics, Deakin University,
Geelong, Australia
truyen.tran@deakin.edu.au

Abstract. We introduce *Neural Choice by Elimination*, a new framework that integrates deep neural networks into probabilistic sequential choice models for learning to rank. Given a set of items to chose from, the elimination strategy starts with the whole item set and iteratively eliminates the least worthy item in the remaining subset. We prove that the choice by elimination is equivalent to marginalizing out the random Gompertz latent utilities. Coupled with the choice model is the recently introduced Neural Highway Networks for approximating arbitrarily complex rank functions. We evaluate the proposed framework on a large-scale public dataset with over $425K$ items, drawn from the Yahoo! learning to rank challenge. It is demonstrated that the proposed method is competitive against state-of-the-art learning to rank methods.

1 Introduction

People often rank options when making choice. Ranking is central in many social and individual contexts, ranging from election [16], sports [17], information retrieval [22], question answering [1], to recommender systems [32]. We focus on a setting known as learning to rank (L2R) in which the system learns to choose and rank items (e.g. a set of documents, potential answers, or shopping items) in response to a query (e.g., keywords, a question, or an user).

Two main elements of a L2R system are rank model and rank function. One of the most promising rank models is listwise [22] where all items responding to the query are considered simultaneously. Most existing work in L2R focuses on designing listwise rank losses rather than formal models of *choice*, a crucial aspect of building preference-aware applications. One of a few exceptions is the Plackett-Luce model which originates from Luce's axioms of choice [24] and is later used in the context of L2R under the name ListMLE [34]. The Plackett-Luce model offers a natural interpretation of making sequential choices. First, the probability of choosing an item is proportional to its worth. Second, once the most probable item is chosen, the next item will be picked from the remaining items in the same fashion.

However, the Plackett-Luce model suffers from two drawbacks. First, the model spends effort to separate items down the rank list, while only the first few items are usually important in practice. Thus the effort in making the right

H. Cao et al. (Eds.): PAKDD 2016 Workshops, LNAI 9794, pp. 15–25, 2016.
DOI: 10.1007/978-3-319-42996-0_2

ordering should be spent on more important items. Second, the Plackett-Luce is inadequate in explaining many competitive situations, e.g., sport tournaments and buying preferences, where the ranking process is reversed – worst items are eliminated first [33].

Addressing these drawbacks, we introduce a probabilistic sequential rank model termed *choice by elimination*. At each step, we remove one item and repeat until no item is left. The rank of items is then the reverse of the elimination order. This elimination process has an important property: Near the end of the process, only best items compete against the others. This is unlike the selection process in Plackett-Luce, where the best items are contrasted against all other alternatives. We may face difficulty in separating items of similarly high quality but can ignore irrelevant items effortlessly. The elimination model thus reflects more effort in ranking worthy items.

Once the ranking model has been specified, the next step in L2R is to design a rank function $f(x)$ of query-specific item attributes x [22]. We leverage the newly introduced *highway networks* [28] as a rank function approximator. Highway networks are a compact deep neural network architecture that enables passing information and gradient through hundreds of hidden layers between input features and the function output. The highway networks coupled with the proposed elimination model constitute a new framework termed *Neural Choice by Elimination (NCE)* illustrated in Fig. 1.

The framework is an alternative to the current state-of-the-arts in L2R which involve tree ensembles [4,5,12] trained with hand-crafted metric-aware

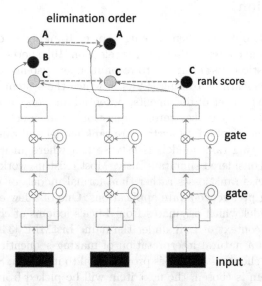

Fig. 1. *Neural choice by elimination* with 4-layer highway networks for ranking three items (A,B,C). Empty boxes represent hidden layers that share the same parameters (hence, recurrent). Double circles are gate that controls information flow. Dark filled circles represent a chosen item at each step – here the elimination order is (B,A,C).

losses [7,21]. Unlike the tree ensembles where typically hundreds of trees are maintained, highway networks can be trained with *dropouts* [27] to produce an implicit ensemble with only one thin network. Hence we aim to establish that *deep neural networks are competitive in L2R*. While shallow neural networks have been used in ranking before [6], they were outperformed by tree ensembles [21]. Deep neural nets are compact and more powerful [3], but they have not been measured against tree-based ensembles for generic L2R problems. We empirically demonstrate the effectiveness of the proposed ideas on a large-scale public dataset from Yahoo! L2R challenge with totally 18.4 thousands queries and 425 thousands documents.

To summarize, our paper makes the following contributions: (i) introducing a new neural sequential choice model for learning to rank; and (ii) establishing that deep nets are scalable and competitive as rank function approximator in large-scale settings.

2   Background

2.1   Related Work

The elimination process has been found in multiple competitive situations such as multiple round contests and buying decisions [14]. *Choice by elimination* of distractors has been long studied in the psychological literature, since the pioneer work of Tversky [33]. These backward elimination models may offer better explanation than the forward selection when eliminating aspects are available [33]. However, existing studies are mostly on selecting a single best choice. Multiple sequential eliminations are much less studied [2]. Second, most prior work has been evaluated on a handful of items with several attributes, whereas we consider hundreds of thousands of items with thousands of attributes. Third, the cross-field connection with data mining has not been made. The link between choice models and Random Utility Theory has been well-studied since Thurstone in the 1920s, and is still an active topic [2,30,31]. Deep neural networks for L2R have been studied in the last two years [10,11,18,25,26]. Our work contributes a formal reasoning of human choices together with a newly introduced highway networks which are validated on large-scale public datasets against state-of-the-art methods.

2.2   Plackett-Luce

We now review Plackett-Luce model [24], a forward selection method in learning to rank, also known in the L2R literature as ListMLE [34]. Given a query and a set of response items $\mathcal{I} = (1, 2, .., N)$, the rank choice is an ordering of items $\pi = (\pi_1, \pi_2, ..., \pi_N)$, where π_i is the index of item at rank i. For simplicity, assume that each item π_i is associated with a set of attributes, denoted as $x_{\pi_i} \in \mathbb{R}^p$. A rank function $f(x_{\pi_i})$ is defined on π_i and is independent of other items. We aim to characterize the rank permutation model $P(\pi)$.

Let us start from the classic probabilistic theory that any joint distribution of N variables can be factorized according to the chain-rule as follows

$$P(\boldsymbol{\pi}) = P(\pi_1) \prod_{i=2}^{N} P(\pi_i \mid \boldsymbol{\pi}_{1:i-1}) \tag{1}$$

where $\boldsymbol{\pi}_{1:i-1}$ is a shorthand for $(\pi_1, \pi_2, .., \pi_{i-1})$, and $P(\pi_i \mid \boldsymbol{\pi}_{1:i-1})$ is the probability that item π_i has rank i given all existing higher ranks $1, ..., i-1$. The factorization can be interpreted as follows: choose the first item in the list with probability of $P(\pi_1)$, and choose the second item from the remaining items with probability of $P(\pi_2|\pi_1)$, and so on. Luce's *axioms of choice* assert that an item is chosen with probability proportional to its *worth*. This translates to the following choice model:

$$P(\pi_i \mid \boldsymbol{\pi}_{1:i-1}) = \frac{\exp\left(f(x_{\pi_i})\right)}{\sum_{j=i}^{N} \exp\left(f(x_{\pi_j})\right)}$$

Learning using maximizing likelihood minimizes the log-loss:

$$\ell_1(\boldsymbol{\pi}) = \sum_{i=1}^{N-1} \left(-f(x_{\pi_i}) + \log \sum_{j=i}^{N} \exp\left(f(x_{\pi_j})\right) \right) \tag{2}$$

3   Choice by Elimination

We note that the factorization in Eq. (1) is not unique. If we permute the indices of items, the factorization still holds. Here we derive a *reverse* Plackett-Luce model as follows

$$P(\boldsymbol{\pi}) = Q(\pi_N) \prod_{i=1}^{N-1} Q(\pi_i \mid \boldsymbol{\pi}_{i+1:N}) \tag{3}$$

where $Q(\pi_i \mid \boldsymbol{\pi}_{i+1:N})$ is the probability that item π_i receives rank i given all existing lower ranks $i+1, i+2, ..., N$.

Since π_N is the most irrelevant item in the list, $Q(\pi_N)$ can be considered as the probability of *eliminating* the item. Thus the entire process is backward elimination: The next irrelevant item π_k is eliminated, given that more extraneous items $(\boldsymbol{\pi}_{i>k})$ have already been eliminated. It is reasonable to assume that *the probability of an item being eliminated is inversely proportional to its worth.* This suggests the following specification

$$Q(\pi_i \mid \boldsymbol{\pi}_{i+1:N}) = \frac{\exp\left(-f(x_{\pi_i})\right)}{\sum_{j=1}^{i} \exp\left(-f(x_{\pi_j})\right)}. \tag{4}$$

Note that, due to specific choices of conditional distributions, distributions in Eqs. (1, 3) are generally not the same. With this model, the log-loss has the following form:

$$\ell_2(\boldsymbol{\pi}) = \sum_{i=1}^{N} \left(f(x_{\pi_i}) + \log \sum_{j=1}^{i} \exp\left(-f(x_{\pi_j})\right) \right) \tag{5}$$

3.1 Derivation Using Random Utility Theory

Random Utility Theory [2,29] offers an alternative that explains the ordering of items. Assume that there exists latent utilities $\{u_i\}$, one per item $\{\pi_i\}$. The ordering $P^*(\boldsymbol{\pi})$ is defined as $\Pr(u_1 \geq u_2 \geq ... \geq u_N)$. Here we show that it is linked to *Gompertz distribution*. Let $u_j \geq 0$ denote the latent random utility of item π_j. Let $v_j = e^{bu_j}$, the Gompertz distribution has the PDF $P_j(u_j) = b\eta_j v_j \exp(-\eta_j v_j + \eta_j)$ and the CDF $F_j(u_j) = 1 - \exp(-\eta_j(v_j - 1))$, where $b > 0$ is the scale and $\eta > 0$ is the shape parameter.

At rank i, choosing the worst item π_i translates to ensuring $u_i \leq u_j$ for all $j < i$. The random utility theory states that probability of choosing π_i can be obtained by integrating out all latent utilities subject to the inequality constraints:

$$Q(\pi_i \mid \boldsymbol{\pi}_{i+1:N}) = \int_0^{+\infty} P_i(u_i) \left[\int_{u_i}^{+\infty} \prod_{j<i} P_j(u_j) du_j \right] du_i$$

$$= \int_0^{+\infty} P_i(u_i) \prod_{j<i} (1 - F_j(u_i)) \, du_i$$

$$= \int_0^{+\infty} b_i \eta_{ii} v_i \exp\left(-v_i \sum_{j \leq i} \eta_{ij} + \sum_{j \leq i} \eta_{ij} \right) du_i$$

Note that we have used η_{ij} instead of η_j since this location parameter is specific to rank i. Defining $\eta_{ij} = \exp(-f(x_{\pi_j}))$ and changing the variable from u_i to v_i gives us:

$$Q(\pi_i \mid \boldsymbol{\pi}_{i+1:N}) = \int_1^{+\infty} \eta_{ii} \exp\left(-v_i \sum_{j \leq i} \eta_{ij} + \sum_{j \leq i} \eta_{ij} \right) dv_i$$

$$= \frac{\eta_{ii} e^{\sum_{j \leq i} \eta_j}}{\sum_{j \leq i} \eta_{ij}} \int_1^{+\infty} \exp\left(-v_i \sum_{j \leq i} \eta_{ij} \right) dv_i$$

$$= \frac{\eta_{ii}}{\sum_{j \leq i} \eta_{ij}} = \frac{\exp(-f(x_{\pi_i}))}{\sum_{j=1}^i \exp(-f(x_{\pi_j}))}.$$

This resembles Eq. (4).

Remark: We note in passing that in case of plain Plackett-Luce, $P(\boldsymbol{\pi}) \equiv P^*(\boldsymbol{\pi})$ if and only if u_{π_j} is drawn from a Gumbel distribution of location $f(x_{\pi_j})$ and scale 1 for all $j = 1, 2, ..., N$ [23,35].

3.2 Linear Time Learning

We show that both the loss and its functional gradient can be computed in linear time. Let $\phi_i = \exp(-f(x_{\pi_i}))$, $Z_i = \sum_{j=1}^i \phi_j = \phi_i + Z_{i-1}$, and

$Y_i = \sum_{j=1}^{i} 1/Z_j$. The loss in Eq. (5) becomes $\ell_2(\boldsymbol{\pi}) = \sum_{i=1}^{N} (f(x_{\pi_i}) + \log Z_i)$ which can be evaluated in linear time. The functional gradient is reduced to $\partial_{f_k}\ell_2 = \gamma_k (1 - \phi_k Y_k)$, which is constant for each k.

4   Neural Highway Networks for Rank Function

Once the rank models have been specified, it remains to define the rank function $f(x)$. We propose the novel use of neural highway networks [28] to approximate $f(x)$, under the new ranking loss functions proposed in Eqs. (2, 5). Highway networks are powerful, compact function approximator that overcomes the major bottleneck of standard deep neural networks: with increasing depth, it is much harder to pass information and gradient between input and output. More specifically, highway networks are a special neural network of L nonlinear projection layers, of which $L-1$ layers are recurrent. At the bottom, the data is projected into a K-dimensional space $z = g(b_H + W_X x)$, where g is an element-wise nonlinear transform. Subsequent layers are recursive same-dimensional projections:

$$z_{l+1} \leftarrow H(z_l) * T(z_l) + z_l * (1 - T(z_l))$$

where $H(z) = g(b_H + W_H z)$, $T(z) \in [0,1]^K$ is an element-wise gating function, and $*$ denotes element-wise product. The gate $T(z)$ allows information to pass freely when $T(z) = 0$ and forces total nonlinear transforms when $T(z) = 1$. A typical implementation is $T(z) = \sigma(b_T + W_T z)$, where σ is the sigmoid function. At the top layer, we have $f(x) = \langle w, z_L \rangle$. Note that when the number of hidden layer is 1, this returns to the standard shallow neural network; and when $T(z) = 1$, the highway network becomes a recurrent network. Let $\boldsymbol{\theta} = (b_T, b_H, W_T, W_H, W_X, w)$ be model parameters, gradient-based learning proceeds as follows:

$$\boldsymbol{\theta} \leftarrow \boldsymbol{\theta} - \frac{\mu}{N} \sum_{k=1}^{N} \frac{\partial \ell_{1,2}}{\partial f(x_{\pi_k})} \frac{\partial f(x_{\pi_k})}{\partial \boldsymbol{\theta}}$$

for learning rate $\mu > 0$, where $\frac{\partial \ell_{1,2}}{\partial f(x_{\pi_k})}$ are functional gradients derived from Eqs. (2, 5).

5   Experimental Evaluation

5.1   Data and Evaluation Metrics

We validate the proposed model using a large-scale Web dataset from the Yahoo! learning to rank challenge [8]. The dataset is split into a training set of $18,425$ queries ($425,821$ documents), and a testing set of $1,520$ queries ($47,313$ documents). We also prepare a smaller training subset, called Yahoo!-small, which has $1,568$ queries and $47,314$ documents. The Yahoo! datasets contain the groundtruth relevance scores (from 0 for irrelevant to 4 for perfectly relevant). There are 519 pre-computed unique features for each query-document pair. We normalize the features across the whole training set to have mean 0 and standard deviation 1.

Two evaluation metrics are employed. The Normalized Discount Cumulative Gain [19] is defined as:

$$NG@T = \frac{1}{N_{max}} \sum_{i=1}^{T} \frac{2^{r_{\pi_i}} - 1}{\log_2(1 + i)}$$

where r_{π_i} is the relevance of item at rank i. The other metric is Expected Reciprocal Rank (ERR) [9], which was used in the Yahoo! learning-to-rank challenge (2011):

$$ERR = \sum_{i} \frac{R(r_{\pi_i})}{i} \prod_{j>i} [1 - R(r_{\pi_j})] \,, \text{s.t.} \, R(r_{\pi_i}) = \frac{2^{r_{\pi_i}} - 1}{16}$$

Both metrics discount for the long list and place more emphasis on the top ranking. Finally, all metrics are averaged across all test queries.

5.2   Model Implementation

The highway nets are configured as follows. Unless stated otherwise, we use ReLU units for transformation $H(z)$. Parameters W_1, W_H and W_T are initialized randomly from a small Gaussian. Gate bias b_T is initialized at -1 to encourage passing more information, as suggested in [28]. Transform bias b_H is initialized at 0. To prevent overfitting, dropout [27] is used, i.e., during training for each item in a mini-batch, input features and hidden units are randomly dropped with probabilities p_{vis} and p_{hid}, respectively. As dropouts may cause big jumps in gradient and parameters, we set max-norm per hidden unit to 1. The mini-batch size is 2 queries, the learning rate starts from 0.1, and is halved when there is no sign of improvement in training loss. Learning stops when learning rate falls below 10^{-4}. We fix the dropout rates as follows: (a) for small Yahoo! data, $p_{vis} = 0$, $p_{hid} = 0.3$ and $K = 10$; (b) for large Yahoo! data, $p_{vis} = 0$, $p_{hid} = 0.2$ and $K = 20$. Figure 2 shows the effect of dropouts on the NCE model on the small Yahoo! dataset.

5.3   Results

Performance of Choice Models. In this experiment we ask whether the new choice by elimination model has any advantage over existing state-of-the-arts (the forward selection method of Plackett-Luce [34] and the popular Rank SVM [20]). Table 1 reports results on the all datasets (Yahoo!-small, Yahoo!-large) on different sequential models. The NCE works better than Rank SVM and Plackett-Luce. Note that due to the large size, the differences are statistically significant. In fact, in the Yahoo! L2R challenge, the top 20 scores (out of more than 1,500 teams) differ only by 1.56 % in ERR, which is less than the difference between Plackett-Luce and choice by elimination (1.62 %).

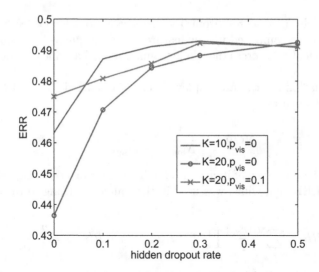

Fig. 2. Effect of dropouts on NCE performance of a 3-layer highway nets on Yahoo! small set. K is number of hidden units, p_{vis} is dropout rate for visible layer.

Table 1. Performance with linear rank functions.

Rank model	Yahoo!-small			Yahoo!-large		
	ERR	NDCG@1	NDCG@5	ERR	NDCG@1	NDCG@5
Rank SVM	0.477	0.657	0.642	0.488	0.681	0.666
Plackett-Luce	0.489	0.683	0.652	0.495	0.699	0.671
Choice by elimination	**0.497**	**0.697**	**0.664**	**0.503**	**0.709**	**0.680**

Neural Nets Versus Gradient Boosting. We also compare the highway networks against the best performing method in the Yahoo! L2R challenge. Since it was consistently demonstrated that gradient boosting trees work best [8], we implement a sophisticated variant of Stochastic Gradient Tree Boosting (SGTB) [13] for comparison. In SGTB, at each iteration, regression trees are grown to fit a random subset of functional gradients $\frac{\partial \ell}{\partial f(x)}$. Grown trees are added to the ensemble with an adaptive learning rate which is halved whenever the loss fluctuates and does not decrease. At each tree node, a random subset of features is used to split the node, following [4]. Tree nodes are split at random as it leads to much faster tree growing without hurting performance [15]. The SGTB is configured as follows: number of trees is 300; learning rate starts at 0.1; a random subset of 50 % data is used to grow a tree; one third of features are randomly selected at each node; trees are grown until either the number of leaves reaches 512 or the node size is below 40.

Table 2 show performance scores of models trained under different losses on the Yahoo!-large dataset. The highway neural networks are consistently com-

Table 2. Comparing highway neural networks against stochastic gradient tree boosting (SGTB) on Yahoo!-large dataset.

Rank function	Placket-Luce			Choice by elimination		
	ERR	NDCG@1	NDCG@5	ERR	NDCG@1	NDCG@5
SGTB	0.497	0.697	0.673	0.506	0.705	0.681
Neutral nets	**0.501**	**0.705**	**0.688**	**0.509**	**0.719**	**0.697**

petitive against the gradient tree boosting, the best performing rank function approximator in this challenge [8].

6   Conclusion

We have presented *Neural Choice by Elimination*, a new framework that integrates deep neural networks into a formal modeling of human behaviors in making sequential choices. Contrary to the standard Plackett-Luce model, where the most worthy items are iteratively selected, here the least worthy items are iteratively eliminated. Theoretically we show that choice by elimination is equivalent to sequentially marginalizing out Thurstonian random utilities that follow Gompertz distributions. Experimentally we establish that deep neural networks are competitive in the learning to rank domain, as demonstrated on a large-scale public dataset from the Yahoo! learning to rank challenge.

References

1. Agarwal, A., Raghavan, H., Subbian, K., Melville, P., Lawrence, R.D., Gondek, D.C., Fan, J.: Learning to rank for robust question answering. In: Proceedings of the 21st ACM International Conference on Information and Knowledge Management, pp. 833–842. ACM (2012)
2. Azari, H., Parks, D., Xia, L.: Random utility theory for social choice. In: Advances in Neural Information Processing Systems, pp. 126–134 (2012)
3. Bengio, Y.: Learning deep architectures for AI. Found. Trends Mach. Learn. **2**(1), 1–127 (2009)
4. Breiman, L.: Random forests. Mach. Learn. **45**(1), 5–32 (2001)
5. Breiman, L.: Bagging predictors. Mach. Learn. **24**(2), 123–140 (1996)
6. Burges, C., Shaked, T., Renshaw, E., Lazier, A., Deeds, M., Hamilton, N., Hullender, G.: Learning to rank using gradient descent. In: Proceedings of the 22nd International Conference on Machine Learning, p. 96. ACM (2005)
7. Burges, C.J., Svore, K.M., Bennett, P.N., Pastusiak, A., Qiang, W.: Learning to rank using an ensemble of lambda-gradient models. In: Yahoo! Learning to Rank Challenge, pp. 25–35 (2011)
8. Chapelle, O., Chang, Y.: Yahoo! learning to rank challenge overview. In: JMLR Workshop and Conference Proceedings, vol. 14, pp. 1–24 (2011)
9. Chapelle, O., Metlzer, D., Zhang, Y., Grinspan, P.: Expected reciprocal rank for graded relevance. In: CIKM, pp. 621–630. ACM (2009)

10. Deng, L., He, X., Gao, J.: Deep stacking networks for information retrieval. In: 2013 IEEE International Conference on Acoustics, Speech and Signal Processing (ICASSP), pp. 3153–3157. IEEE (2013)
11. Dong, Y., Huang, C., Liu, W.: RankCNN: when learning to rank encounters the pseudo preference feedback. Comput. Stan. Interfaces **36**(3), 554–562 (2014)
12. Friedman, J.H.: Greedy function approximation: a gradient boosting machine. Ann. Stat. **29**(5), 1189–1232 (2001)
13. Friedman, J.H.: Stochastic gradient boosting. Comput. Stat. Data Anal. **38**(4), 367–378 (2002)
14. Fu, Q., Lu, J., Wang, Z.: 'Reverse' nested lottery contests. J. Math. Econ. **50**, 128–140 (2014)
15. Geurts, P., Ernst, D., Wehenkel, L.: Extremely randomized trees. Mach. Learn. **63**(1), 3–42 (2006)
16. Gormley, I.C., Murphy, T.B.: A mixture of experts model for rank data with applications in election studies. Ann. Appl. Stat. **2**(4), 1452–1477 (2008)
17. Henery, R.J.: Permutation probabilities as models for horse races. J. R. Stat. Soc. Ser. B **43**(1), 86–91 (1981)
18. Huang, P.-S., He, X., Gao, J., Deng, L., Acero, A., Heck, L.: Learning deep structured semantic models for web search using clickthrough data. In: Proceedings of the 22nd ACM International Conference on Information and Knowledge Management, pp. 2333–2338. ACM (2013)
19. Järvelin, K., Kekäläinen, J.: Cumulated gain-based evaluation of IR techniques. ACM Trans. Inf. Syst. (TOIS) **20**(4), 446 (2002)
20. Joachims, T.: Optimizing search engines using clickthrough data. In: Proceedings of the Eighth ACM SIGKDD International Conference on Knowledge Discovery and Data Mining, pp. 133–142. ACM, New York (2002)
21. Li, P., Burges, C., Wu, Q., Platt, J.C., Koller, D., Singer, Y., Roweis, S.: McRank: learning to rank using multiple classification and gradient boosting. In: Advances in Neural Information Processing Systems (2007)
22. Liu, T.-Y.: Learning to Rank for Information Retrieval. Springer, Berlin (2011)
23. McFadden, D.: Conditional logit analysis of qualitative choice behavior. In: Frontiers in Econometrics, pp. 105–142 (1973)
24. Plackett, R.L.: The analysis of permutations. Appl. Stat. **24**, 193–202 (1975)
25. Severyn, A., Moschitti, A.: Learning to rank short text pairs with convolutional deep neural networks. In: Proceedings of the 38th International ACM SIGIR Conference on Research and Development in Information Retrieval, pp. 373–382. ACM (2015)
26. Song, Y., Wang, H., He, X.: Adapting deep ranknet for personalized search. In: Proceedings of the 7th ACM International Conference on Web Search and Data Mining, pp. 83–92. ACM (2014)
27. Srivastava, N., Hinton, G., Krizhevsky, A., Sutskever, I., Salakhutdinov, R.: Dropout: a simple way to prevent neural networks from overfitting. J. Mach. Learn. Res. **15**, 1929–1958 (2014)
28. Srivastava, R.K., Greff, K., Schmidhuber, J.: Training very deep networks (2015). arXiv preprint: arXiv:1507.06228
29. Thurstone, L.L.: A law of comparative judgment. Psychol. Rev. **34**(4), 273 (1927)
30. Tran, T., Phung, D., Venkatesh, S.: Thurstonian Boltzmann machines: learning from multiple inequalities. In: International Conference on Machine Learning (ICML), Atlanta, USA, 16–21 June 2013

31. Tran, T., Phung, D.Q., Venkatesh, S.: Sequential decision approach to ordinal preferences in recommender systems. In: Proceedings of the 26th AAAI Conference, Toronto, Ontario, Canada (2012)

32. Truyen, T., Phung, D.Q., Venkatesh, S.: Probabilistic models over ordered partitions with applications in document ranking and collaborative filtering. In: Proceedings of SIAM Conference on Data Mining (SDM), Mesa, Arizona, USA. SIAM (2011)

33. Tversky, A.: Elimination by aspects: a theory of choice. Psychol. Rev. **79**(4), 281 (1972)

34. Xia, F., Liu, T.Y., Wang, J., Zhang, W., Li, H.: Listwise approach to learning to rank: theory and algorithm. In Proceedings of the 25th International Conference on Machine Learning, pp. 1192–1199. ACM (2008)

35. Yellott, J.I.: The relationship between Luce's choice axiom, Thurstone's theory of comparative judgment, and the double exponential distribution. J. Math. Psychol. **15**(2), 109–144 (1977)

Attribute Selection and Classification of Prostate Cancer Gene Expression Data Using Artificial Neural Networks

Sreenivas Sremath Tirumala[✉] and A. Narayanan

Auckland University of Technology, Auckland, New Zealand
ssremath@aut.ac.nz

Abstract. Artificial Intelligence (AI) approaches for medical diagnosis and prediction of cancer are important and ever growing areas of research. Artificial Neural Networks (ANN) is one such approach that have been successfully applied in these areas. Various types of clinical datasets have been used in intelligent decision making systems for medical diagnosis, especially cancer for over three decades. However, gene expression datasets are complex with large numbers of attributes which make it more difficult for AI approaches to classification and prediction. Prostate Cancer dataset is one such dataset with 12600 attributes and only 102 samples. In this paper, we propose an extended ANN based approach for classification and prediction of prostate cancer using gene expression data. Firstly, we use four attribute selection approaches, namely Sequential Floating Forward Selection (SFFS), RELIEFF, Sequential Backward Feature Section (SFBS) and Significant Attribute Evaluation (SAE) to identify the most influential attributes among 12600. We use ANNs and Naive Bayes for classification with complete sets of attributes as well as various sets obtained from attribute selection methods. Experimental results show that ANN outperformed Naive Bayes by achieving a classification accuracy of 98.2 % compared to 62.74 % with the full set of attributes. Further, with 21 selected attributes obtained with SFFS, ANNs achieved better accuracy (100 %) for classification compared to Naive Bayes. For prediction using ANNs, SFFS was able achieve best results with 92.31 % of accuracy by correctly predicting 24 out of 26 samples provided for independent sample testing. Moreover, some of the gene selected by SFFS are identified to have a direct reference to cancer and tumour. Our results indicate that a combination of standard feature selection methods in conjunction with ANNs provide the most impressive results.

Keywords: Prostate cancer classification · Artificial neural networks · Feature selection methods · Gene expression data analysis

1 Introduction

Artificial Intelligence (AI) approaches for medical diagnosis and prediction of cancer are important and ever growing areas of research. Artificial Neural Networks (ANNs) is one such approach that have been successfully applied in these

© Springer International Publishing Switzerland 2016
H. Cao et al. (Eds.): PAKDD 2016 Workshops, LNAI 9794, pp. 26–34, 2016.
DOI: 10.1007/978-3-319-42996-0_3

areas. Various types of clinical datasets have been used in intelligent decision making systems for medical diagnosis, especially cancer dfor over three decades. However, gene expression datasets are complex with large numbers of attributes which make it more difficult for AI approaches to classification and prediction. The importance of using AI techniques in bio-informatics has been known for some time [1]. Artificial Neural Networks (ANNs) have been implemented for classification and prediction of various types of cancers like [2], colorectal [3], Lung [4], colon [5] etc. Most of these implementation are performed using gene expression datasets [6]. Classification of complex non-linear data like gene expression data is a challenging task due to its high dimensionality especially when the number of samples are far less number of attributes in the dataset. With such datasets, analysing the importance of attributes and identifying the significance of an attribute become more difficult. Earlier research on using ANNs for gene expression analysis was limited to mainly single-layered ANNs due to non-availability of powerful hardware. One such early work emphasizes the importance of identifying a set of significant genes among the thousands of genes in the dataset [7].

Among various types of cancer, prostate cancer is the second leading cancer for men. Some of the previous work on prostate cancer is confined to early detection and progress of prostate cancer using clinical data of the patient [8,9]. The only noted work on prostate gene expression data is done by Singh and others which provides an analysis on the impact of differences in the gene expression and the development of prostate tumour [10]. Recently there has been notable work on cancer gene expression dataset classification using Deep Learning which proves the complexity involved in classification of gene expression data [11]. However that work is limited to classification and lacks experimental details.

The contribution of this paper is in identifying significant attributes (genes) from the gene expression dataset that have direct influence on classification as well as prediction of prostate cancer.

This paper is organized as follows. Section 2 provides a brief explanation of attribute selection approaches used in this research along with results. The first part of Sect. 3 provides the experimental setup detailing ANN topology and parameters used in the experiments followed by comparative analysis of classification results using various attribute sets obtained from Sect. 2. Experimental results of predicting prostate cancer with unseen sample testing is also presented in this section. Section 4 provides a brief analysis on the obtained results followed by Conclusion and Future Work in Sect. 5.

2   Attribute Selection

The Gene expression dataset of prostate cancer consists of 102 samples with 52 normal and 50 tumour cases [10]. There are 12600 attributes (genes) for each sample. Due to its complexity, it is a difficult as well as time consuming process to classify using this data set. In this type of situation, one method is to apply feature selection techniques to choose a few significant attributes without compromising the knowledge. Firstly, the dataset is standardized using $v' = (v - \mu)/\sigma$ where v' is the new value, v is the original value, μ is the mean of attribute and σ is the standard deviation. On this standardized data, we applied four different feature selection algorithms, namely, Sequential Floating Forward Selection (SFFS), Sequential Backward Floating Selection (SBFS), RELIEFF and Significance Attribute Evaluation (SAE). For the purpose of this research, feature and attribute are used synonymously, but more generally features can include groups of attributes obtained, say, through principal component analysis (PCA). No attempt was made to use PCA in this research.

SFFS is based on Sequential Forward Search (SFS) first proposed in 1994 [12]. Since then, SFFS has gone through several enhancements for improving performance and quality [13]. In SFS, the process initially starts with an empty set and uses a selection criterion, usually mean squared error or misclassification rate to minimize overall feature subsets. The main drawback of SFS is its inability to remove a feature once it is selected in spite of any reduction in its importance when compared with the current set of attributes.

SFFS is an extension of SFS with an ability to conduct a floating search and remove insignificant features from the selected subset. In SFFS, the attribute selection is similar to SFS. In SFFS, attribute selection starts with an empty set of features $S = 0$ and significant features are added with respect to S. In the process, from S the least significant feature x is selected such that $S - x$ is better than $S.4$. This process is continued till the formation of $F1(S)$ with significant features. Then, the initial feature selection process is started again and the next subset $F2(S)$ is obtained. Comparing $F1$ and $F2$ will give the best subset of that size. This entire process is continued until enough subsets are evaluated.

In Sequential Backward Floating Selection (SBFS) the feature selection is applied by eliminating the least significant features starting with the complete feature set, which is opposite to SFFS. As the name implies, the direction of search is backward. The significance of RELIEFF selection algorithms is its ability to identify the attribute dependency with its heuristic guidance algorithm before eliminating an insignificant attribute [14]. The attribute selection in Significant Attribute Evaluation (SAE) is based on probabilistic conditions [15]. The condition used in this selection process is based on assigned significant values of the attributes as a two-way association function for the class it belongs to. Further, the overall attribute-class association is the commutative of all values of the attribute and its association with its class.

The selection experiments are carried out with prostate cancer gene expression dataset using all four feature selection methods, 10 times for each method. The results along with the number of attributes selected by each approach are presented as Table 1 and the complete list of attributes is presented in Table 2. The number of attributes selected by SFFS, RELIEFF, SBFS and SAE are 21, 11, 42 and 10 respectively. The highest number of attributes (44) is selected by SBFS whereas the least number of attributes (10) by SAE. The significance of these attributes is tested with respect to the classification accuracy and prediction which is presented in the next Section.

Table 1. Attribute selection

No.	Selection approach	No. of attributes
1	-	12600
2	SFFS	21
3	RELIEFF	11
4	SBFS	42
5	SAE	10

Table 2. List of selected attributes

Approach	Attributes
SFFS (21)	0009 0040 0049 0062 0118 0186 0199 0210 0230 0373 0381 0939 1071 1201 2517 2729 4247 5195 8828 9142 10427
RELIEFF (11)	1601 6323 7187 7790 8036 8662 8669 8996 9783 10167 11702
SBFS (42)	0095 0940 1211 1335 1571 1782 1906 2179 2578 2699 2809 3304 3837 3888 4059 4074 4977 5221 5411 5933 6273 6277 6534 6599 7083 7087 7689 8240 8668 8749 8978 9482 9715 9884 10277 10415 10450 10702 10905 11081 11586 12106 12288
SAE (10)	4298 6395 6553 7180 8783 9105 9783 10071 10427 12086

3   Experiment Results

3.1   Experimental Setup

To determine the best possible ANN topology for classification and prediction, we started the experiment with an arbitrary topology and implemented various other topologies, from a single-layered ANN to five-layered ANN, with different combinations of hidden nodes for with the full gene expression dataset (12600 attributes). Both Matlab (version 2015b) and Weka (version 3.7) are used for carrying the experiments. Matlab is used for optimal topology determination and all ANN experiments. Both Matlab and Weka were used for Attribute selection and classification accuracy comparison. The reason for using two different toolkits is to eliminate software based issues (if any, especially in the case of initialization) and for effective comparison. The dataset is divided as 70 %, 20 % and 10 % for training, validation and testing respectively. The ANN is trained with Scale Conjugate Gradient (SCG).

Each experiment is performed 10 times for 500 epochs, with learning rate and momentum at a constant value of 0.3 and 0.1 respectively. The experimental results are presented as Table 3. We started with a single-layered ANN with 30 hidden nodes and the classification accuracy achieved with this is 93.1 %. For a three-layered ANN with 30, 40, 50 nodes in the hidden layers, the classification accuracy is 92.3 % whereas when the hidden node sequence is changed to 50, 40, 30, the accuracy is increased by 2.8 % to 95.1 %. From these results, it is evident

Table 3. Classification results

No.	Hidden layers	Hidden nodes	Accuracy (%)
1	1	30	93.1
2	2	30,30	91.1
3	3	30,40,50	92.3
4	3	50,30,40	95.1
5	3	50,30,50	97
6	**3**	**30,30,30**	**98.2**
7	4	30,30,30,30	97
8	5	30,30,30,30,30	96.1
9	5	50,40,30,40,50	96.1
10	5	50,30,30,30,50	89.2
11	4	50,30,30,50	79.4

that an ANN with 3 hidden layers and 30, 30, 30 hidden nodes (symmetric node count) produces the best classification accuracy of 98.2 % with complete dataset of 12600 attributes. However, when the number of hidden layers is increased to four (30, 30, 30, 30), the classification accuracy fell to 97 %.

The influence of symmetric and asymmetric node count and the number of hidden layers with respect to the classification accuracy was previously discussed for deep neural networks using layer-wise training (deep learning) [16]. It is interesting to observer that similar results are obtained with respect to traditional multi-layer ANNs using SGD algorithm for training instead of layer-wise training. The configuration of ANNs that produced best accuracy (12600 input, $30 \times 30 \times 30$ hidden, one output) is used for rest of the classification and prediction.

3.2   Classification

The classification experiments are carried out using various sets of attributes obtained from different feature selection methods presented in earlier section. We used the same ANNs configuration (three-layered symmetric node count of 30, 30, 30, 70 % training, 20 % validation and 10 % testing) which achieved best accuracy in the previous section. The experimental results with classification accuracy and average root-mean-square error (RMSE) is presented as Table 4.

With full set of attributes ANN was able to achieved 98.2 % of accuracy as determined in the previous section. The overall best accuracy of 100 % is achieved by ANNs with SFFS (21 attributes) which is 1.8 % more than the results obtained with all 12600 attributes (98.2} and 2.5 % more than the results using another ANN based approach (97.5 %) [11]. With SAE (least number of attributes) ANNs classification accuracy is 92.2 % whereas with SBFF (maximum selected attributes) it is 94.1 %. We run the same experiments for classification using

Table 4. Classification results using ANN

No.	Selection method	Accuracy (%)	Average RMSE
1	-(12600)	98.2	0.0124
2	**SFFS (21)**	**100**	**0.0116**
3	RELIEFF (11)	95.2	0.0434
4	SBFS (42)	94.1	0.1492
5	SAE (10)	92.2	0.0487

Naive Bayes for a comparative analysis with ANN classification accuracy and the results are presented in Table 4.

With the full set of attributes, ANN was able to achieve 98.2 % accuracy. The overall best accuracy of 100 % is achieved by ANNs with SFFS (21 attributes), which is 1.8 % more than the results obtained with all 12600 attributes (98.2 %) and 2.5 % more than the results using another ANN based approach (97.5 %) [11]. With SAE (least number of attributes) ANNs classification accuracy is 92.2 % whereas with SBFF (maximum selected attributes) it is 94.1 %. We run the same experiments for classification using Naive Bayes for a comparative analysis with ANN classification accuracy and the results are presented in Table 5.

Table 5. Classification - ANNs vs Naive Bayes

No.	Approach	ANN	Naive Bayes
1	-(12600)	98.2	62.74
2	**SFFS (21)**	**100**	86.27
3	RELIEFF (11)	95.2	84.31
4	SBFS (42)	94.1	63.71
5	SAE (10)	92.2	**94.11**

With the full set of attributes, ANNs achieved an accuracy of 98.2 % whereas Naive Bayes is only 62.74 %. With SFFS attribute set with which ANNs achieved the best results (100 %), Naive Bayes could manage only 86.27 %. However, the best accuracy for Naive Bayes (94.11 %) is achieved with SAE attribute set (least number of attributes) where ANNs classification accuracy is 92.2 % for the same. With SBFS (42 attributes) ANN and Naive Bayes achieved 94.1 % and 63.71 % of classification accuracy respectively.

3.3   Prediction Using Unseen Sample Testing

As detailed in the earlier section, ANNs achieved better accuracy for classification than Naive Bayes. In this section, we try to evaluate ANNs for predicting whether the given sample is tumour or normal. We isolated 26 (25 % of full dataset) samples from the dataset and trained our ANN with the remaining 76 samples. From the 76 samples, 75 % is allocated for training and 25 % for cross-validation. Each isolated sample is fed individually as test data for prediction. Each experiment is performed 10 times with 10 different sets of withheld samples for 300 epochs and the results are tabulated in Table 6.

Table 6. Results - unseen sample testing (26 samples)

No.	Selection method	Correctly predicted	% of Accuracy
1	- (12600)	22	84.62
2	**SFFS (21)**	**24**	**92.31**
3	RELIEFF (11)	22	84.62
4	SBFS (42)	18	69.23
5	SAE (10)	23	88.46

From the results shown in Table 6, SFFS continued to dominate with high accuracy of 92.31 % by correctly predicting 24 out of 26 test samples. The second best prediction accuracy of 88.46 % is obtained with SAE attribute set. REDLIFF achieved 84.62 % same as results with complete 12600 attribute set followed by SBFS in the last place with 69.23 % similar to its position in classification experiments.

4   Discussion

From the experimental results for both classification and prediction, SBSF produces significantly worse results than all other methods ($T = 3.73$, ≤ 0.05). SBFS with 42 attributes achieved significantly less accuracy than SAE with 10 attributes for both classification and prediction. It is noteworthy to observe the accuracy differences between SAE (10 attributes) and RELIEFF (11 attributes) RELIEFF (95.2 %) achieved better classification accuracy than SAE (92.2 %) with ANNs but for prediction, SAE was able to identify 23 cases correctly (88.46 %), 1 case more than RELIEFF (22 cases with accuracy of 84.62 %). There is only one common attribute (9783) that is present in both SAE and RELIEFF. It is interesting to note that SAE has an attribute (10427) which is present in SFFS (but not in RELIEFF or SBFS) which has achieved best results in our experiments. With investigation about this attribute in The National Centre for Biotechnology Information (NCBI) database, it is concluded that the gene referred to by this attribute (10427) has a direct reference to prostate tumour [17]. Preliminary investigation on the genes (attributes) selected by SFFS (21) show that the majority of these gene has a direct reference to various types of cancers and cancer related tumours.

5   Conclusion and Future Direction

This paper proposes an Artificial Neural Network (ANN) approach enhanced with feature selection for use in gene expression analysis, classification and prediction of prostate cancer. We used various attribute selection approaches to identify the most important attributes that influence the classification accuracy and prediction rate for prostate cancer gene expression dataset. The experimental results show that Sequential Floating Forward Selection (SFFS) was able to identify most effective attributes with which we achieved 100 % accuracy for classification with ANNs. Further, with SFFS attributes, our ANN approach was able to achieve 92.31 % of accuracy by correctly predicting 24 out of 26 samples provided for independent sample testing. Further, some of the gene selected by SFFS are identified to have a direct reference to cancer/tumour. Attribute selection approaches used in this experiment are statistically based methods. It would be interesting to use machine learning and evolutionary computation based attribute selection approaches for gene expression datasets that may be able to combine the best aspects of two or more feature selection approaches. Another aspect is to identify the attribute sensitivity and possible biological relationships to extract more knowledge on significance and influence of each attributes selected using these approaches. Finally, using cluster analysis to group and identify relationship between attributes may be another direction of research that could possibly lead to comparisons with PCA-based approaches.

References

1. Narayanan, A., Keedwell, E., Olsson, B.: Artificial intelligence techniques for bioinformatics. Appl. Bioinf. **1**, 191–222 (2002)
2. Baker, J.A., Kornguth, P.J., Lo, J.Y., Williford, M.E., Floyd Jr., C.E.: Breast cancer: prediction with artificial neural network based on bi-radsstandardized lexicon. Radiology **196**(3), 817–822 (1995)
3. Bottaci, L., Drew, P.J., Hartley, J.E., Hadfield, M.B., Farouk, R., Lee, P.W., Macintyre, I.M., Duthie, G.S., Monson, J.R.: Artificial neural networks applied to outcome prediction for colorectal cancer patients in separate institutions. Lancet **350**(9076), 469–472 (1997)
4. Zhou, Z.-H., Jiang, Y., Yang, Y.-B., Chen, S.-F.: Lung cancer cell identification based on artificial neural network ensembles. Artif. Intell. Med. **24**(1), 25–36 (2002)
5. Ahmed, F.E.: Artificial neural networks for diagnosis and survival prediction in colon cancer. Mol. Cancer **4**(1), 29 (2005)
6. Khan, J., Wei, J.S., Ringner, M., Saal, L.H., Ladanyi, M., Westermann, F., Berthold, F., Schwab, M., Antonescu, C.R., Peterson, C., et al.: Classification and diagnostic prediction of cancers using gene expressionprofiling and artificial neural networks. Nat. Med. **7**(6), 673–679 (2001)
7. Narayanan, A., Keedwell, E.C., Gamalielsson, J., Tatineni, S.: Single-layer artificial neural networks for gene expression analysis. Neurocomputing **61**, 217–240 (2004)
8. Snow, P.B., Smith, D.S., Catalona, W.J.: Artificial neural networks in the diagnosis and prognosis of prostate cancer: a pilot study. J. Urol. **152**(5 Pt 2), 1923–1926 (1994)

9. Djavan, B., Remzi, M., Zlotta, A., Seitz, C., Snow, P., Marberger, M.: Novel artificial neural network for early detection of prostate cancer. J. Clin. Oncol. **20**(4), 921–929 (2002)
10. Singh, D., Febbo, P.G., Ross, K., Jackson, D.G., Manola, J., Ladd, C., Tamayo, P., Renshaw, A.A., D'Amico, A.V., Richie, J.P., Lander, E.S., Loda, M., Kantoff, P.W., Golub, T.R., Sellers, W.R.: Gene expression correlates of clinical prostate cancer behavior. Cancer Cell **1**, 203–209 (2002)
11. Fakoor, R., Ladhak, F., Nazi, A., Huber, M.: Using deep learning to enhance cancer diagnosis and classification. In: Proceedings of the International Conference on Machine Learning (2013)
12. Pudil, P., Novovičová, J., Kittler, J.: Floating search methods in feature selection. Pattern Recogn. Lett. **15**, 1119–1125 (1994)
13. Ververidis, D., Kotropoulos, C.: Sequential forward feature selection with low computational cost. In: 2005 13th European Signal Processing Conference, pp. 1–4. IEEE (2005)
14. Kononenko, I., Simec, E., Robnik-Sikonja, M.: Overcoming the myopia of inductive learning algorithms with RELIEFF. Appl. Intell. **7**, 39–55 (1997)
15. Ahmad, A., Dey, L.: A feature selection technique for classificatory analysis. Pattern Recogn. Lett. **26**(1), 43–56 (2005)
16. Tirumala, S.S., Narayanan, A.: Hierarchical data classification using deep neural networks. In: Arik, S., Huang, T., Lai, W.K., Liu, Q. (eds.) ICONIP 2015. LNCS, vol. 9489, pp. 492–500. Springer, Heidelberg (2015). doi:10.1007/978-3-319-26532-2_54
17. Li, Y., Graham, C., Lacy, S., Duncan, A., Whyte, P.: The adenovirus E1A-associated 130-kD protein is encoded by a member of the retinoblastoma gene family and physically interacts with cyclins A and E. Genes Dev. **7**(12a), 2366–2377 (1993)

An Improved Self-Structuring Neural Network

Rami M. Mohammad[1], Fadi Thabtah[2(✉)], and Lee McCluskey[1]

[1] University of Huddersfield, Huddersfield, UK
{rami.mohammad,t.l.mccluskey}@hud.ac.uk
[2] Nelson Marlborough Institute of Technology, Nelson, New Zealand
fadi.fayez@nmit.ac.nz

Abstract. Creating a neural network based classification model is traditionally accomplished using the trial and error technique. However, the trial and error structuring method nornally suffers from several difficulties including overtraining. In this article, a new algorithm that simplifies structuring neural network classification models has been proposed. It aims at creating a large structure to derive classifiers from the training dataset that have generally good predictive accuracy performance on domain applications. The proposed algorithm tunes crucial NN model thresholds during the training phase in order to cope with dynamic behavior of the learning process. This indeed may reduce the chance of overfitting the training dataset or early convergence of the model. Several experiments using our algorithm as well as other classification algorithms, have been conducted against a number of datasets from University of California Irvine (UCI) repository. The experiments' are performed to assess the pros and cons of our proposed NN method. The derived results show that our algorithm outperformed the compared classification algorithms with respect to several performance measures.

Keywords: Classification · Neural network · Phishing · Pruning · Structure

1 Introduction

Artificial Neural Network (ANN) methods proved their merit in several classification domains [1]. However, one downside of any neural network (NN) based classification models is that their outcomes are difficult to interpret and they are considered as a black-box. We believe that this particular drawback can have a positive impact on application domains when the outcome's predictive accuracy is vital to the domain users and often more important than the understanding of how the NN model works [4].

An important issue that gained the attention of many researchers is the NN structuring process. Although selecting a suitable number of hidden neurons and determining the value of some parameters, i.e. learning rate, momentum value and epoch size, showed to be crucial when constructing any NN model [4]. Still, there is no clear mechanism for determining such parameters values at preliminary

© Springer International Publishing Switzerland 2016
H. Cao et al. (Eds.): PAKDD 2016 Workshops, LNAI 9794, pp. 35–47, 2016.
DOI: 10.1007/978-3-319-42996-0_4

stages, and most model designers rely on trial and error technique. The trial and error technique might be suitable for domains where rich prior experience and a NN expert are available, though, it often involves a tedious process since prior knowledge and experienced human experts are hard to get in practice. Also, the trial and error technique has been criticized of being a time-consuming process [3]. A poorly structured NN model may cause the classifier to underfit the training dataset. Whereas, overexageration in restructuring the classifier entirely to suit every data attribute in the input dataset may cause the classifier to be overfitted.

One possible solution to avoid the overfitting problem is restructuring the NN model by tuning certain parameters, adding new neurons to the hidden layer or even in some cases inserting a new layer to the network. A NN with a limited numbers of hidden neurons may not derive a satisfactory model accuracy. Whereas, a NN with too many hidden nodes normally overfits the training dataset. We argue that at a certain iteration during the training phase, the current produced model cannot be further improved, thus the structuring process should be terminated. Therefore, an acceptable error margin should be specified during or prior building the NN model, which itself is a challenging task. This is since it is difficult to determine in advance what is the acceptable error rate and this also may vary from one application data to another. The extreme cases of this problem occur when (a) the model designer sets the error rate to an unreachable threshold which consequently causes the model to trape in a local minima or (b) the model designer sets the error rate to a value that can be reached too quickly.

Overall, automating the structuring process of NN models is a timely issue and it might displace some of the burden from the system designer. However, as stated earlier automating the structure of the NN models does not merely means inserting new neuron(s) to the hidden layer because the more hidden neurons does not guarantees that the accuracy will improve. Hence, it is important to enhance the NN performance by tuning certain parameters such as the learning rate before adding a new neuron to the hidden layer. Sadly, selecting the learning rate value is also a trial and error process. Yet, the optimal learning rate value is still concealed.

In this article, we propose a method that simplifies the structure of the NN classifiers aiming to overcome some of the aforementioned issues. Our method has been named Self-Structuring Neural Network (iSSNN). Particularly, iSSNN will make the training process more dynamic by adjusting on the need particular model's thresholds such as the learning rate and the number of epoch. The classifiers derived from the iSSNN algorithm are assumed to be general enough to be derived from the training dataset and to generalise output(s) on test dataset.

2   Literature Review

The traditional trial and error method is commonly used in structuring ANNs. However, several attempts have been devoted to automate the ANN structuring process such as constructive, pruning and constructive-pruning algorithms.

Constructive Algorithms

This approach starts with a simple NN structure, i.e. one hidden layered NN with a single neuron in the hidden layer, and recursively new parameters such as hidden layers, hidden neurons, and connections, are added to the initial structure until reaching a satisfactory result. After each addition, the entire network or only the recently added parameter is retrained. Constructive approach is relatively easy for inexperienced users because they are normally asked to specify few initial parameters, for example the number of neurons in the input layer and epoch size and then new parameters are added to the network. This approach is computationally efficient since it searches for small structures. However, constructive approach has some hurdles that should carefully be addressed including the user has to decide when to add a new parameter, when to stop the addition process, and when to terminate training and when to produce the network.

Dynamic Node Creation (DNC) [2] is most likely the first constructive algorithm. This algorithm adds neurons in the hidden layer one by one whenever the mean error rate on the training dataset starts to flatten until the network achieves good generalization. After each addition, the algorithm retrains the entire network. Although DNC is simple, it usually produces complicated structures since it keeps adding hidden neurons to achieve a predefined desired error rate defined earlier by the designer.

The Cascade-Correlation algorithm (CC-alg) [3] generates NNs with multiple hidden layers each of which consists of only one hidden neuron where each neuron is linked to previously added neurons. However, the generalization ability of the produced NN may decrease if the number of the hidden layers increases. Several improvements on the CC-alg have been done to facilitate adding more than one neuron in each hidden layer such as [3].

Pruning Algorithms

Unlike constructive approach, the pruning approach starts with an oversized NN structure, i.e. a multi hidden layered NN with a large number of hidden neurons in each hidden layer. Later on, some parameters, i.e. connections, hidden neurons, and hidden layers are removed from the network. After each training process, the user removes some parameters from the network and the new structure is retrained so that the remaining parameters can compensate the functions played by the removed parameters. If the network performance improves, the user removes more parameters and retrains the network again. However, if the network performance is not improved, the user restores what have been deleted and tries to remove other parameters. This process is repeated recursively until achieving the final network. Usually, only one parameter is removed in each pruning phase. Overall, this approach is time consuming since the user does not know a priori how big the initial NN structure should be for a specific problem.

Constructive-Pruning Algorithms

This approach comprises two phases, a constructive and a pruning. During the training phase new hidden layers, hidden neurons, and connections are added.

The constructive phase may result in a ridiculously complicated structure. Therefore, a pruning phase is employed to simplify the network structure and at the same time preserves the network performance. The pruning phase can run simultaneously with the constructive phase, or it can be started as soon as the training phase is accomplished.

3   Improved Self-Structuring Neural Network Algorithm

The pseudocode of the proposed algorithm is shown in Fig. 1 and here under we elaborate in each step.

```
Input
        Upload the minimal dataset and divide it to Training, Testing and Validation
        Integer T_i specifying the number of epochs
        Maximum number of possible hidden neurons
Output
        Optimal number of neurons in the hidden layer
        Optimal learning rate value
        Connection weights between input, hidden and output layers
Initialize
1       Number of neurons in the input layer = number of input features;
2       Number of neurons in the output layer = 1
3       Number of neurons in the hidden layer = 1;
4       Weights = random numbers ranging from -0.5 to +0.5;
5       Learning rate LR= 0.3;
6       Momentum value = 0.2
7       Desired Error DER = 50%;
Start
8       Train the network to find the calculated error-rate CER;
9       If CER < DER then {
10 A: Set DER= CER;
11      Train the network;
12      Update the LR after each training epoch;
13      Check the early stopping condition;
14      If (DER Achieved && iteration< T_i) then
15            Go to A;
16      Else {
17            Add a new neuron to the hidden layer;
18            Train the network;
19            If (DER Achieved && iteration< T_i)
20                  Go to A;
21            Else
22                  Produce the Network:
```

Fig. 1. iSSNN pseudocode

Preliminary Phase

This phase involves several steps including:

1. The number of neurons in the input layer is set to the number of the features offered in the training dataset *(line 1)*.
2. The number of neurons in the output layer is set to one since iSSNN aims to create binary classification models *(line 2)*. In other words, we will create a single neuron that might hold two possible values.
3. The number of neurons in the hidden layer is to be determined implicitly by the algorithm. The algorithm normally starts with one hidden neuron. Then, it creates the simplest NN structure that consists of only one neuron in the hidden layer *(line 3)*. This neuron is connected to all neurons in the input and output layers.

4. Small non-zero random values will be assigned to each connection weight *(line 4)*.
5. The learning rate value commonly ranges from ≈0 to ≈1 as in [5]. Following the default value of WEKA [6], the learning rate and momentum value are assumed 0.3 and 0.2 respectively *(line 5) and (line 6)*. However, the learning rate value is adjusted several times during the network training process.
6. The initial desired error-rate *(DER)* is set to 50% *(line 7)*. This value will be used to assess if the algorithm can find a possible solution. The model designer specifies the maximum number of epochs and the maximum number of allowed hidden neurons.
7. The input dataset is divided into training, testing, and validation sets. The training set will be used to learn the model and update weights; the testing set will be used to assess the overall performance of the derived classifier. Finally, the validation set plays an important role in producing the final model as we will see later.

Warming-up Phase

In this phase *(line 8–9)*, iSSNN decides whether to proceed with creating a new classifier or not and computes the calculated error-rate *(CER)*, aiming to determine what is the *DER* to be achieved in the next training phase. If iSSNN finds a *CER* less than the initial *DER* before reaching the maximum number of epochs, then it assumes that the current structure can further be improved and therefore, iSSNN resets the epoch, and assumes that the *DER* to be achieved in the next training phase is the current *CER*. Then, the iSSNN moves to the "training phase" (Sect. 3). On the other hand, if the *CER* is larger than the *DER*, then the algorithm will be terminated *(line 24)*. The *CER* is equivalent to Mean Square Error *(MSE)* and is calculated as per Eq. 1 where A_k is the predicted value for example k; and D_k is the real value associated with example k in a training dataset with size n.

$$CER = \frac{1}{n} \sum\nolimits_{k=0}^{n} (A_k - D_k)^2 \qquad (1)$$

Training Phase

In this phase *(line 10–13)*, iSSNN algorithm continues building and adjusting the network until the *CER* is less than the *DER* or the maximum number of epochs is reached. Each training epoch starts by updating the learning rate based on the *CER* achieved in the previous epoch.

After each training epoch, iSSNN compares the *CER* at time t with that at $t - 1$, if the error has decreased, the learning rate is slightly increased by a specific ratio φ in order to accelerate the error-rate reduction process and converge quickly to the desired solution. In this case, the weights are updated. On the other hand, if the error has increased or has not changed, iSSNN decreases the learning rate by φ' since we might be approaching one possible solution and we need to slow down and evaluate the solution deeply. In this case, the weights are not updated.

Commonly, φ and φ' are set to 0.1 and 0.5 respectively as in [7]. The reason that φ is smaller than φ' is the fact that we do not want to make a large jump that may cause the algorithm to converge from the possible solution. However, as soon as the algorithm approaches a possible solution we need to examine that solution thoroughly and therefore the learning rate is normally decreased.

Generally, the trial and error based NN structuring approach assumes that the number of neurons in the hidden layer and learning rate are fixed values that are not changed during the training phase. However, iSSNN algorithm follows a different approach in determining the number of neurons in the hidden layer based on learning curves since iSSNN leaves the network expansion as a last option and keeps pushing on training to possibly improve the NN performance before adding any new neuron.

After each training epoch, the iSSNN algorithm calculates the error on the validation dataset. When the error on the validation dataset starts to increase, this is a sign that the current classifier has begun to overfit the training data, and therefore the training phase should halt. Nevertheless, the validation dataset may have several local minima; thus, if we stop training at the iteration with the first error increase, we may lose some other better feasible solutions since the error-rate may decrease again at later iterations. Therefore, iSSNN algorithm tracks the error on the validation dataset and when the lastly achieved error is smaller than the minimum achieved error so far, the generalisation ability of the model has improved, and thus iSSNN saves the weights and continues the training process. However, when the lastly achieved error is larger than the minimum achieved error, the algorithm continues the training process without saving the weights. Finally, if the lastly achieved error is larger than the minimum achieved error by α, then the algorithm terminates the training process (early stopping). This is since we assume that α might cause the model to diverge from the ideal solution.

A recent study on early stopping [8] revealed that in most cases, early stopping is triggered when $\alpha = 50\%$. Equation 2 clarifies how iSSNN algorithm handles early stopping where ε is the lastly achieved error, and ε' is the minimum error.

$$IF \begin{cases} \varepsilon < \varepsilon' \xrightarrow{weights\,Saved} Continue\,training \\ (\varepsilon > \varepsilon')\,and\,(\varepsilon < [(1+\alpha) * \varepsilon']) \xrightarrow{weights\,not\,Saved} Continue\,training \\ Otherwize \rightarrow Training\,terminated \end{cases} \quad (2)$$

Improvement Phase

In the training phase, when iSSNN obtains a $CER < DER$ before reaching the maximum epoch, this could be an indication that the model can be further improved without adding any neurons to the hidden layer *(line 14–15)*. Therefore, iSSNN maintains the learning rate and weights achieved so far; resets the epoch, assumes that the *DER* to be achieved in the next "training phase" is the *CER*, and goes back to the training phase. Otherwise, the algorithm goes to "Adding a New Neuron Phase" *(line 16)*.

Adding a New Neuron Step

iSSNN algorithm arrives at this step if it cannot achieve the desired *DER* and reaches either the maximum allowed epoch or the early stopping condition. In this case, we assume that the current structure has been squeezed to the limit and the network's ability of processing the information is insufficient. Therefore, iSSNN adds a new neuron to the hidden layer *(line 17)*. Then, it

- connects the new neuron to all input and output neurons
- assigns small non-zero value to its weight
- maintains the learning rate and weights achieved so far
- resets the epoch.

Yet, inserting a new neuron to the hidden layer does not mean that this neuron is added permanently into the network, we must first assess whether the new neuron improves the network performance or not. Hence, the algorithm continues training the network *(line 18)*, and if after adding a new neuron, the *DER* is achieved, the algorithm

- maintains the learning rate and weights, resets the epoch
- assumes that the *DER* to be achieved in the next training phase is the *CER*
- goes back to the "training phase" *(line 19–20)*.

Otherwise, the algorithm moves to "Producing the Final Network Phase" *(line 21)*. The main concern in this phase is that the number of hidden neurons can freely evolve resulting in a complicated structure. Thus, the algorithm allows the system designer to set the maximum number of hidden neurons to minimize this risk.

Producing the Final Network Phase

When a neuron is added and the network performance has not improved, the iSSNN

- removes the added neuron
- resets the learning rate and the weights as they were before adding the new neuron
- terminates the training process
- generate final network is produced *(line 22)*.

The most obvious network parameters to evolve in the iSSNN algorithm are the learning rate, the weights, and the number of hidden neurons. TANH activation function has been used for the input layer, whereas, the bipolar hard limit activation function has been used for the hidden layer.

4   Evaluation

Several experiments are conducted to evaluate the performance of iSSNN algorithm. The experimental evaluation compares the iSSNN with Decision Tree (C4.5) [9], Bayesian Network (BN) [10], Logistic Regression (LR) [11], and the traditional Feed Forward Neural Network (FFNN) algorithm. FFNN assumes that the number of neurons in the input layers equals the number of attributes in the training dataset, whereas the number of neurons in the output layer equals the number of classes. The number of neurons in the hidden layer is the average number of neurons in the layers [6] and is calculated as per Eq. (3).

$$\#hidden\,neurons = \frac{\#input\,neurons + number\,of\,output\,neurons}{\#\,of\,layers} \quad (3)$$

Other algorithms were selected since they use different learning strategies in producing the classifiers. For all these algorithms, we used the default parameter settings of WEKA [6]. Whereas, for iSSNN algorithm, two input values should be entered from the system designer, i.e. number of epochs and maximum number of possible hidden neurons. There is no rule of thumb in which one can decide on these values [5], and therefore, following some recent studies which employ NN to create classification models [12–15], we set the maximum number of possible neurons to 10. These above studies utilised different epoch sizes and the most commonly used epoch size values were 100, 200, 500, and 1000.

Four experiments are conducted, in which the maximum number of possible hidden neurons is 10, and epoch size has been set to 100, 200, 500, and 1000 in experiments 1, 2, 3, and 4 respectively. The iSSNN algorithm has been implemented in Java and all considered classification algorithms have been implemented in WEKA. All experiments were conducted in a computer system with CPU Pentium Intel® CoreTM i5-2430M @ 2.40 GHz, RAM 4.00 GB. The platform is Windows 7 64-bit Operating System.

Ten different binary classification datasets from the UCI [16] have been chosen. We have picked small, medium and large datasets with several numbers of attributes for fair selection. Table 1 shows the datasets description, i.e. name, number of attributes, number of instances, number of missing values, and class distribution for each dataset. Some datasets hold categorical values and the iSSNN algorithm requires converting these categorical values into numerical values. iSSNN algorithm allocates either 1 or −1 to class values since the activation function in the hidden layer is a bipolar hard limit. So, any class variable holds values other than 1 and −1 will be converted to 1 and −1 for experimental purposes. In order to differentiate input attributes from class variables, we assign 0.5 and −0.5 for the binary attributes, and 0.5, 0, and −0.5 for trinary attributes. Other attributes holding numerical values are left without any changes.

The iSSNN algorithm splits the training dataset into training, testing and validation datasets. The hold-out validation technique is used in our experiments. Thus, all datasets will be divided into 80 % for training and 20 % for testing. Moreover, when creating the iSSNN classifiers the training datasets will be further divided into 80 % for training and 20 % for validation.

Table 1. UCI dataset characteristics

Dataset	Number of attributes	Number of instances	Missing values	Class distribution
Breast	10	699	16	66 % 34 %
Labor	17	57	326	35 % 65 %
Vote	17	435	392	61 % 39 %
Pima	9	786	0	65 % 35 %
Tic-Tac	10	958	0	35 % 65 %
Liver	7	345	0	42 % 58 %
Sonar	61	208	0	47 % 53 %
Hepatitis	20	155	167	21 % 79 %
Ionosphere	35	351	0	36 % 64 %
kr-vs-kp	37	3196	0	52 % 48 %

Four evaluation measures based on the confusion matrix have been employed in our experiments as per Table 2.

Table 2. Confusion matrix

Actual value	Predicted value	
	Positive	*Negative*
Positive	*TP*	*FN*
Negative	*FP*	*TN*

where True Positive (TP) is the number of positive examples correctly classified as positive, False Negative (FN) is the number of positive examples incorrectly classified as negative, False Positive (FP) is the number of negative examples incorrectly classified as positive and True Negative (TN) is the number of negative examples correctly classified as negative. The iSSNN algorithm is compared with other classification algorithms in terms of one error-rate as per Eq. 4.

$$\text{error-rate} = 1 - \text{Accuracy}(\%) \tag{4}$$

where "Accuracy(%)" is the proportion of instances that have correct classification from the size of the dataset and is calculated as per Eq. 5.

$$\text{Accuracy}(\%) = \frac{\text{TP} + \text{TN}}{\text{TP} + \text{FP} + \text{TN} + \text{FN}} \tag{5}$$

5   Experimental Results

Table 3 shows the error-rate produced by iSSNN and other considered algorithms against the 10 UCI datasets. The figures in the table indicate that iSSNN outperforms the remaining algorithms in most cases and using different epoch size set. For instance, when epoch size was set to 500, the won-lost-tie records of iSSNN against C4.5, BN, LR and FFNN are 9-0-1, 5-2-3, 5-4-1 and 5-2-3 respectively. In fact, the average error rate performance of the iSSNN using the different epoch size is somehow consistent. The average error of iSSNN begun to slightly deteriorates when the epoch size has increased with one exception when we set the epoch size to 1000.

Other algorithms have slightly outperformed iSSNN in certain epoch size experiments. For example, when the epoch size was initially set to 100, LR algorithm has outperformed the proposed algorithm with a record of 6-2-2, and FFNN has tied error rate performance with a record of 4-4-4 against iSSNN. Furthermore, when we increased the epoch size to 200 the iSSNN algorithm began to improve to reach high competitiveness with LR, and FFNN algorithms. Then, when the epoch size increased to 500, the iSSNN outperformed the rest of the considered algorithms on average with reference to error rate as shown clearly in Fig. 2.

Figure 2 depicts the average error rate derived by all classifiers. Our algorithm produced classifiers that have lower average error rate by 0.57 %, 1.07 %, 5.90 % and 8.23 % than LR, FFNN, BN and C4.5 algorithms respectively. These results have a good sign that NN based algorithms, i.e. FFNN and iSSNN; generate higher predictive classifiers than C4.5 and BN. One possible reason is the fact that these algorithms have the ability to deal with fault tolerance situations, i.e. their performance does not significantly affected if some data are missing in the training dataset. That explains the high error-rate of C4.5 in some datasets such as "Breast", "Labor", and "Hepatitis". Knowing that, C4.5 utilises a probabilistic methods to handle missing data.

One notable result from Table 3 and Fig. 2 is that the average error-rate produced by LR's classifier is slightly better than those generated by iSSNN particularly when the epoch sizes were set to very low or very high value(s).

Table 3. Error-rate of iSSNN and other considered algorithms (%)

Dataset	C4.5	BN	LR	FFNN	iSSNN-100	iSSNN-200	iSSNN-500	iSSNN-1000
Breast	7.14	3.57	2.86	4.29	3.57	3.57	3.57	3.57
Labor	27.27	9.09	9.09	9.09	9.09	9.09	9.09	9.09
Liver	40.58	39.13	28.99	31.88	39.13	31.88	34.78	34.78
Ionosphere	20.00	12.86	18.57	15.71	20.00	17.14	17.14	15.71
Pima	24.03	17.53	18.83	25.97	19.48	18.18	20.13	20.13
Tic-Tac	16.15	29.69	1.57	3.15	2.08	3.15	1.44	3.56
Sonar	19.05	23.81	16.67	9.52	14.29	11.52	9.52	9.52
Hepatitis	32.26	9.68	16.12	16.12	16.12	19.35	9.68	16.12
Vote	5.75	11.49	1.15	4.60	3.45	4.60	4.60	3.45
kr-vs-kp	0.47	12.52	2.19	0.78	2.03	0.47	0.47	0.47
Average	19.27	16.94	11.61	12.11	12.92	11.90	11.04	11.64

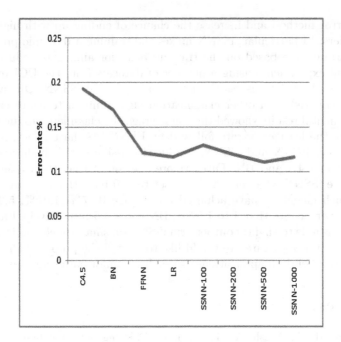

Fig. 2. ErrorRate from iSSNN and considered algorithms

Overall, iSSNN was able to produce competitive results on different epoch sizes. That can be attributed to the training procedure of iSSNN. To elaborate, iSSNN keeps pushing on the learning rate to improve the NN performance as much as possible by adjusting the desired error-rate several times before adding a new hidden neuron. The learning rate in iSSNN is not static but it changes after each training epoch. If the error-rate achieved at epoch i is smaller than the error at epoch $i - 1$, the iSSNN increases the learning rate in order to converge quickly to the possible solutions. However, if the error-rate at epoch i is higher than the error-rate at epoch $i - 1$ the iSSNN decrease the learning rate since we might approach one possible solution and the iSSNN needs to slow down and evaluate that solution. Yet, if the iSSNN cannot achieve the desired error-rate and it reaches the maximum number of epochs or the early stopping condition then the iSSNN adds a new hidden neuron.

In addition, the mechanism of producing the weights in iSSNN is another reason of producing good classifiers since the weights are only saved when the performance of the network on the validation dataset has improved.

6   Conclusions

In this article, we proposed an improved self-structuring neural network algorithm called iSSNN that simplifies structuring NN classifiers. Our algorithm tunes model parameters during the training phase to reduce the deficiencies of trail and error method and increase the chance of ending up with high predictive classifiers. In particular, iSSNN makes the training a dynamic process and adjusts learning rate based on the training behavior aiming to reduce overfitting. Several experiments using a number of datasets from the UCI repository have been conducted to assess the performance of the iSSNN. Our algorithm has been compared with other classification algorithms in terms of error-rate. The experimental results showed that on average the classifiers produced by the iSSNN have the least error-rate followed by FFNN. As matter fact, NN based algorithms, i.e. FFNN and iSSNN, produced classifiers with higher predictive accuracy than C4.5 and BN. Furthermore, we found that the classifiers produced by the iSSNN when epoch size is set to 500 have the least error-rate on average. Such classifiers have achieved on average 0.57%, 1.07%, 5.90% and 8.23% lower error-rate than LR, FFNN, BN and C4.5 respectively. Finally, LR algorithm was able to slightly outperform iSSNN on small epoch and large epoch experiments. In near future, we would like to extend the proposed algorithm to handle multi label data applications especially bioinformatics and text mining.

References

1. Abdelhamid, N., Ayesh, A., Thabtah, F.: Phishing detection based associative classification data mining. Expert Syst. Appl. **41**(13), 5948–5959 (2014)
2. Ash, T.: Dynamic node creation in backpropagation networks. Connect. Sci. **1**(4), 365–375 (1989)
3. Fahlman, S.E., Lebiere, C.: The cascade-correlation learning architecture. In: Advances in Neural Information Processing Systems, pp. 524–532 (1990)
4. Ma, L., Khorasani, K.: A new strategy for adaptively constructing multilayer feedforward neural networks. Neurocomputing **51**(1), 361–385 (2003)
5. Basheer, I.A., Hajmeer, M.: Artificial neural networks: fundamentals, computing, design, and application. J. Microbiol. Methods **43**(1), 3–31 (2000)
6. Hall, M., et al.: Waikato Environment for Knowledge Analysis (2011). http://www.cs.waikato.ac.nz/ml/weka/
7. Duffner, S., Garcia, C.: An online backpropagation algorithm with validation error-based adaptive learning rate. In: de Sá, J.M., Alexandre, L.A., Duch, W., Mandic, D.P. (eds.) ICANN 2007. LNCS, vol. 4668, pp. 249–258. Springer, Heidelberg (2007)
8. Riley, M., Karl, J., Chris, T.: A study of early stopping, ensembling, and patchworking for cascade correlation neural networks. IAENG Int. J. Appl. Math. **40**(4), 307–316 (2010)
9. Quinlan, J.: Data mining tools See5 and C5.0 (1998)
10. Friedman, N., Geiger, D., Goldszmidt, M.: Bayesian network classifiers. Mach. Learn. - Spec. Issue Learn. Probab. Represent. **29**(2–3), 131–163 (1997)
11. Witten, I.H., Frank, E., Hall, M.A.: Data Mining: Practical Machine Learning Tools and Techniques with Java Implementations, 3rd edn. Morgan Kaufmann, Boston (2011)
12. Hinton, G., et al.: Deep neural networks for acoustic modeling in speech recognition. IEEE Signal Process. Mag. **29**(6), 82–97 (2012)

13. Ganatra, A., Kosta, Y.P., Panchal, G., Gajjar, C.: Initial classification through back propagation in a neural network following optimization through GA to evaluate the fitness of an algorithm. Int. J. Comput. Sci. Inf. Technol. **3**(1), 98–116 (2011)
14. Insung, J., Wang, G.-N.: Pattern classification of back-propagation algorithm using exclusive connecting network. World Acad. Sci. **36**(1), 189–193 (2007)
15. Mohammad, R.M., Thabtah, F., McCluskey, L.: Predicting phishing websites using neural network trained with back-propagation. In: ICAI, Las Vigas, pp. 682–686 (2013)
16. Lichman, M.: School of Information and Computer Sciences, University of California, Irvine (2013). http://archive.ics.uci.edu/ml/index.html

Imbalanced ELM Based on Normal Density Estimation for Binary-Class Classification

Yulin He[1]([✉]), Rana Aamir Raza Ashfaq[1,2], Joshua Zhexue Huang[1], and Xizhao Wang[1]

[1] College of Computer Science and Software Engineering,
Shenzhen University, Shenzhen 518060, China
[2] Department of Computer Science, Bahauddin Zakariya University,
Multan, Pakistan
csylhe@126.com, {yulinhe,aamir,zx.huang,xzwang}@szu.edu.cn

Abstract. The **im**balanced **E**xtreme **L**earning **M**achine based on kernel density estimation (imELM-kde) is a latest classification algorithm for handling the imbalanced binary-class classification. By adjusting the real outputs of training data with intersection point of two *probability density functions* (*p.d.f.*s) corresponding to the predictive outputs of majority and minority classes, imELM-kde updates ELM which is trained based on the original training data and thus improves the performance of ELM-based imbalanced classifier. In this paper, we analyze the shortcomings of imELM-kde and then propose an improved version of imELM-kde. The Parzen window method used in imELM-kde leads to multiple intersection points between *p.d.f.*s of majority and minority classes. In addition, it is unreasonable to update the real outputs with intersection point, because the *p.d.f.*s are estimated based on the predictive outputs. Thus, in order to improve the shortcomings of imELM-kde, an **im**balanced ELM based on **n**ormal **d**ensity **e**stimation (imELM-nde) is proposed in this paper. In imELM-nde, the *p.d.f.*s of predictive outputs corresponding to majority and minority classes are computed with normal density estimation and the intersection point is used to update the predictive outputs instead of real outputs. This makes the training of probability density estimation-based imbalanced ELM simpler and more feasible. The comparative results show that our proposed imELM-nde performs better than unweighted ELM and imELM-kde for imbalanced binary-class classification problem.

Keywords: Extreme learning machine · Imbalanced classification · Probability density function · Kernel density estimation · Normal density estimation

1 Introduction

Extreme **L**earning **M**achine (ELM) [3,5–7] is a fast and simple training algorithm for **S**ingle hidden-**L**ayer **F**eed-forward neural **N**etwork (SLFN), which randomly

© Springer International Publishing Switzerland 2016
H. Cao et al. (Eds.): PAKDD 2016 Workshops, LNAI 9794, pp. 48–60, 2016.
DOI: 10.1007/978-3-319-42996-0_5

assignes the input-layer weights and hidden-layer biases and analytically determines the output-layer weights by solving *Moore-Penrose* generalized inverse [12] of hidden-layer output matrix. The theoretically proofs guarantee the universal approximate capability [4] and optimal generalization performance [8, 10] of ELM. The lower computational complexity and better generalization performance make that ELM obtains a wide range of applications [1, 9, 16, 19], where the imbalanced classification with ELM is a very attractive issue in recent years.

The ELM-based imbalanced classification algorithms can be divided into two categories: weighted ELM and probability density estimation-based ELM. The well-known weighted ELM methods include total error rate-based ELM [13], weighted regularized ELM [2], Zong *et al.*'s weighted ELM [20], and fuzzy ELM [18]. These methods assignes the weight for the inputs of each sample in training data set according to different weighting schemes, e.g., calculating the inverse of number of samples belonging to a given class, modifying the inverse of number of samples with the golden standard, and designing the weight based on the training error of unweighted ELM, etc. Probability density estimation-based ELM is a latest strategy for developing the imbalanced ELM classification algorithm. The representative work is the **im**balanced **E**xtreme **L**earning **M**achine based on **k**ernel **d**ensity **e**stimation (imELM-kde) [17] which mainly focuses on the imbalanced binary-class classification. Yang *et al.* [17] analyzed the relationship between ELM and naive Bayesian classifier and got that the output of ELM can approximate the posterior probability of naive Bayesian classifier. Thus, imELM-kde used the Parzen window method [11] to estimate the *probability density functions (p.d.f.s)* corresponding to the predictive outputs of majority and minority classes and then retrained ELM based on the updated training data by adjusting the real outputs with intersection of two *p.d.f.s*. The experimental results in comparison with existing weighted ELMs demonstrated the feasibility and superiority of imELM-kde.

However, the further analysis shows that there are two main shortcomings for imELM-kde. One is the multiple intersections and another is to update the real outputs with intersection point. Because the *p.d.f.* obtained with kernel density estimation usually has multiple peaks, it causes there are multiple intersections for two *p.d.f.s* when the predictive outputs of minority class with ELM are seriously destroyed. Meanwhile, it is time-consuming to find the optimal intersection from multiple intersections. In addition, the performance of Parzen window method severely depends on the selection of *bandwidth* which is an necessary parameter for kernel density estimation [15]. However, the authors can't clearly discuss which intersection should be used to update the real outputs and how to determine the *bandwidth* for kernel density estimation in [17]. Furthermore, it is unreasonable to update the real outputs with intersection in imELM-kde, because the *p.d.f.s* are estimated based on the predictive outputs rather than real outputs. Thus, in order to improve the shortcomings of imELM-kde mentioned above, an **im**balanced ELM based on **n**ormal **d**ensity **e**stimation (imELM-nde) is proposed in this paper. The imELM-nde uses the normal density estimation to compute the *p.d.f.s* corresponding to the predictive outputs of majority and minority classes. This makes the selection of intersection simpler and guarantees that there is only one intersection between the means of normal *p.d.f.s.* In addition, the imELM-nde uses the intersection to update the predictive outputs of training data instead of real outputs. The experimental results in comparison with unweighted ELM and imELM-kde show that our proposed imELM-nde obtains the better imbalanced classification performances.

The remainder of this paper is organized as follows. In Sect. 2, we provide a brief introduction to imELM-kde. In Sect. 3, we analyze the shortcomings of imELM-kde and present the proposed imELM-nde algorithm. In Sect. 4, we report experimental comparisons that demonstrate the feasibility and effectiveness of imELM-nde. Finally, we give our conclusions in Sect. 5.

2   Imbalanced ELM Based on Kernel Density Estimation

In this section, we firstly describe the unweighted ELM and then introduce the imbalanced ELM based kernel density estimation (imELM-kde). In this paper, all the learning algorithms are discussed based on the binary-class classification problem.

2.1   Unweighted ELM

Assume there is a training data set S having N distinct samples (x_n, t_n), where $x_n = (x_{n1}, x_{n2}, \cdots, x_{nd})$, $t_n = (1,0)$ (x_n belongs to the first class) or $t_n = (0,1)$ (x_n belongs to the second class), $n = 1, 2, \cdots, N$, $d = 1, 2, \cdots, D$, D is the number of inputs of x_n. We want to train a SLFN based on the given training data set S. The unweighted ELM [7] firstly initializes the input-layer weights and hidden-layer biases with random numbers in interval $[0,1]$ and then calculates the output-layer weights according to the following formula[1]:

$$\beta = H^\dagger T, \quad T = [t_1, t_2, \cdots, t_N]^T, \tag{1}$$

where $H^\dagger$ is the *Moore-Penrose* generalized inverse of the hidden layer output matrix

$$H = \begin{bmatrix} h(x_1) \\ h(x_2) \\ \vdots \\ h(x_N) \end{bmatrix} = \begin{bmatrix} g(w_1 x_1 + b_1) & g(w_2 x_1 + b_2) & \cdots & g(w_L x_1 + b_L) \\ g(w_1 x_2 + b_1) & g(w_2 x_2 + b_2) & \cdots & g(w_L x_2 + b_L) \\ \vdots & \vdots & \ddots & \vdots \\ g(w_L x_N + b_L) & g(w_2 x_N + b_L) & \cdots & g(w_L x_N + b_L) \end{bmatrix},$$

$g(v) = \frac{1}{1+e^{-v}}$ is sigmoid activation function,

$$W = \begin{bmatrix} w_1 \ w_2 \cdots w_L \end{bmatrix} = \begin{bmatrix} w_{11} & w_{21} & \cdots & w_{L1} \\ w_{12} & w_{22} & \cdots & w_{L2} \\ \vdots & \vdots & \ddots & \vdots \\ w_{1D} & w_{2D} & \cdots & w_{LD} \end{bmatrix} \quad \text{and} \quad b = [b_1, b_2, \cdots, b_L]^T$$

---

[1] For simplicity, we don't use the ridge regression-based ELM [6] in this paper. All the probability density estimation-based ELMs discussed below are designed based on ELM without the regularization factor $C > 0$.

are respectively the input-layer weight matrix and the hidden-layer bias vector, L is the number of hidden-layer nodes in SLFN. For an unseen sample $x = (x_1, x_2, \cdots, x_d)$, the unweighted ELM predicts its output $y = (y_1, y_2)$ as:

$$y = h(x)\beta = h(x)H^\dagger T. \tag{2}$$

If $y_1 > y_2$, the unweighted ELM judges x belongs to the first class; otherwise, x belongs to the second class.

2.2   imELM-kde

When the class distribution of a given training data set is imbalanced, the learning algorithms including unweighted ELM mentioned above have the tendency to favor the majority class because they are all trained by assuming the balanced class distribution or equal misclassification cost [20]. In order to handle the imbalanced classification with ELMs effectively, several ELM variants have been designed, e.g., weighted ELMs [2,13,18,20] and probability density estimation-based ELM [17]. The former assigns the weights for inputs with different weighting schemes and the latter adjusts the outputs with probability density estimation approach.

Designing ELM based on probability density estimation, e.g., imELM-kde [17], is of particular interest in this paper. **Algorithm 1**[2] gives the detailed procedure of imELM-kde. The principle of imELM-kde is that there is an approximately equivalent relationship between the predictive output of unwieghted ELM and the posterior probability of naive Bayesian classifier, i.e., $f_m(x, t) \approx p(t_m | x)$, $m = 1, 2$, where $f_m(x, t)$ is the output of the m-th output-layer node and $p(t_m | x)$ is the posterior probability of x belonging to the m-th class. Thus, the determination of class label for x can be conducted by using the posterior probability which is represented with the output of ELM. There are two output-layer nodes in SLFN and then we can estimate two posterior probabilities p_1 and p_2 based on $[f_1(x_1, t), f_1(x_2, t), \cdots, f_1(x_N, t)]$ and $[f_2(x_1, t), f_2(x_2, t), \cdots, f_2(x_N, t)]$, respectively. Hence, it is possible to judge the class label for x according to the intersection s of p_1 and p_2. s can be deemed as the theoretically optimal breakpoint [17] when the class distribution is balanced. However, the optimal breakpoint is always pushed towards the minority class when the class distribution is imbalanced. That is to say, the classification performance of minority class will be seriously destroyed if the classification is carried out with the current intersection s. In order to improve the performance of classifier on minority class, the $p.d.f.s.$ p_1 and p_2 should be moved towards the optimal breakpoint with the shift $0.5 - s$, where the optimal breakpoint is 0.5 when we use 0 and 1 to represent the class labels for samples in training data set S.

---

[2] In [17], the authors didn't provide the specific discussion regarding how to map the predictive outputs into a one-dimensional space. Here, we used the mapping method in our proposed inELM-nde to deal with this issue.

Algorithm 1. imELM-kde

1: **Input:** A binary-class training data set $S =$ $\left\{(x_n, t_n) \in R^D \times R^2 \,|\, x_n = (x_{n1}, x_{n2}, \cdots, x_{nd}), t_n = (t_{n1}, t_{n2}), t_{nm} \in \{0, 1\}\right.$ (In this study, 0 and 1 respectively represent the majority and minority classes), $n = 1, 2, \cdots, N;\, d = 1, 2, \cdots, D;\, m = 1, 2\}$; the number L of hidden-layer nodes.

2: **Output:** An imbalanced classification algorithm imELM-kde.

3: **Step 1:** Train an unweighted ELM classifier F on training data set S, where there are two output-layer nodes in F.

4: **Step 2:** Acquire the predictive output $y_n = (y_{n1}, y_{n2})$ for each x_n in S with classifier F.

5: **Step 3:** Obtain two *p.d.f.*s p_1 and p_2 based on $\left(y'_{11}, y'_{21}, \cdots, y'_{N_1,1}\right)$ and $\left(y'_{12}, y'_{22}, \cdots, y'_{N_2,2}\right)$ by using kernel density estimation approach, i.e., Parzen window method, where $y'_{n_1,1} \in (y_{11}, y_{21}, \cdots, y_{N1})$ and $y'_{n_2,2} \in (y_{12}, y_{22}, \cdots, y_{N2})$ are the predictive outputs of samples belonging to the first and second classes, respectively; $n_1 = 1, 2, \cdots, N_1$, $n_2 = 1, 2, \cdots, N_2$, and $N_1 + N_2 = N$.

6: **Step 4:** Find the intersection s of two *p.d.f.*s and calculate the shift $u = 0.5 - s$.

7: **Step 5:** Update the real output $t_{n1} \leftarrow t_{n1} + u$ and $t_{n2} \leftarrow t_{n2} + u$ for each x_n and then retrain ELM classifier F based on the updated training data set. The retrained ELM classifier is imELM-kde.

---

3 Imbalanced ELM Based on Normal Density Estimation

In this section, we firstly analyze the shortcomings of imELM-kde and then present an imbalanced ELM based on normal density estimation (imELM-nde) to improve the shortcomings of imELM-kde.

3.1 Analysis to imELM-kde

Although the comparative experiments on 32 KEEL[3] imbalanced data sets reported the better performance of imELM-kde [17], we find that there are two following main shortcomings in imELM-kde.

– Multiple intersections. Given N observations $(v_1, v_2, \cdots, v_N)$ of random variable V, the kernel density estimation uses the Parzen window method to estimate the *p.d.f.* $p(v)$ for V as:

$$p(v) = \frac{1}{N} \sum_{n=1}^{N} \frac{1}{\sqrt{2\pi}h} \exp\left[-\frac{(v - v_n)^2}{2h^2}\right], \tag{3}$$

where $h > 0$ is the bandwidth parameter which severely impacts the estimation performance of Parzen window [15]. The large h will make the estimation smooth and the small one will lead to a rough estimation [14]. In imELM-kde, the authors didn't clearly discuss how to determine this parameter. In the following experiment, we let $h = N^{-\frac{3}{4}}$. We select 2 representatively imbalanced data sets, i.e., *ecoli3* and *glass1*, from the KEEL data sets used in [17]

---

[3] KEEL-dataset repository. http://www.keel.es/.

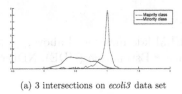 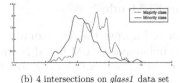

(a) 3 intersections on *ecoli3* data set

(b) 4 intersections on *glass1* data set

Fig. 1. Multiple intersections of two *p.d.f.*s in imELM-kde. ELM F in Algorithm 1 has 30 hidden-layer nodes and the input-layer weights and hidden-layer biases are initialized with the random numbers in interval $[0, 1]$.

and estimate *p.d.f.*s of predictive outputs corresponding to majority class and minority classes. Figure 1 shows the multiple intersections of two *p.d.f.*s. From these two pictures, we can clearly see that there are 3 and 4 intersections for *ecoli3* and *glass1* data sets, respectively. The multiple intersections of *p.d.f.*s are caused by the kernel density estimation which leads to the multiple peaks of *p.d.f.*s. Here, the problem is which intersection should be chose and can bring about the good classification performance for imELM-kde. [17] can't provide us a specific method to select the optimal intersection. In addition, it is difficult to calculate the intersections of *p.d.f.*s. Assume there is another *p.d.f.* $p'(v)$ which is also estimated with Parzen window method based on N' observations $(v'_1, v'_2, \cdots, v'_N)$:

$$p'(v) = \frac{1}{N'} \sum_{n=1}^{N'} \frac{1}{\sqrt{2\pi}h'} \exp\left[-\frac{(v - v'_n)^2}{2h'^2}\right]. \tag{4}$$

We can find that it is hard to solve the v which makes $p(v) = p'(v)$. The analytic solution of v can't be obtained. We have to use some optimization methods to find such v subjected to $p(v) = p'(v)$. This will cause the significant increase of computational complexity.

– Adjustment to real output with intersection. Assume the optimal intersection s have been obtained. It is unreasonable to use the shift $u = 0.5 - s$ to update the real outputs of training data, because the *p.d.f.*s p_1 and p_2 in Algorithm 1 are estimated based on the predictive outputs $(y'_{11}, y'_{21}, \cdots, y'_{N_1,1})$ and $(y'_{12}, y'_{22}, \cdots, y'_{N_2,2})$. The intersection s reflects the distributions of predictive outputs rather than real outputs $(t_{11}, t_{21}, \cdots, t_{N1})$ and $(t_{12}, t_{22}, \cdots, t_{N2})$. That is to say, the intersection represents the movements of *p.d.f.*s corresponding to predictive outputs. However, imELM-kde uses this intersection s to guide the movement of real outputs. Assume we have estimated the *p.d.f.*s p'_1 and p'_2 based on $(t_{11}, t_{21}, \cdots, t_{N1})$ and $(t_{12}, t_{22}, \cdots, t_{N2})$ and the optimal intersection s' of p'_1 and p'_2 has been found. We can get that the possibility of $s' \neq s$ is very little because $\|p'_1 - p_1\|^2 \nrightarrow 0$ and $\|p'_2 - p_2\|^2 \nrightarrow 0$ for the given domain. Thus, it will limit the performance of imELM-kde by using the intersection of *p.d.f.*s corresponding to predictive outputs to update the real outputs.

3.2   imELM-nde

In order to improve the shortcomings of imELM-kde mentioned above, we propose an imbalanced ELM based **N**ormal **D**ensity **E**stimation (NDE). NDE estimates the *p.d.f.* for random variable V as

$$q(v) = \frac{1}{\sqrt{2\pi}\sigma} \exp\left[-\frac{(v-\mu)^2}{2\sigma^2}\right], \tag{5}$$

where $\mu = \frac{1}{N}\sum\limits_{n=1}^{N} v_n$ is the mean value and $\sigma^2 = \frac{1}{N-1}\sum\limits_{n=1}^{N}(v_n-\mu)^2$ is the variance. In fact, we can find that NDE assumes the random variable V obeys a normal distribution with mean value μ and variance σ^2. Let

$$q_1(v) = \frac{1}{\sqrt{2\pi}\sigma_1} \exp\left[-\frac{(v-\mu_1)^2}{2\sigma_1^2}\right], \mu_1 = \frac{1}{N_1}\sum\limits_{n_1=1}^{N_1} y'_{n_1,1}, \sigma_1^2 = \frac{1}{N_1-1}\sum\limits_{n=1}^{N_1}(y'_{n_1,1}-\mu_1)^2 \tag{6}$$

and

$$q_2(v) = \frac{1}{\sqrt{2\pi}\sigma_2} \exp\left[-\frac{(v-\mu_2)^2}{2\sigma_2^2}\right], \mu_2 = \frac{1}{N_2}\sum\limits_{n_2=1}^{N_2} y'_{n_2,2}, \sigma_2^2 = \frac{1}{N_2-1}\sum\limits_{n_2=1}^{N_2}(y'_{n_2,2}-\mu_2)^2. \tag{7}$$

represent the normal density functions which are estimated based on $(y'_{11}, y'_{21}, \cdots, y'_{N_1,1})$ and $(y'_{12}, y'_{22}, \cdots, y'_{N_2,2})$, respectively. NDE guarantees that $q_1(v)$ and $q_2(v)$ have at most one intersection within interval $[\mu_1, \mu_2]$ $(\mu_2 \geq \mu_1)$ or $[\mu_2, \mu_1]$ $(\mu_1 \geq \mu_2)$. The intersection of $q_1(v)$ and $q_2(v)$ can be calculated as follows. Let $q_1(v) = q_2(v)$, i.e.,

$$\frac{1}{\sqrt{2\pi}\sigma_1} \exp\left[-\frac{(v-\mu_1)^2}{2\sigma_1^2}\right] = \frac{1}{\sqrt{2\pi}\sigma_2} \exp\left[-\frac{(v-\mu_2)^2}{2\sigma_2^2}\right]. \tag{8}$$

We can transform Eq. (8) into

$$\left(\sigma_2^2 - \sigma_1^2\right)v^2 - \left(2\mu_1\sigma_2^2 - 2\mu_2\sigma_1^2\right)v + \mu_1^2\sigma_2^2 - \mu_2^2\sigma_1^2 - \sigma_1^2\sigma_2^2\mathrm{In}\left(\frac{\sigma_2}{\sigma_1}\right) = 0 \tag{9}$$

and then get the solutions of Eq. (9) as

$$\begin{cases} v_1 = \dfrac{\left(\mu_1\sigma_2^2 - \mu_2\sigma_1^2\right) + \sigma_1\sigma_2\sqrt{(\mu_1-\mu_2)^2 - \left(\sigma_2^2-\sigma_1^2\right)\mathrm{In}\left(\frac{\sigma_2}{\sigma_1}\right)}}{\left(\sigma_2^2-\sigma_1^2\right)} \\ v_2 = \dfrac{\left(\mu_1\sigma_2^2 - \mu_2\sigma_1^2\right) - \sigma_1\sigma_2\sqrt{(\mu_1-\mu_2)^2 - \left(\sigma_2^2-\sigma_1^2\right)\mathrm{In}\left(\frac{\sigma_2}{\sigma_1}\right)}}{\left(\sigma_2^2-\sigma_1^2\right)} \end{cases}. \tag{10}$$

Without loss of generality, we assume $\mu_1 < \mu_2$ and $\sigma_1^2 < \sigma_2^2$. Then, we can get that $\mu_1 < v_1 < \mu_2$ and $\mu_1 < v_2 < \mu_2$ don't hold simultaneously.

We can respectively derive the following inequalities from $\mu_1 < v_1 < \mu_2$ and $\mu_1 < v_2 < \mu_2$:

$$(\mu_2 - \mu_1)\sigma_1^2 < \sigma_1\sigma_2\sqrt{(\mu_1 - \mu_2)^2 - (\sigma_2^2 - \sigma_1^2)\ln\left(\frac{\sigma_2}{\sigma_1}\right)} < (\mu_2 - \mu_1)\sigma_2^2 \quad (11)$$

and

$$(\mu_2 - \mu_1)\sigma_1^2 < -\sigma_1\sigma_2\sqrt{(\mu_1 - \mu_2)^2 - (\sigma_2^2 - \sigma_1^2)\ln\left(\frac{\sigma_2}{\sigma_1}\right)} < (\mu_2 - \mu_1)\sigma_2^2. \quad (12)$$

We can easily find that Eqs. (11) and (12) are contradictory and Eq. (12) doesn't hold because $-\sigma_1\sigma_2\sqrt{(\mu_1 - \mu_2)^2 - (\sigma_2^2 - \sigma_1^2)\ln\left(\frac{\sigma_2}{\sigma_1}\right)} < 0$ (Note that $(\mu_2 - \mu_1)\sigma_1^2 > 0$ and $(\mu_2 - \mu_1)\sigma_2^2 > 0$).

The above-mentioned analysis demonstrates that there is only one intersection located in the interval $[\mu_1, \mu_2]$ or $[\mu_2, \mu_1]$ if $q_1(v)$ and $q_2(v)$ have the intersection between their mean values. The following Eq. (13) gives the calculation formula of intersection sv:

$$\begin{cases} sv = v_1, & \text{if } \mu_1 < \mu_2 \\ sv = v_2, & \text{if } \mu_1 > \mu_2 \end{cases} \quad (13)$$

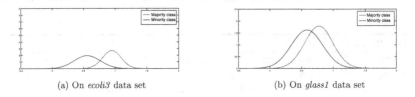

(a) On *ecoli3* data set   (b) On *glass1* data set

Fig. 2. Single intersection of two *p.d.f.*s in imELM-nde. ELM F in Algorithm 2 has 30 hidden-layer nodes and the input-layer weights and hidden-layer biases are initialized with the random numbers in interval $[0, 1]$.

Based on the obtained intersection as shown in Eq. (13), Algorithm 2 depicts the detailed procedure of imELM-nde. The main differences between Algorithm 1 and Algorithm 2 are the density estimation method and output updating strategy. We also plot the *p.d.f.*s for *ecoli3* and *glass1* data sets with NDE method and present the pictures in Fig. 2. We can find that there is only one intersection between the mean values of majority and minority classes. It is convenient for imELM-nde to use this intersection to update the predictive outputs. In addition, we can analytically calculate the intersection, so it is time-saving and doesn't bring about the significant increase of computational complexity. With respect to the output updating, we provide a diagram (Fig. 3) to depict the movement of different *p.d.f.*s in imELM-nde. From Fig. 3, we can see that the objective of movement is to make the area of A smaller, where $A = \{(v, qv) \, | v \in \mathbb{R}, qv \leq q_1(sv) \text{ or } qv \leq q_2(sv)\}$.

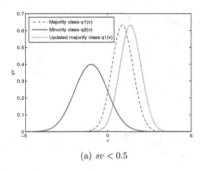 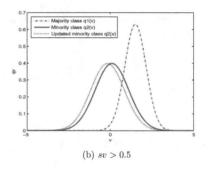

(a) $sv < 0.5$ (b) $sv > 0.5$

Fig. 3. Movements of *p.d.f.* guided by intersection sv ($\mu_1 > \mu_2$ and $q_1 (sv) = q_2 (sv)$)

4   Experimental Comparisons

In this paper, we select 6 imbalanced data sets from the KEEL data sets used in [17] and compare the classification performance of imELM-nde with unweighted ELM and imELM-kde. The details of these 6 imbalanced data sets can be found form [17]. The experimental results are summarized in Table 1, where the accuracy and time are acquired with the procedure of 10-times 10-fold cross-validation. The intersection information of imELM-kde and imELM-nde are obtained based on the whole training data set, i.e., we use the whole training

---

Algorithm 2. imELM-nde

1: **Input:**   A   binary-class   training   data   set $S = \left\{ (x_n, t_n) \in R^D \times R^2 \,|\, x_n = (x_{n1}, x_{n2}, \cdots, x_{nd}) , t_n = (t_{n1}, t_{n2}) , t_{nm} \in \{0, 1\} , n = 1, 2, \cdots, N; d = 1, 2, \cdots, D; m = 1, 2 \right\}$; the number L of hidden-layer nodes.

2: **Output:** An imbalanced classification algorithm imELM-nde.

3: **Step 1:** Train an unweighted ELM classifier F on training data set S, where there are two output-layer nodes in F.

4: **Step 2:** Acquire the predictive output $y_n = (y_{n1}, y_{n2})$ for each x_n in S with classifier F.

5: **Step 3:** Obtain two *p.d.f.*s q_1 and q_2 based on $(y'_{11}, y'_{21}, \cdots, y'_{N_1,1})$ and $(y'_{12}, y'_{22}, \cdots, y'_{N_2,2})$ by using normal density estimation approach as shown in Eq. (5).

6: **Step 4:** Calculate the intersection sv with Eq. (13).

7: **Step 5:** Update the predictive output y_{n1} and y_{n2} based on the following rules: if $\mu_1 < \mu_2$,

$$\begin{cases} y_{n2} \leftarrow y_{n2} + (0.5 - sv) \, , \text{ if } sv < 0.5 \\ y_{n1} \leftarrow y_{n1} - (sv - 0.5) \, , \text{ if } sv > 0.5 \end{cases} ; \qquad (14)$$

otherwise,

$$\begin{cases} y_{n1} \leftarrow y_{n1} + (0.5 - s') \, , \text{ if } sv < 0.5 \\ y_{n2} \leftarrow y_{n2} - (sv - 0.5) \, , \text{ if } sv > 0.5 \end{cases} . \qquad (15)$$

Then, retrain ELM classifier F based on the updated training data set. The retrained ELM classifier is imELM-nde.

Table 1. Comparison of different ELMs on 6 imbalanced data sets

Dataset	L	Unweighted ELM				imELM-kde					imELM-nde						
		TrainAcc	TestAcc	TrainTime	TestTime	Intersections	TrainAcc	TestAcc	TrainTime	TestTime	Intersection	μ_1	μ_2	TrainAcc	TestAcc	TrainTime	TestTime
abalone9-18	20	0.952±0.003	0.948±0.011	0.019	0.003	0.737, 1.329	0.959±0.003	0.956±0.018	0.263	0.000	0.747	0.962	0.378	0.964±0.003	0.958±0.019	0.136	0.003
cleveland-0_vs_4	30	0.972±0.013	0.942±0.060	0.009	0.000	0.787, 1.407	0.969±0.014	0.927±0.072	0.285	0.000	0.758	0.965	0.556	0.974±0.014	0.945±0.059	0.114	0.000
ecoli-0-1-3-7_vs_2-6	20	0.980±0.005	0.943±0.086	0.263	0.000	0.868, 1.174	0.968±0.016	0.946±0.088	0.275	0.000	0.806	0.983	0.351	0.975±0.007	0.957±0.077	0.119	0.000
ecoli3	30	0.932±0.009	0.908±0.033	0.008	0.000	0.840, 1.217	0.944±0.006	0.917±0.024	0.272	0.000	0.761	0.949	0.558	0.944±0.006	0.928±0.039	0.113	0.000
glass-0-1-6_vs_2	30	0.916±0.013	0.888±0.108	0.005	0.000	0.737, 1.377	0.893±0.076	0.899±0.060	0.297	0.000	0.650	0.933	0.320	0.920±0.014	0.907±0.071	0.161	0.000
glass1	30	0.802±0.015	0.687±0.065	0.008	0.000	0.716, 1.102, 1.118, 1.291	0.763±0.083	0.705±0.093	0.294	0.000	0.663	0.778	0.596	0.803±0.018	0.733±0.070	0.111	0.000

data set to train the unweighted ELM and then estimate the $p.d.f.$s of predictive outputs with different probability density estimation methods. The meanings of μ_1 and μ_2 in Table 1 can refer to Eqs. (6) and (7).

The input-layer weights and hidden-layer biases of all ELMs in this comparison are initialized with the random numbers in interval $[0, 1]$. For imELM-kde and imELM-nde, the unweighted ELM and retained ELM have the same input-layer weights and hidden-layer biases. We let the number L of hidden-layer nodes range from 10 to 100 in step of 10 and list L which can bring about the best testing accuracy for imELM-nde in Table 1. Unweighted ELM, imELM-kde, and imELM-nde are implemented using Matlab 7.1 on a Thinkpad SL410K PC with Windows 8 running on a Pentium Dual-core T4400 2.20 GHz processor with 4 GB RAM.

From the comparative results in Table 1, we can see that our proposed imELM-nde obtains the higher testing accuracies on 6 selected imbalanced data sets in comparison with unweighted ELM and imELM-kde, and the training time of imELM-nde is lower than imELM-kde. The main reasons that imELM-nde obtains the lower training time and higher testing accuracy than imELM-kde are estimating the $p.d.f.$s with NDE method and updating the predictive outputs with intersection, respectively. NDE makes imELM-nde can calculate intersection directly without any optimization method. In this experiment, we use Newton iteration method to find the intersections of $p.d.f.$s in imELM-kde. Table 1 gives the details of imELM-kde and imELM-nde intersections on different data sets. imELM-kde has multiple intersections, while imELM-nde only one intersection between the mean values μ_1 and μ_2. In [17], the authors don't consider the multiple intersections of imELM-kde and thus they can't describe which intersection should be used to predict. In our experiment, we select the intersection which can generate the best trainging accuracy as the optimal intersection for the prediction of imELM-kde. The higher generalization performance of imELM-nde is related to the adjustment of predictive outputs instead of real outputs. It is more reasonable that using the intersection to guide the movement of $p.d.f.$s which are estimated based on the predictive outputs.

Above all, our proposed imELM-nde indeed improves the classification performance of imELM-kde on 6 imbalanced binary-class data sets, including lower training times and higher testing accuracies in Table 1.

5   Conclusions

In this paper, we proposed an imbalanced ELM learning algorithm which is based on normal density estimation (imELM-nde) to handle the imbalanced binary-class classification problem. In comparison with imbalanced ELM based on kernel density estimation (imELM-kde), imELM-nde has only one intersection between the mean values of normal $p.d.f.$s corresponding to the predictive outputs of majority and minority classes. The analytic solution of intersection doesn't significantly increase the computational complex of imELM-nde. in addition, imELM-nde used the intersection to update the predictive outputs of unweighted ELM rather than real outputs and then retained unweighted

ELM with the updated training data set. The comparative results on selected imbalanced data sets demonstrated the feasibility and effectiveness that using normal density estimation to improve the generalization performance of *p.d.f.* estimation-based ELM.

Acknowledgments. This work is supported by China Postdoctoral Science Foundations (2015M572361 and 2016T90799), Basic Research Project of Knowledge Innovation Program in Shenzhen (JCYJ201503241400368 25), and National Natural Science Foundations of China (61503252, 61473194, 71371063, and 61473111).

References

1. Chacko, B.P., Krishnan, V.R.V., Raju, G., Anto, P.B.: Handwritten character recognition using wavelet energy and extreme learning machine. Int. J. Mach. Learn. Cybern. **3**(2), 149–161 (2012)
2. Deng, W., Zheng, Q., Chen, L.: Regularized extreme learning machine. In: Proceddings of 2009 IEEE Symposium on Computational Intelligence and Data Mining, pp. 389–395 (2009)
3. Fu, A.M., Dong, C.R., Wang, L.S.: An experimental study on stability and generalization of extreme learning machines. Int. J. Mach. Learn. Cybern. **6**(1), 129–135 (2015)
4. Huang, G.B., Chen, L., Siew, C.K.: Universal approximation using incremental constructive feedforward networks with random hidden nodes. IEEE Trans. Neural Netw. **17**(4), 879–892 (2006)
5. Huang, G.B., Wang, D.H., Lan, Y.: Extreme learning machines: a survey. Int. J. Mach. Learn. Cybern. **2**(2), 107–122 (2011)
6. Huang, G.B., Zhou, H., Ding, X., Zhang, R.: Extreme learning machine for regression and multiclass classification. IEEE Trans. Syst. Man Cybern. Part B Cybern. **42**(2), 513–529 (2012)
7. Huang, G.B., Zhu, Q.Y., Siew, C.K.: Extreme learning machine: theory and applications. Neurocomputing **70**(1), 489–501 (2006)
8. Lin, S.B., Liu, X., Fang, J., Xu, Z.B.: Is extreme learning machine feasible? A theoretical assessment (Part II). IEEE Trans. Neural Netw. Learn. Syst. **26**(1), 21–34 (2015)
9. Liu, P., Huang, Y.H., Meng, L., Gong, S.Y., Zhang, G.P.: Two-stage extreme learning machine for high-dimensional data. Int. J. Mach. Learn. Cybern. (2014). doi:10.1007/s13042-014-0292-7
10. Liu, X., Lin, S.B., Fang, J., Xu, Z.B.: Is extreme learning machine feasible? A theoretical assessment (Part I). IEEE Trans. Neural Netw. Learn. Syst. **26**(1), 7–20 (2015)
11. Parzen, E.: On estimation of a probability density function and mode. Ann. Math. Stat. **33**(3), 1065–1076 (1962)
12. Serre, D.: Matrices: Theory and Applications. Springer, New York (2002)
13. Toh, K.A.: Deterministic neural classification. Neural Comput. **20**(6), 1565–1595 (2008)
14. Wand, M.P., Jones, M.C.: Kernel Smoothing. CRC Press, Boca Raton (1994)
15. Wang, X.Z., He, Y.L., Wang, D.D.: Non-Naive Bayesian classifiers for classification problems with continuous attributes. IEEE Trans. Cybern. **44**(1), 21–39 (2014)

16. Wu, J., Wang, S.T., Chung, F.L.: Positive and negative fuzzy rule system, extreme learning machine and image classification. Int. J. Mach. Learn. Cybern. **2**(4), 261–271 (2011)
17. Yang, J., Yu, H., Yang, X., Zuo, X.: Imbalanced extreme learning machine based on probability density estimation. In: Bikakis, A., Zheng, X. (eds.) MIWAI 2015. LNCS, vol. 9426, pp. 160–167. Springer, Heidelberg (2015). doi:10.1007/978-3-319-26181-2_15
18. Zhang, W.B., Ji, H.B.: Fuzzy extreme learning machine for classification. Electron. Lett. **49**(7), 448–450 (2013)
19. Zhao, H.Y., Guo, X.Y., Wang, M.W., Li, T.L., Pang, C.Y., Georgakopoulos, D.: Analyze EEG signals with extreme learning machine based on PMIS feature selection. Int. J. Mach. Learn. Cybern. (2015). doi:10.1007/s13042-015-0378-x
20. Zong, W., Huang, G.B., Chen, Y.: Weighted extreme learning machine for imbalance learning. Neurocomputing **101**, 229–242 (2013)

Multiple Seeds Based Evolutionary Algorithm for Mining Boolean Association Rules

Mir Md. Jahangir Kabir$^{(\boxtimes)}$, Shuxiang Xu, Byeong Ho Kang,
and Zongyuan Zhao

School of Engineering and ICT, University of Tasmania, Hobart, Australia
{mmjkabir,Shuxiang.Xu,Byeong.Kang,
Zongyuan.Zhao}@utas.edu.au

Abstract. Most of the association rule mining algorithms use a single seed for initializing a population without paying attention to the effectiveness of an initial population in an evolutionary learning. Recently, researchers show that an initial population has significant effects on producing good solutions over several generations of a genetic algorithm. There are two significant challenges raised by single seed based genetic algorithms for real world applications: (1) solutions of a genetic algorithm are varied, since different seeds generate different initial populations, (2) it is a hard process to define an effective seed for a specific application. To avoid these problems, in this paper we propose a new multiple seeds based genetic algorithm (MSGA) which generates multiple seeds from different domains of a solution space to discover high quality rules from a large data set. This approach introduces m-domain model and m-seeds selection process through which the whole solution space is subdivided into m-number of same size domains and from each domain it selects a seed. By using these seeds, this method generates an effective initial population to perform an evolutionary learning of the fitness value of each rule. As a result, this method obtains strong searching efficiency at the beginning of the evolution and achieves fast convergence along with the evolution. MSGA is tested with different mutation and crossover operators for mining interesting Boolean association rules from different real world data sets and compared the results with different single seeds based genetic algorithms.

Keywords: Multiple seeds based genetic algorithm · Boolean association rules · Initial population · Conditional probability · Evolutionary learning

1 Introduction

Data mining techniques are the most important and useful tool for extracting novel, interesting and valid patterns and knowledge from a large amount of data. The objective of data mining processes is to build an efficient descriptive and predictive model of a large dataset which will not only explain it but will also be able to generalize to new data sets [1]. Mining association rules play a vital role in advancing the scientific knowledge, development and applications of data mining techniques. Association rules are used to define and represent the dependencies between item sets in a large data set. If A and B are two item sets and $A \cap B = \emptyset$, then an association rule can be represented by the

© Springer International Publishing Switzerland 2016
H. Cao et al. (Eds.): PAKDD 2016 Workshops, LNAI 9794, pp. 61–72, 2016.
DOI: 10.1007/978-3-319-42996-0_6

following form A → B. Different measures such as support and confidence values are used to indicate the quality of a rule. High quality rules have high support and confidence values. Classical algorithms extract rules from a dataset based on a user defined support and confidence values [2, 3]. Search strategies are approaches used to discover the high quality rules. It can be categorized into two groups: deterministic and stochastic. Most of the deterministic methods are based on a support-confidence framework, and are proposed by Apriori, ECLAT, MAFIA [4, 5]. These methods raise two major issues: (1) Users need to define a suitable threshold value for getting high quality rules from a large data set although they have no knowledge regarding that data set and (2) these methods generate an exponential search space of size 2^n, where n is the number of item sets [2, 6, 7]. Due to the exponential solution space, the computational cost of deterministic approaches are expensive [8]. Therefore, designing effective and efficient deterministic methods is not often suitable [1].

Inspired by Charles Darwin's evolutionary approach, the Genetic Algorithm (GA) was first invented by Holland and promoted by Goldberg. This algorithm is a stochastic approach rather than an exhaustive one. In real world applications, due to the presence of a huge number of misleading and trivial rules, almost all large scale problems become non-monotonic. In these cases, GA performs better than other association rule mining algorithms for large scale problems due to its effectiveness and efficiency [1, 9]. GA is best known for being a robust and a global search technique, which can search an extremely large space within a short amount of time and obtain globally optimum solutions. GAs have been successfully applied to a broad spectrum of problems including machine learning, multiobjective optimization problems and multimodal function optimization.

In real world applications, data sets also contain categorical values as well as quantitative or numeric values [10]. Because of this reason, several studies have been proposed for mining Boolean association rules (BARs) from data sets with categorical values [6, 7, 11]. Most of these algorithms use single seed to initialize the population. For global optimization, GAs usually use a metaheuristic method, but relatively few research papers are published based on the techniques of the generation of initial populations. Traditionally, pseudo random chromosomes are used to generate an initial population. Current research shows that initial populations have significant effects of producing good solutions over several generations [12]. Some researchers [13] use quasi random sequences to generate initial populations for GA. These sequences, which do not imitate random points are successfully used in computer simulations, quasi random searches and numerical integration.

Most of the association rule mining algorithms which are based on GA, use single seed chromosome for generating an initial set of solutions. These algorithms suffer from the following major challenges: (1) Different seed chromosomes generate different initial populations. Because of this reason different seed chromosomes yield different results. (2) It is a hard process to define a good seed for a specific application. (3) Defining seed is not an automatic process rather it is manual since the maximum range of a seed chromosome varies from data sets to data sets.

To explore more search space and exploit it for further generation, a large number of research papers have been done, introducing new methods and genetic operators. As these methods and operators are problem specific, so the researchers [14] introduced an approach named dynamic diversity control in a genetic algorithm (DDCGA) for increasing the diversity in the chromosomes of a population. The basic idea of this process is to generate the multiple archives by gathering high quality chromosomes from different initial seeds of a simple genetic algorithm. Through this technique, the diversity of the population is increased and the evolutionary process can explore more search space [14].

Motivated by the features of the diversity control approach, in this study we propose a new genetic algorithm, named multiple seeds based genetic algorithm (MSGA), which is based on multiple seeds to initialize the population. To deal with the challenges raised by a single seed based approach, this proposed method subdivides the whole solution space into m-regions and randomly selects high quality seed chromosomes from each region. After selection of m-seeds from m-regions, this approach generates initial population from each seed using a Euclidean distance method. As a result, at the beginning of the evolutionary process MSGA obtains strong searching ability and generates an optimum result.

Main Contributions: In order to address the major challenges and issues raised by single seed based genetic algorithm, we present a novel framework named MSGA (Multiple Seeds Based Genetic Algorithm) for obtaining strong search ability. The novel features of this method are as follows:

(C1) m-Domain Model. Our proposed method subdivides the whole solution space into a m-number of same size domains. The purpose of dividing the whole solution space is to get seeds from each domain and to maintain diversity for generating an initial population.

(C2) m-Seeds Selection Process. Our proposed approach uses the m-seeds selection process where n-number of chromosomes are generated from each domain. From the members of a domain, this process selects only one high fitness value chromosome. This chromosome is used as a seed for that domain.

(C3) Initialize Population based on m-Seeds. Based on a seed chromosome, the next step is to generate n-number of individuals by randomly changing any position of a seed chromosome. Through this technique, m seeds generate $m \times n$ number of individuals. These individuals will use as an initial population for MSGA.

(C4) Method Implementation and Evaluation. The main aim of this study is to show the effectiveness and performance of using multiple seeds based method over a single seed based method, applying different genetic operators for finding high quality rules from different data sets. For this reason, in this study we use a conditional probability [7] as a fitness function for evaluating a rule.

To demonstrate the feasibility of our proposed method, we have conducted a number of experiments to mine a reduced set of interesting association rules by optimizing conditional probability using different crossover and mutation operators and compare the result with different single seeds based approaches. Experimental results show that, a multiple seeds based method demonstrates satisfactory performance over different single seeds based methods.

Paper Outline. The remainder of this study is organized as follows: MSGA (Multiple Seeds Based Genetic Algorithm) is presented in Sect. 2. Experimental results and analysis are followed in Sect. 3. Finally, the conclusion of the proposed approach is given in Sect. 4.

2 Methodology

2.1 Multiple Seeds Based Genetic Algorithm

The major focus of this research is to apply the multiple seeds based generation mechanism to generate diversified initial population with good coverage into the evolutionary process, which will generate a large amount of high quality rules. This process also helps to automate selection of a seed chromosome without depending on a dataset. As we discussed in Sect. 1, researchers [12] shows with an example that an initial population has significant effects on evolutionary learning for several generations. Traditional genetic algorithm uses a single seed to generate an initial population. The basic idea of a single seed based genetic algorithm (SSGA) is to randomly select a chromosome from a large solution space for generating an initial population. Because of random selection, SSGA could face premature convergence problem and extract a

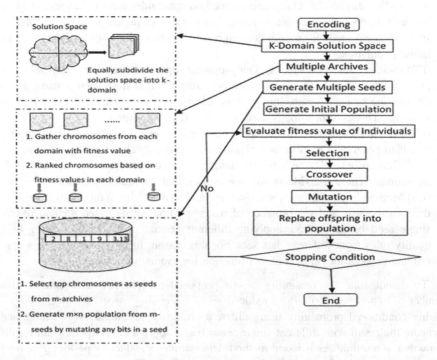

Fig. 1. The architecture of MSGA

small number of high quality rules from a large data set. On the otherhand, some seeds may have a low fitness value but could generate a large number of high quality rules since it explores a huge area of a large solution space. From random selection of a seed chromosome and generating an initial population based on that chromosome cannot guarantee whether that population cover whole solution space or not. As an initial population has significant effects on obtaining best results after several generations, so the population diversity including good coverage of a large solution space is important for the generation of an initial population for balancing the exploration and exploitation search. Thus, a global optimum can be achieved.

The basic idea of this research is to equally divide the whole solution space into m-domain. From each domain, this method generates n-number of individuals. The individuals which are randomly generated from a domain are stored in an archive. Therefore, m-domains generate m-archives. Chromosomes of each archive are ranked based on the fitness values of those chromosomes. A chromosome of a high fitness value has higher rank than the chromosome of a low fitness value. From each archive, top ranked chromosome is selected as a seed. By mutating any bits of a seed, each seed generates n-number of individuals. Therefore, m seeds generate m × n individuals which is used as an initial population for multiple seeds based genetic algorithm. The architecture of MSGA is shown in Fig. 1.

2.2 Distance Measure and Multiple Archive Design

In different types of combinatorial problems, distance measures are strongly problems depended. In this study, we use real encoding technique, i.e. Euclidean distance method to measure the distance between two chromosomes. Suppose X and Y are two chromosomes and the length of each of those chromosomes is denoted by L. The convergence of a population during the evolutionary learning is described by the following distance measure:

$$d(P) = \frac{1}{n} \sum_{i=0}^{n-1} \sum_{j=1}^{n-1} (D(I_i, I_j))^2 \tag{1}$$

where n is the size of a population, I_i and I_j are i-th and j-th individual, and D is the distance between two individuals.

To find the high quality association rules from a large solution space, this approach subdivides the whole solution space into m-domains. In the following, we will briefly describe the encoding technique of an association rule, subdividing the whole solution space into m-domains, chromosome generation from each domain, selecting seeds from domains, and generating an initial population from multiple seeds.

Encoding: Our proposed model follows the Michigan strategy of encoding each association rule into a single chromosome. Given an association rule of k length means that, a rule contains k items. Figure 2 shows the configuration of the chromosome

n	$item_1$	$item_2$	...	$item_n$	$item_{n+1}$	.	$item_k$

Fig. 2. A chromosome of an association rule of k length

which contains k-genes, i.e. k number of items. The first place of the chromosome contains a number which acts as an indicator for separation of the antecedent from the consequent. So, the k-rule represents a chromosome of length k + 1. For example a rule is A → B, where antecedent A contains $item_1$ to $item_n$ and the consequent B contains $item_{n+1}$ to $item_k$, where $0 < n < k$ and $item_1 ... item_k \in$ set of items, I.

Division of a Solution Space: For dividing the whole solution space into m-domains, this approach considers each chromosome as a position in an L dimensional solution space. To do this, it measure the distance between initial to end item sets, which is the maximum distance in a solution space. Each item in a data set D is assigned by a unique identifier. For example, if a data set contains n items then $item_1$, $item_2$, . . ., $item_n$ are assigned by ID $1, 2, . . . n$. In order to measure the distance between two chromosomes, we ignore the first position that is an indicator of a chromosome of an association rule of Fig. 2. For an association rule of k-length, the initial and end chromosomes are defined by the following figures (Figs. 3 and 4).

1	2	3	....	k

Fig. 3. An initial chromosome

n-(k-1)	n-(k-2)	...	n-1	n

Fig. 4. An end chromosome

Note that the order of the chromosome ID is important for defining the initial and end chromosomes. After calculating the Euclidean distance between an initial and end chromosome, next step is to equally divide the whole distance into m-regions. If the total distance is d, then the range (r) of each domain is calculated by the following equation, r = d/m. Based on the ranges, the whole solution space of a data set is subdivided into m equal size domains as shown in Fig. 5.

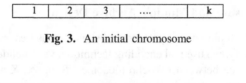

0>range≤r	r>range≤2r	2r>range≤3r	....	(m-1)r>range≤ mr
$Domain_1$	$Domain_2$	$Domain_3$		$Domain_m$

Fig. 5. Ranges of m-domains

Chromosome Generation from Each Domain: The following factors which are listed in Table 1 are the influential coefficients which are used for designing an archive. These factors will be described in this section along with the technique used for generating individuals. In experimental analysis (Sect. 3), we compared the results with different single seed based genetic algorithms. The cage size of an archive depends on the population size and the number of archives. Each domain is assigned an archive. The member chromosomes of an archive are the members of the assigned domain. Whether a generated chromosome is the member of the assigned domain or not depends on the Euclidean distance between a generated and an initial chromosome. This approach randomly generates chromosomes and calculates the distance from the initial chromosome. Based on the distance and specified ranges of the domains (see Fig. 5), it inserts the chromosomes to the specific archives. For example, if a dataset has five items a, b, c, d, e and each item is assigned with an unique ID, i.e. $\{a = 1, b = 2, c = 3, d = 4, e = 5\}$. Then the initial and final chromosome is (1, 2, 3) and (3, 4, 5), respectively. The Euclidean distance between initial and end chromosome is 3.46. If we consider four domains, then the calculated range of each domain is, $d/m = 3.46/4 = 0.865$. Therefore, the four domains can be defined as, $0 > domain_1 \leq 0.865, 0.865 > domain_2 \leq 1.73$, $1.73 > domain_3 \leq 2.595$ and $2.595 > domain_4 \leq 3.46$. The population of an archive is sorted with respect to its chromosome fitness values and assign $n/n \ldots 1/n$ value to each chromosome based on the fitness value. So the best chromosome of an archive obtains n/n that is assigned as a top ranked chromosome, whereas the worse chromosome of that archive gains $1/n$. Therefore, with this approach, a better chromosome of a domain has more chance to perform as a seed chromosome.

Table 1. Factors for designing an archive

Factors	
Policy for archive population	Distance
Cage size of an archive	Population size/m
Population rank policy	Fitness
Population size	Varied

Generating an Initial Population from m-Seeds: An effective initial population is generated from m-seeds. A top ranked chromosome from each archive is selected as a seed. Therefore, m archives generate m seeds. Note that, a seed cannot guarantee that this chromosome will have a high fitness value in a domain from where it is generated. Each seed uses a mutation function to produce an n individual, where the mutation probability is 1. Therefore, m seeds generate m × n individuals. These individuals are used as an initial population for the multiple seeds based genetic algorithm.

According to the above description, the multiple seeds based genetic algorithm for discovering BARs is summarized through the following flowchart:

PROCEDURE: **MSGA**	
Input:	Data set D, population_size, no_of_archives, sp (selection probability), cp (crossover probability), mp (mutation probability), k (rule length)
Output:	A population consists of the positive association rules with conditional probability = 1
(0)	Mapping categorical attributes of a data set D into Boolean attributes
(1)	archives[no_of_archives] ← generate_archives(initial chrom, end chrom, no_of_archives)
(2)	seed_chromosomes[no_of_archives] ← seed_generation (archives)
(3)	**begin** i ← 0
(4)	pop[i] ← population initialization (seed_chromosomes, population_size, no_of_archives)
(5)	**while** not reach_generation_number (pop[i]) **do**
(6)	**begin** temp_pop[0] ← 0
(7)	**for** ∀*chromosome* ∈ pop[i] **do**
(8)	**if** selection(chromosome, sp) **then**
(9)	temp_pop[0] ← chromosome
(10)	temp_pop[0] ← crossover(temp_pop[0], cp)
(11)	**for** ∀*chromosome* ∈ temp_pop[0] **do**
(12)	temp_pop[0] ← mutation(chromosome, mp)
(13)	i ← i+1
(14)	**end**
(15)	**return** pop[i]
(16)	**end**

3 Experimental Results

For analysing the performance of the proposed method, several experiments were carried out on different real world data sets. To evaluate the proposed approach and compare the results with single seeds based simple genetic algorithms, we considered two real world data sets, which were taken from the UCI machine learning repository (http://archive.ics.uci.edu/ml/datasets.html).

Table 2. The specifications of data sets

	Breast cancer	Solar flare
Attributes	51	50
Records	277	1066

As mentioned in Sect. 1, we mapped categorical attributes of a data set into Boolean attributes. The specifications of these mapped data sets are summarized in Table 2 where the number of Boolean attributes and records of a data set are represented by "Attributes" and "Records", respectively.

Table 3 shows the parameters which are used for running the MSGA and a single seed based simple genetic algorithm (SSGA). As described in Sect. 2, multiple seeds are generated from multiple archives and these seeds are applied to generate an effective initial population for mining high quality association rules, each having a condition probability between 80 %–100 %. Traditionally, a simple genetic algorithm randomly generates a single seed for initializing a population for evolutionary learning. In order to analyse the performance of MSGA over a single seed based simple genetic algorithm, in this experiment we separately used those seeds which are generated by MSGA for initializing a population. The effects of different mutation and crossover operators on the initial population for evolutionary learning for generating high quality association rules are examined in two different real world data sets. For developing the different experiments, the average results of three runs are considered for each data set.

Table 3. The parameters used for running the MSGA

MSGA	Population Size (popsize): 100, Selection Probability (sp): 0.95, Crossover Probability (cp): 0.85, Mutation Probability (mp): 0.01, Rule Length (k): 3, No. of Generations: 55, No. of Archives: 4
SSGA	Population Size (popsize): 100, Selection Probability (sp): 0.95, Crossover Probability (cp): 0.85, Mutation Probability (mp): 0.01, Rule Length (k): 3, No. of Generations: 55

Since an initial population has a significant effect on generating a best population in further generation, from the experimental results it can say that single seeds based genetic algorithms generate a smaller number of positive association rules, which are shown in Figs. 6 and 7. Form the experimental figures we see that some seeds generate a large number of rules for some mutation and crossover operators, but for other crossover operators these seeds generate a smaller number of rules for the same mutation operators. On the other hand, the results obtained by the MSGA present better or similar high quality rules for different mutation and crossover operators for all data sets than the rules obtained by single seeds based genetic algorithms.

For the Breast Cancer data set, seed 1 and seed 4 have fitness values of 1 and 0.21, respectively. From Fig. 6, we see that seed 1 based genetic algorithm generates a large number of high quality rules using insertion (INS) mutation and uniform crossover operators with respect to other single seeds based genetic algorithms. Whereas, seed 4 based genetic algorithm performs better than other seeds based genetic algorithms using displacement (DISP), inversion (INV), scramble (SCM) mutation and uniform crossover operators. From the above analysis it can conclude that, a genetic algorithm based on a single seed having a high fitness value cannot guarantee that it will generate a large number of high quality rules using different mutation and crossover operators for all data sets. This is also true for a lower fitness value based seed chromosome. On the other hand, MSGA which comprised all seeds to generate an initial population has a significant effect for further generation of best population and this approach presents better or similar high quality rules using different mutation and crossover operators for all data sets, which are shown in Figs. 6 and 7.

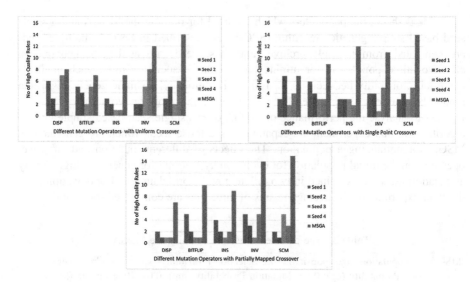

Fig. 6. Performance of different seeds and MSGA for different mutation and crossover operators for a Breast Cancer data set. (Color figure online)

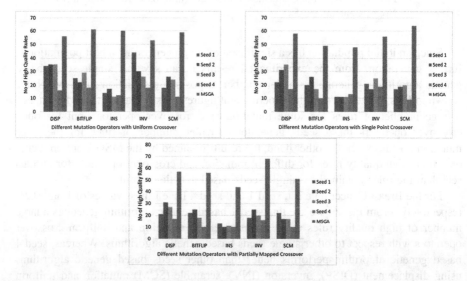

Fig. 7. Performance of different seeds and MSGA for different mutation and crossover operators for a Solar Flare data set. (Color figure online)

Several experiments were carried out for analysing the convergence of the proposed method and single seeds based genetic algorithms for Breast Cancer data set. The convergence of different single seeds and MSGA using different mutation and crossover operators are shown in Fig. 8. From these figures, it can conclude that all the algorithms scale quite linearly, however in most of the cases MSGA converge fast than different single seeds based methods.

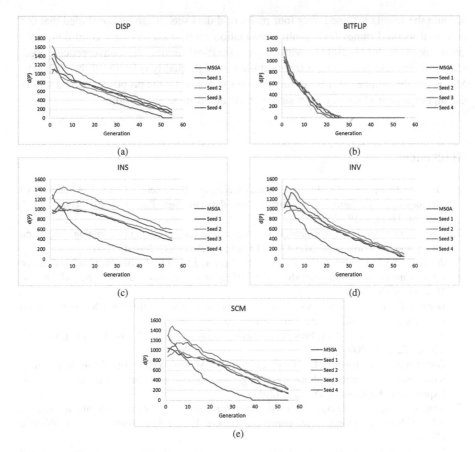

Fig. 8. The convergence of MSGA and different seeds based GAs for different mutation operators with uniform crossover for a Breast Cancer data set. (Color figure online)

4 Conclusions

In this paper we have proposed MSGA, a new evolutionary algorithm which is generating multiple seeds from an m-domain solution space for producing an effective initial population for further evolutionary learning to mine a large number of high quality association rules from categorical data sets. This approach introduces an m-domain model, m-seeds selection method and m-seeds based initialization approach to the evolutionary model in order to discover all the high quality rules and to improve the searching ability and convergence speed. Moreover, this study shows the effectiveness and performance of using multiple seeds based approach over single seeds based methods, applying different genetic operators for finding high quality association rules from different data sets.

MSGA is successfully applied with different mutation and crossover operators in mining interesting BARs from categorical data sets and compared the results with different single seeds based genetic algorithms under the same conditions. Taking into account the results obtained over four real world data sets, it can be concluded that our proposed method mines high quality association rules, each having a condition probability between 80 %–100 %, with a good trade-off among the convergence speed, search ability and presenting a large number of high quality rules in all the data sets. Moreover, the number of rules for all data sets obtained by the proposed method shows the higher search efficiency than single seeds based genetic algorithms.

References

1. Mukhopadhyay, A., Maulik, U., Bandyopadhyay, S., Coello, C.A.C.: A survey of multiobjective evolutionary algorithms for data mining: Part I. IEEE Trans. Evol. Comput. **18**(1), 4–19 (2014)
2. Hipp, J., Güntzer, U., Nakhaeizadeh, G.: Algorithms for association rule mining—a general survey and comparison. ACM SIGKDD Explor. Newsl. **2**(1), 58–64 (2000)
3. del Jesus, M.J., Gámez, J.A., González, P., Puerta, J.M.: On the discovery of association rules by means of evolutionary algorithms. Wiley Interdisc. Rev. Data Min. Knowl. Discov. **1**(5), 397–415 (2011)
4. Borgelt, C.: Efficient implementations of apriori and eclat. In: IEEE ICDM Workshop on Frequent Item Set Mining Implementations, pp. 280–296 (2003)
5. Zaki, M.J.: Scalable algorithms for association mining. IEEE Trans. Knowl. Data Eng. **12**(3), 372–390 (2000)
6. Qodmanan, H.R., Nasiri, M., Minaei-Bidgoli, B.: Multi objective association rule mining with genetic algorithm without specifying minimum support and minimum confidence. Expert Syst. Appl. **38**(1), 288–298 (2011)
7. Yan, X., Zhang, C., Zhang, S.: Genetic algorithm-based strategy for identifying association rules without specifying actual minimum support. Expert Syst. Appl. **36**(2), 3066–3076 (2009)
8. Kabir, M.M.J., Xu, S., Kang, B.H., Zhao, Z.: Comparative analysis of genetic based approach and apriori algorithm for mining maximal frequent item sets. In: IEEE Congress on Evolutionary Computation (CEC), pp. 39–45 (2015)
9. Martin, D., Rosete, A., Alcala-Fdez, J., Herrera, F.: A new multiobjective evolutionary algorithm for mining a reduced set of interesting positive and negative quantitative association rules. IEEE Trans. Evol. Comput. **18**(1), 54–69 (2014)
10. Kabir, M.M.J., Xu, S., Kang, B.H., Zhao, Z.: A new evolutionary algorithm for extracting a reduced set of interesting association rules. In: Arik, S., Huang, T., Lai, W.K., Liu, Q. (eds.) ICONIP 2015. LNCS, vol. 9490, pp. 133–142. Springer, Heidelberg (2015). doi:10.1007/978-3-319-26535-3_16
11. Shenoy, P., Srinivasa, K., Venugopal, K., Patnaik, L.: Dynamic association rule mining using genetic algorithms. Intell. Data Anal. **9**(5), 439–453 (2005)
12. Maaranen, H., Miettinen, K., Penttinen, A.: On initial populations of a genetic algorithm for continuous optimization problems. J. Glob. Optim. **37**(3), 405–436 (2007)
13. Maaranen, H., Miettinen, K., Mäkelä, M.M.: Quasi-random initial population for genetic algorithms. Comput. Math. Appl. **47**(12), 1885–1895 (2004)
14. Chang, P.C., Huang, W.H., Ting, C.J.: Dynamic diversity control in genetic algorithm for mining unsearched solution space in TSP problems. Expert Syst. Appl. **37**(3), 1863–1878 (2010)

Machine Learning for Sensory Data Analysis (MLSDA)

Predicting Phone Usage Behaviors with Sensory Data Using a Hierarchical Generative Model

Chuankai An[✉] and Dan Rockmore

Computer Science Department, Dartmouth College, Hanover, NH 03755, USA
{chuankai,rockmore}@cs.dartmouth.edu

Abstract. Using a sizable set of sensory data and related usage records on Android devices, we are able to give a reasonable prediction of three imporant aspects of phone usage: messages, phone calls and cellular data. We solve the problem via an estimation of a user's daily routine, on which we can train a hierarchical generative model on phone usages in all time slots of a day. The model generates phone usage behaviors in terms of three kinds of data: the state of user-phone interaction, occurrence times of an activity and the duration of the activity in each occurrence. We apply the model on a dataset with 107 frequent users, and find the prediction error of generative model is the smallest when compare with several other baseline methods. In addition, CDF curves illustrate the availability of generative model for most users with the distribution of prediction error for all test cases. We also explore the effects of time slots in a day, as well as size of training and test sets. The results suggest several interesting directions for further research.

Keywords: Phone usage prediction · Generative model

1 Introduction

Smartphone applications can record data from diverse sensors and components in the device, such as an accelerometer or Bluetooth. The popularity of smartphone usage makes it possible to collect large amounts of sensory data, from which it is possible to predict user behavior. Examples include the prediction of mobile application usage [21] and daily track between different locations [6]. Some usage records, such as phone calls, alarms, and GPS are highly and clearly related to human behavior. Those behaviors are in turn correlated with a person's daily routine. Communication behaviors (e.g. sent messages, phone calls, cellular data) are of particular interest since they are related to the business model of the data carriers and service providers. With an in depth knowledge of user behaviors, or a good predictive algorithm for such behaviors, service providers can offer plans personalized for the usage pattern. For example, a better ad push notification service would not disturb certain ongoing events and thereby enhance user experience. The question we ask in this paper is, can we extract and predict the patterns making up a daily routine from large numbers of sensory records?

© Springer International Publishing Switzerland 2016
H. Cao et al. (Eds.): PAKDD 2016 Workshops, LNAI 9794, pp. 75–87, 2016.
DOI: 10.1007/978-3-319-42996-0_7

Traditional methods for solving "prediction problems" (e.g. linear regression) treat categorical (but still numerical) features as numerical values without inner simultaneous or chronological connections. In this work we take for granted that daily routine is the basic and intrinsic foundation of behavior prediction. The traditional prediction methods do not organize all features in the natural way as they are generated in daily life. For example, binary output or values in $[0, 1]$ of Logistic regression might not reflect the accurate value of usage behavior in a wide range (even as the amount of data increases dramatically).

Current work on mobile device usage mining does not give a direct route to predicting user behaviors with an understanding of daily routine. In the literature there is primarily a focus on the prediction of the next event in the near future, such as the next used application or next geographic position or route [6,16]. Some methods [26] require external information, such as a large community of people to find similar user profiles. In our method, the prediction for a user does not rely on outside datasets so that the lack of similar user groups will not weaken the result.

Some papers on human dynamic activity mining [17,18] apply Markov models to describe the change between "active" and "passive" states and estimate the number of events for each class of states. Often there is a lack of enough numbers of states to fit mobile usage data (see Fig. 2). Another group of work [7,8,11,19,20] focuses on the intervals between consecutive events in communications, but there is little in depth analysis of the cumulative attributes in some phone usage behaviors, such as the conversation length of phone calls. In this paper, we are concerned more with the length of total conversation than the intervals between phone calls.

Our method addresses the phone usage prediction problem with a hierarchical generative model of three levels. The first one is state transition. Human circadian rhythm affects the frequency of activities on phones. We divide a day into smaller time slots and classify them into different states, such as sleep, passive and active. The second parameter is the number of occurrences for some activity in each time slot. The third is the duration of each occurrence. Once we learn the necessary parameters in those three levels, a generative model will simulate the user's usages on a phone in order to make a prediction. We apply our generative model on a dataset from Android Device Analyzer [24]. The results show that the generative model performs well with the smallest error among several methods. Briefly, the contributions of this paper are:

- A hierarchical generative model to predict phone usage behaviors, which extends the current focus on event intervals to event duration.
- Demonstration of the effectiveness of the generative model in large practical datasets of sensory data (given enough states in the Markov model to describe state-to-state transition).
- Enabling better personalized mobile service based on user behavior.
- Exploration of the best setting of parameters in the generative model with control experiments.

The rest of the paper is organized as follows: Sect. 2 reviews the related work. Section 3 defines the problem. Section 4 introduces the model with several algorithms. Section 5 reports the details of experiment and analyzes the results. Section 6 concludes the paper with key findings and ideas for future work.

2   Related Work

Many researchers are mining general patterns of smartphone usages [2,10,12,25]. Verkasalo [23] concludes and proposes frameworks of measurement for mobile usage records. Falaki [4] conducts a survey to illustrate the diversity of smartphone usage and predicts energy cost based on the pattern.

Prediction of certain phone usage behavior is a hot topic. Hollmen and Tresp [9] detects fraud mobile communication using hidden layers in a generative model. Farrahi and Gatica-Perez [5,6] uses an LDA model to track routines about locations. Liao et al. [14–16] selects features based on usage relations and predicts the next used application with temporal features. Xu et al. [26] finds similar users in a large dataset to predict a user's app usage. Our framework extends the range of prediction for more kinds of behaviors on smart devices.

Poisson process has been used to analyze and model human dynamics in [1,3,22]. Several papers [8,11,19,20] discuss the model of intervals between communication behaviors such as the exponential distribution and self-related model. Generative models also perform well in wide areas. Alceu [7] applies the RSC generative model on social media comment activity to match patterns of inter-arrival time. Kleinberg [13] divides the burst of documents streams into hierarchical sub-events to simulate the process. Malmgren proposes a Cascading Non-homogeneous Poisson Process Model (CNPP) in [17,18] to extract personal patterns in email communications with two states. Enlightened by the above work, we extend the meaning of states and add one level to the CNPP model to describe patterns in daily phone usage, and use generative model to predict future usage.

3   Problem Definition

Consider a set of users $u_1, u_2...u_n$, with time-stamp sensory records on phones. The records will reflect the change of device setting or the user-phone interaction. Each record can be described as $R = (D, T, U, A)$. D is the day when the usage happens. T is the time of the day. U represents the usage and system settings of a certain sensor or component, such as messages, screen locks, network connections. A means the attributes and values of U. The paper [25] introduces possible values of U and corresponding A. One sample record is "2012-01-21T08:16:50.533+1300;audio|volume|alarm;7". It shows the alarm volume.

Our goal is to predict the phone usage in the future t days based on the given records of $u_1, u_2...u_n$. Though we can predict other sensory data in the similar way, we focus on three kinds of behaviors: the number of sent messages M, the total duration of phone call (call in and out) C and the size of cellular data (rx and tx) D. They occupy the main part of bills on phone communication and represent daily usage on the phone. They reflect a user's connectivity in a social network. To predict phone usages using a generative model, we should define and learn states of user-phone interaction, then explore the distribution of messages M, phone call C and cellular data D in each state based on some pattern.

4   Behavior Prediction

4.1   Patterns in Phone Usage Behavior

Dividing a day into 48 even time slots, we count the average number of event occurrences for many days. Here are figures with patterns of one user as an example. Figure 2 shows the number of records for all kinds of phone usage and sensors, the number of received and sent messages, the total phone call duration, the size of cellular data of one sample user. In general, the user interacts with phones more actively in some time slots. For example, Fig. 2(a) shows that the device will collect more records from 9 am to 10 pm. At night, especially from midnight to 7 am, the number of records decreases sharply. When the user is sleeping, the device might collect records about itself rather than the user (e.g., records about networking). The different and uneven distributions for all users suggest a differentiation of states. The transition of phone-usage states in a day becomes the first layer in the following generative model. We need at least three states since in Fig. 2(b), the number of messages can be zero, small or large (and bursty), which correspond to the sleep, passive, active states in our model.

4.2   Hierarchical Generative Model

Figure 1 illustrates the process of generating a kind of event (e.g., phone call). A day is divided into several time slots. The state of phone usage S_i of the ith time slot can be described with one of the three states, which are sleep, passive, and active. Given the state of phone usage, the model generates the times of

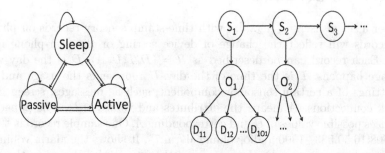

Fig. 1. Generative model includes three levels, which are S states of time slots, O times of occurrences, duration D of one occurrence. The state changes in time order through sleep, passive, and active.

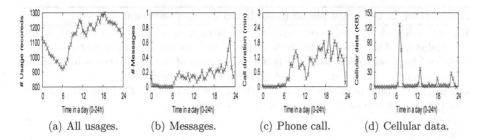

(a) All usages.   (b) Messages.   (c) Phone call.   (d) Cellular data.

Fig. 2. The pattern of usage at time slots in a day.

occurrence O_i of the event in each slot based on a random seed and probability distribution learned from training set. Then the model generates the duration D_{ij} in ith time slot for jth occurrence of the event if the event lasts for a period of time (e.g., the duration of a phone call). After the generation in the first time slot, a transition matrix between usage states will lead the process to the next time slot with the usage state S_2. The model can generate prediction for any length of time in the future. Different values of parameters can describe the diversity in user behaviors.

Algorithm 1 shows how to generate the usage records for a certain behavior. Some instantaneous behaviors such as messages only need to generate occurrence times. A transition matrix of states determines the current state with a uniform random variable in the interval $[0, 1]$. In each state S, assume the time of occurrences is in distribution of $\Psi_O(S)$. We can generate a random value with $\Psi_O(S)$ as the prediction. Finally, for each occurrence, with the distribution of duration $\Psi_D(S)$ under a certain state, a generated random value represents the duration for each occurrence in the similar way. We can sum up the results of duration for all days in the future to get the prediction results. The model simulates user behaviors in the three layers, where parameters in statistical distributions determine the expectation of output prediction. Section 4.3 will introduce how to learn the input transition matrix and parameters of several distribution.

4.3   Parameter Estimation

State Transition. According to uneven distribution of usage behaviors in Fig. 2, we define three states of user-phone interaction. Sleep means that the user does not use the phone but it remains on. Passive and active correspond to the normal and peak periods of occurrence times and duration.

Given all usage records in the training set, Algorithm 2 shows the way to identify states for all time slots. For all usage records in each time slot, we count the user-phone usage related behaviors to build a feature vector. The elements in the feature vector are in Table 1. If during a slot there is no occurrence of any event which we aim to predict, the state is sleep. Then for the other time slots, apply the k-means algorithm to cluster them into two classes, passive and active. The distance metric in k-means is Manhattan Distance.

Algorithm 1. Generate phone usage behaviors as prediction.

Input: N length of prediction days, $Slot\_num$ number of slots in a day, S_0 is the
  initial state of the first slot in the first day, T denotes the transition matrix of three
  states (sleep, passive, active), Ψ_O is the distribution of occurrence times in a certain
  state, and Ψ_D is the distribution of duration in a certain state.

Output: O_{ij} times of occurrence in the jth slot of the ith day, D_{ijk} the kth duration
  of the usage behavior in the jth slot of the ith day.

  $i \leftarrow 0$
  while $i < N$ **do**
    $i \leftarrow i + 1$
    $j \leftarrow 0$
    while $j < Slot\_num$ **do**
      $j \leftarrow j + 1$
      if $S_j \neq$ sleep **then**
        $O_{ij} \leftarrow$ RAND$(\Psi_O(S_j))$
        for each kth occurrence in O_{ij} **do**
          $D_{ijk} \leftarrow$ RAND$(\Psi_D(S_j))$
        end for
      end if
      $state\_seed \leftarrow$ RAND$()$
      $(T\_sleep, T\_passive) \leftarrow$ transition(T, S_j)
      $S_{next} \leftarrow$ decide$(T\_sleep, T\_passive, state\_seed)$
    end while
  end while

Once we know the states of all time slots in training set, we can compute the
transition probabilities based on the frequency of change between two neighbors.
A probability will be set as (tiny) α if it is zero to avoid endless self-looping in
some state. We treat a day as four time periods, night (0 am–6 am), morning
(6 am–noon), afternoon (noon–6 pm), and evening (6 pm–0 am). For each time
period, a 3×3 transition matrix describes the threshold of transition between

---

Algorithm 2. Classify time slots into three states.

Input: Set of records in all slots $TS = \{TS_1, TS_2...TS_n\}$, State = {sleep, passive,
  active}, Set of behaviors to predict U = {messages, phone call, cellular data}

Output: $TS_i.state$ state of each slot.

  for each time slot TS_i in TS **do**
    $f_i \leftarrow$ count_feature(TS_i)
  end for
  for each feature f_i **do**
    if no occurrence of any event in U **then**
      $TS_i.state \leftarrow$ sleep
    end if
  end for
  Undefined $\leftarrow \{TS_i - TS_i.state \neq$ sleep$\}$
  k-means-cluster(Undefined)

---

any two states, so a uniform random seed can determine the next state. An even distribution among three states can generate the initial state S_0 in Algorithm 1.

Occurrence Times Distribution. Given the series of occurrence times $O_1, O_2, ..., O_n$ in all time slots within the same usage state, a suitable distribution may describe it. It matches the definition of Poisson distribution as Eq. 1. By solving the MLE problem with likelihood function as Eq. 1, we can get λ for each state, which works as the Ψ_O in Algorithm 1.

$$P(X = O) = \frac{\lambda^O e^{-\lambda}}{O!} \quad L(\lambda) = \prod_{i=1}^{n} \frac{e^{-\lambda}\lambda^{O_i}}{O_i!} \tag{1}$$

$$P(x; \mu, \sigma) = \frac{1}{\sigma\sqrt{2\pi}} e^{-\frac{(\ln x - u)^2}{2\sigma^2}} \tag{2}$$

Duration Distribution. Duration of an occurrence for an event means how long does it last or how much resources does it get, such as the length of a phone call and the data flow in a period of connection to cellular network. The intervals of consecutive events should obey an exponential distribution, but the interval of two neighbors is not the duration that we concern. So here we do not use exponential distribution to model the length of duration. Since the duration should be always positive value and the dataset we use shows the fact that people tend to have short conversions, we choose a log-normal distribution to describe the distribution of durations. Given the probability density function (Eq. 2) of the log-normal distribution and the observed duration list $D_1, D_2...D_n$, by MLE method we will know μ and σ, which determine the Ψ_D in Algorithm 1. If the durations in training set do not obey a log-normal distribution, we limit the errors by naive methods such as the latest observation. Moreover, to avoid prediction of an infinite duration we set limits on the maximum duration in each occurrence and in the sum of each day.

5   Experiment Results

5.1   Datasets

The original datasets are recorded by the application called Device Analyzer [24,25], which contains records of more than $10,000$ users. We filter the datasets with several thresholds, such as the length of period when the app is recording data, the average number of records related to messages, phone calls and networking per month. Usage records of more than two months make it possible for predictions month to month. Enough records (270 per month) about communication indicate a user will interact with the device frequently, so the usage records are more likely collected from a user's main device. We discard the datasets in which some records miss the accurate time and date by formatting check. We end up with 107 users whose records are complete and correct for a period of time. The records reflect the attributes of start/shut-down, power, airmode, audio, cpu, video, image, memorycard, phone, screen, time, messages, wifi, networking, bluetooth, root, contacts, location, alarm and other sensors. The shortest length of records is 59 days and the longest is 632 days. The total number of all kinds of usage records (e.g. sensory data, device settings, and communication) for a user varies from 587, 817 to 22, 906, 385.

The Device Analyzer records many details about sensors, device settings and usage behaviors. We select those which are caused by the user or change the user's behavior to build feature lists, then classify all time slots with the values in each feature list as Table 1. More kinds of sensory data can be added into the list if the sensors are deployed on all users' devices. Since we cannot equip all devices with more sensitive and advanced sensors, the list only includes features that almost all devices can record. We should also realize that the other sensors, such as accelerometer and GPS module might be helpful to reflect user's behaviors.

Table 1. Elements in a feature list.

1	number of apps start by a user	2	sum of rx data by cellular network
3	sum of tx data by cellular network	4	times of cellular network connection
5	number of phone calls	6	total length of phone call
7	length of the time when the screen is on	8	number of screen switch (on/off)
9	number of devices found by bluetooth	10	number of received messages
11	number of sent messages	12	number of bell rings

5.2 Performance

We compare the average prediction errors among 107 users of their sent messages, phone call duration, size of cellular data with several following baselines. The datasets are divided into training sets and test sets. The size of test set for all users is 30 days, which means we predict the usage behaviors for about a month in the future. Each day is divided into 48 time slots, which means a time slot lasts half an hour. The experiments are running offline in a server so we do not focus on time complexity. All experiments about generative models are executed multiple times.

(1) Naive. Treat the latest records in training set as the prediction.
(2) Average. Average the value in previous months as the prediction.
(3) Drift method. Predict with the first and the latest observations.
(4) Similar one. Choose the value of the past month which has the smallest feature list distance to the test case.
(5) Simple linear regression. Only consider the values of target usage behaviors.
(6) Lasso algorithm. Treat the feature list as the input.
(7) No-states (CNPP). Run the generative model with only two states.

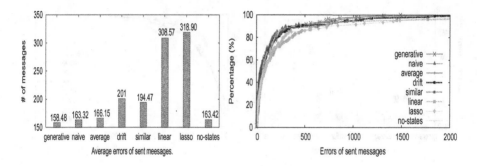

Fig. 3. Errors and CDF curves of #sent messages.

In Fig. 3, the average errors of 107 users' sent messages in the future 30 days vary from 158.48 to 318.90. The generative model performs the best here with smallest error, and Lasso method has the largest error. The naive method, average method and no-states method have almost the same errors about 165 messages/month. The generative model is slightly better. This illustrates the utility of the generative model and the distinguished user-phone interaction states. The generative model can avoid the rare peak in message usage, so it is better than naive or average. The three states facilitate the model to describe the distribution of occurrences and durations more accurately. In terms of the other methods, they ignore the inner relationship between user states and features and the target message behavior, so they have much larger error than the generative model. On the right, CDF curves show the distribution of errors among all users. The generative model stays with several other methods in the beginning part and comes to the top when error reaches 500. For the generative model, more than 65 % users have errors less than 100 messages/month, about 80 % errors are less than 200 messages/month, it has the smallest maximum errors among all methods. All users in the dataset frequently use their devices, some of them may changes their routine or have unexpected burst so all models face instances of large errors. However, for the majority of users, the generative model performs well and avoids more huge error cases than other methods.

In Fig. 4, the average errors of 107 users' phone call durations in the future 30 days range from 504.9 to 1091.11 (min). The generative model has the smallest error. The second and third best methods are no-states and average. The generative model and its no-states version allocate a tiny possibility for the rarely observed data so they are not sensitive to long-time phone call communication, thus they work better with the average method than the others. In the right figure of CDF curves, the generative model is at the top among all methods with more than 60 % of users having errors less than 500 min/month and 80 % of users having errors less than 640 min/month. Though the log-normal distribution that we choose to describe duration distribution needs to be improved, the generative model still performs better than other methods. It proves the advantages of the generative model, including a seemingly deeper identification of daily routine and robustness with seldom usage patterns.

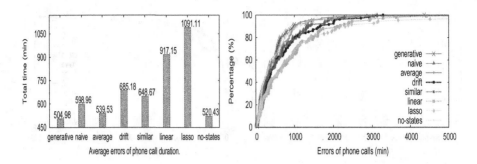

Fig. 4. Errors and CDF curves of phone call duration.

In Fig. 5, the average of 107 users' cellular data size in the future 30 days changes from 1605 to 2105 (MB). The generative model still has the smallest error. No-states, naive, similar methods are comparatively better than others. For the generative model, though more than 60 % cases have errors less than 500 MB/month and about 80 % cases have errors less than 650 MB/month, there are about 9 % of cases with errors more than 1000 MB. The large errors in data flow prediction exist in all methods, because some users will receive or send huge data packets in the future without similar history, and the size of data flow is unlimited. As a result, the generative model stays on the top in the beginning, but it mixes with other curves at the end due to the minority huge data errors. Though the generative model is not the best in the beginning, with less huge-error cases, it still beats the other methods in terms of average error. Moreover, the log-normal distribution might not fit well with the rare unexpected large dataflow since it estimates the large data flow with small possibility. Cellular data flow usually happens in the environment of movement or a place without Wi-Fi. The generative model lacks more details about user routine, which limits the performance of cellular data prediction. However, in total the generative model is better than the other methods due to the hierarchical framework.

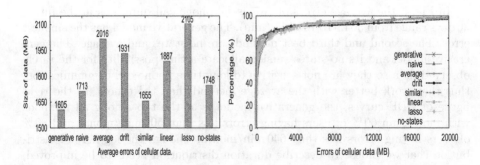

Fig. 5. Errors and CDF curves of cellular data size.

Sent messages, phone call duration and cellular data size represent three types of usage behaviors respectively. They are no-duration behavior such as sent messages, occurrence with limited duration such as phone calls, occurrence with unlimited duration such as cellular data. For the third type of usage behaviors, we should find more ways to limit the prediction and model the unexpected burst.

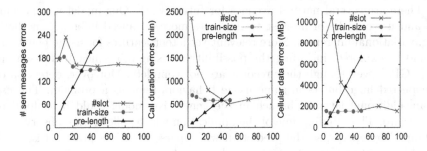

Fig. 6. Effects of three parameters on three usage behaviors.

5.3   Effect of Factors

Figure 6 illustrates the effect of three parameters, number of time slots in a day, length of training set and length of prediction in the future. The horizontal axis represents either the number of smaller time slots in a day, or the days in training set and test set. The vertical axis shows errors of a certain usage behavior. The number of time slots in a day changes from 4 to 96, with fixed 30 days as the size of test set and the rest records as training sets. The size of training sets for each user varies from 5 to 50 days with fixed records of 30 days as the test sets and 48 time slots in a day. To see the effect of prediction length, we put 50 days' records aside as the test sets, and run the generative model with time slots of 48, then compare the errors in the first 5, 10 to 50 days of test sets. When the number of time slots increases, the errors of three usage behaviors decrease first and fluctuates after 48. If we divide a day into a few slots, the differences between sleep, passive and active states diminish. In contrast, too many time slots will result in a sparse feature list. Like time slots, when the training sets are small, the generative model lacks enough records. When the training sets become large, perhaps the previous usage pattern is not inherited by the test sets. So medium size training sets perform well. The errors are approximately proportional to the increase of prediction length from 5 to 50, since the model accumulates errors day by day.

6   Conclusion

In this paper, we illustrate daily patterns in mobile usage and sensory records and build a hierarchical generative model with multiple user-phone interaction states. The model predicts three usage behaviors with acceptable errors for the majority of users. Given the simple distributions of occurrence and duration, our improved accuracy over various baselines demonstrates the value of our revised model on large real datasets. We explore the effects of several parameters in the prediction process to guide a suitable choice of timeslots as well as size of training and test sets. The prediction of phone usage behavior by a generative model may be useful for personalizing service.

There are several natural avenues for future work. Our model is very simple and it would be of interest to integrate more advanced inference methods (e.g. variational inference). More relevant yet latent features for usage behaviors should be explored, including the possibility of using more meaningful sensors (e.g., GPS) even though their records are not complete. Moreover, detection of unexpected huge bursts in some usage behaviors remains a problem. The use of an additional layer or branch in the generative model could be helpful in this regard. The running time of the application which collects the sensory data is limited by energy, so the prediction with sparse data is a practical issue. A suitable sampling method may be the key point for this.

References

1. Cho, J., Garcia-Molina, H.: Estimating frequency of change. ACM Trans. Internet Technol. (TOIT) **3**(3), 256–290 (2003)
2. Do, T.M.T., Blom, J., Gatica-Perez, D.: Smartphone usage in the wild: a large-scale analysis of applications and context. In: ICMI, pp. 353–360. ACM (2011)
3. Eckmann, J., Moses, E., Sergi, D.: Entropy of dialogues creates coherent structures in e-mail traffic. Proc. Nat. Acad. Sci. USA **101**(40), 14333–14337 (2004)
4. Falaki, H., Mahajan, R., Kandula, S., Lymberopoulos, D., Govindan, R., Estrin, D.: Diversity in smartphone usage. In: MobiSys, pp. 179–194. ACM (2010)
5. Farrahi, K., Gatica-Perez, D.: What did you do today?: discovering daily routines from large-scale mobile data. In: Proceedings of MM, pp. 849–852. ACM (2008)
6. Farrahi, K., Gatica-Perez, D.: Probabilistic mining of socio-geographic routines from mobile phone data. Sel. Top. Signal Process. **4**(4), 746–755 (2010)
7. Ferraz Costa, A., Yamaguchi, Y., Juci Machado Traina, A., Traina Jr., C., Faloutsos, C.: RSC: Mining and modeling temporal activity in social media. In: KDD, pp. 269–278. ACM (2015)
8. Hidalgo, R.C.A.: Conditions for the emergence of scaling in the inter-event time of uncorrelated and seasonal systems. Phys. A: Stat. Mech. Appl. **369**(2), 877–883 (2006)
9. Hollmén, J., Tresp, V.: Call-based fraud detection in mobile communication networks using a hierarchical regime-switching model. In: Advances in Neural Information Processing Systems, pp. 889–895 (1999)
10. Jin, Y., et al.: Characterizing data usage patterns in a large cellular network. In: SIGCOMM Workshop on Cellular Networks, pp. 7–12. ACM (2012)
11. Juan, D.-C., Li, L., Peng, H.-K., Marculescu, D., Faloutsos, C.: Beyond poisson: modeling inter-arrival time of requests in a datacenter. In: Tseng, V.S., Ho, T.B., Zhou, Z.-H., Chen, A.L.P., Kao, H.-Y. (eds.) PAKDD 2014, Part II. LNCS, vol. 8444, pp. 198–209. Springer, Heidelberg (2014)

12. Kang, J.M., Seo, S.S., Hong, J.W.K.: Usage pattern analysis of smartphones. In: Network Operations and Management Symposium, pp. 1–8. IEEE (2011)

13. Kleinberg, J.: Bursty and hierarchical structure in streams. Data Min. Knowl. Disc. **7**(4), 373–397 (2003)

14. Liao, Z.X., Lei, P.R., Shen, T.J., Li, S.C., Peng, W.C.: Mining temporal profiles of mobile applications for usage prediction. In: ICDMW, pp. 890–893. IEEE (2012)

15. Liao, Z.X., Li, S.C., Peng, W.C., Yu, P.S., Liu, T.C.: On the feature discovery for app usage prediction in smartphones. In: ICDM, pp. 1127–1132. IEEE (2013)

16. Liao, Z.X., Pan, Y.C., Peng, W.C., Lei, P.R.: On mining mobile apps usage behavior for predicting apps usage in smartphones. In: CIKM, pp. 609–618. ACM (2013)

17. Malmgren, R.D., Hofman, J.M., Amaral, L.A., Watts, D.J.: Characterizing individual communication patterns. In: KDD, pp. 607–616. ACM (2009)

18. Malmgren, R.D., Stouffer, D.B., Motter, A.E., Amaral, L.A.: A poissonian explanation for heavy tails in e-mail communication. Proc. Nat. Acad. Sci. **105**(47), 18153–18158 (2008)

19. Vaz de Melo, P.O.S., Faloutsos, C., Assunção, R., Loureiro, A.: The self-feeding process: a unifying model for communication dynamics in the web. In: WWW, pp. 1319–1330 (2013)

20. Melo, P.O., Faloutsos, C., Assunçao, R., Alves, R., Loureiro, A.A.: Universal and distinct properties of communication dynamics: how to generate realistic inter-event times. TKDD **9**(3), 24 (2015)

21. Shin, C., Hong, J.H., Dey, A.K.: Understanding and prediction of mobile application usage for smart phones. In: Ubicomp, pp. 173–182. ACM (2012)

22. Sia, K.C., Cho, J., Cho, H.K.: Efficient monitoring algorithm for fast news alerts. IEEE Trans. Knowl. Data Eng. **19**(7), 950–961 (2007)

23. Verkasalo, H.: Analysis of smartphone user behavior. In: Mobile Business and 2010 Ninth Global Mobility Roundtable (ICMB-GMR), pp. 258–263. IEEE (2010)

24. Wagner, D.T., Rice, A., Beresford, A.R.: Device analyzer: large-scale mobile data collection. ACM SIGMETRICS Perform. Eval. Rev. **41**(4), 53–56 (2014)

25. Wagner, D.T., Rice, A., Beresford, A.R.: Device analyzer: understanding smartphone usage. In: Stojmenovic, I., Cheng, Z., Guo, S. (eds.) MOBIQUITOUS 2013. LNICST, vol. 131, pp. 195–208. Springer, Heidelberg (2014)

26. Xu, Y., et al.: Preference, context and communities: a multi-faceted approach to predicting smartphone app usage patterns. In: ISWC, pp. 69–76. ACM (2013)

Comparative Evaluation of Action Recognition Methods via Riemannian Manifolds, Fisher Vectors and GMMs: Ideal and Challenging Conditions

Johanna Carvajal[1,3], Arnold Wiliem[1], Chris McCool[2], Brian Lovell[1], and Conrad Sanderson[1,3,4(✉)]

[1] University of Queensland, Brisbane, Australia
[2] Queensland University of Technology, Brisbane, Australia
[3] NICTA, Brisbane, Australia
conrad.sanderson@nicta.com.au
[4] Data61, CSIRO, Canberra, Australia

Abstract. We present a comparative evaluation of various techniques for action recognition while keeping as many variables as possible controlled. We employ two categories of Riemannian manifolds: symmetric positive definite matrices and linear subspaces. For both categories we use their corresponding nearest neighbour classifiers, kernels, and recent kernelised sparse representations. We compare against traditional action recognition techniques based on Gaussian mixture models and Fisher vectors (FVs). We evaluate these action recognition techniques under ideal conditions, as well as their sensitivity in more challenging conditions (variations in scale and translation). Despite recent advancements for handling manifolds, manifold based techniques obtain the lowest performance and their kernel representations are more unstable in the presence of challenging conditions. The FV approach obtains the highest accuracy under ideal conditions. Moreover, FV best deals with moderate scale and translation changes.

1 Introduction

Recently, there has been an increasing interest on action recognition using Riemannian manifolds. Such recognition systems can be roughly placed into two main categories: **(i)** based on linear subspaces (LS), and **(ii)** based on symmetric positive definite (SPD) matrices. The space of m-dimensional LS in $\mathbb{R}^n$ can be viewed as a special case of Riemannian manifolds, known as Grassmann manifolds [1].

Other techniques have been also applied for the action recognition problem. Among them we can find Gaussian mixture models (GMMs), bag-of-features (BoF), and Fisher vectors (FVs). In [2,3] each action is represented by a combination of GMMs and then the decision making is based on the principle of selecting the most probable action according to Bayes' theorem [4]. The FV representation can be thought as an evolution of the BoF representation, encoding

© Springer International Publishing Switzerland 2016
H. Cao et al. (Eds.): PAKDD 2016 Workshops, LNAI 9794, pp. 88–100, 2016.
DOI: 10.1007/978-3-319-42996-0_8

additional information [5]. Rather than encoding the frequency of the descriptors for a given video, FV encodes the deviations from a probabilistic version of the visual dictionary (which is typically a GMM) [6].

Several review papers have compared various techniques for human action recognition [7–11]. The reviews show how this research area has progressed throughout the years, discuss the current advantages and limitations of the state-of-the-art, and provide potential directions for addressing the limitations. However, none of them focus on how well various action recognition systems work across same datasets *and* same extracted features. An earlier comparison of classifiers for human activity recognition is studied [12]. The performance comparison with seven classifiers in one single dataset is reported. Although this work presents a broad range of classifiers, it fails to provide a more extensive comparison by using more datasets and hence its conclusions may not generalise to other datasets.

So far there has been no systematic comparison of performance between methods based on SPD matrices and LS. Furthermore, there has been no comparison of manifold based methods against traditional action recognition methods based on GMMs and FVs in the presence of realistic and challenging conditions. Lastly, existing review papers fail to compare various classifiers using the same features across several datasets.

Contributions. To address the aforementioned problems, in this work we provide a more detailed analysis of the performance of the aforementioned methods under the same set of features. To this end, we test with three popular datasets: KTH [13], UCF-Sports [14] and UT-Tower [15]. For the Riemannian representations we use nearest-neighbour classifiers, kernels as well as recent kernelised sparse representations. Finally, we quantitatively show when these methods break and how the performance degrades when the datasets have challenging conditions (translations and scale variations). For a fair comparison across all approaches, we will use the same set of features, as explained in Sect. 2. More specifically, a video is represented as a set of features extracted on a pixel basis. We also describe how we use this set of features to obtain both Riemannian features: (1) covariance features that lie in the space of SPD matrices, and (2) LS that lie in the space of Grassmann manifolds. In Sects. 3 and 4, we summarise learning methods based Riemannian manifolds as well as GMMs and FVs. The datasets and experiment setup are described in Sect. 5. In Sect. 6, we present comparative results on three datasets under ideal and challenging conditions. The main findings are summarised in Sect. 7.

2   Video Descriptors

Here, we describe how to extract from a video a set of features on a pixel level. The video descriptor is the same for all the methods examined in this work. A video $\mathcal{V} = \{I_t\}_{t=1}^T$ is an ordered set of T frames. Each frame $I_t \in \mathbb{R}^{r \times c}$ can be represented by a set of feature vectors $F_t = \{f_p\}_{p=1}^{N_t}$. We extract the following $d = 14$ dimensional feature vector for each pixel in a given frame t [2]:

$$\boldsymbol{f} = [\, x, \, y, \, \boldsymbol{g}, \, \boldsymbol{o} \,]^{\top} \tag{1}$$

where x and y are the pixel coordinates, while $\boldsymbol{g}$ and $\boldsymbol{o}$ are defined as:

$$\boldsymbol{g} = \left[\, |J_x|, \, |J_y|, \, |J_{yy}|, \, |J_{xx}|, \, \sqrt{J_x^2 + J_y^2}, \, \text{atan}\frac{|J_y|}{|J_x|} \,\right] \tag{2}$$

$$\boldsymbol{o} = \left[\, u, \, v, \, \frac{\partial u}{\partial t}, \, \frac{\partial v}{\partial t}, \, \left(\frac{\partial u}{\partial x} + \frac{\partial v}{\partial y}\right), \, \left(\frac{\partial v}{\partial x} - \frac{\partial u}{\partial y}\right) \,\right] \tag{3}$$

The first four gradient-based features in (2) represent the first and second order intensity gradients at pixel location (x, y). The last two gradient features represent gradient magnitude and gradient orientation. The optical flow based features in (3) represent: the horizontal and vertical components of the flow vector, the first order derivatives with respect to time, the divergence and vorticity of optical flow [16], respectively. Typically only a subset of the pixels in a frame correspond to the object of interest ($N_t < r \times c$). As such, we are only interested in pixels with a gradient magnitude greater than a threshold τ [17]. We discard feature vectors from locations with a small magnitude, resulting in a variable number of feature vectors per frame.

For each video $\mathcal{V}$, the feature vectors are pooled into set $\mathcal{F} = \{\boldsymbol{f}_n\}_{n=1}^{N}$ containing N vectors. This pooled set of features $\mathcal{F}$ can be used directly by methods such as GMMs and FVs. Describing these features using a Riemannian Manifold setting requires a further step to produce either a covariance matrix feature or a linear subspace feature.

Covariance matrices of features have proved very effective for action recognition [17,18]. The empirical estimate of the covariance matrix of set $\mathcal{F}$ is given by:

$$C = \frac{1}{N} \sum_{n=1}^{N} \left(\boldsymbol{f}_n - \overline{\mathcal{F}}\right)\left(\boldsymbol{f}_n - \overline{\mathcal{F}}\right)^{\top} \tag{4}$$

where $\overline{\mathcal{F}} = \frac{1}{N} \sum_{n=1}^{N} \boldsymbol{f}_n$ is the mean feature vector.

The pooled feature vectors set $\mathcal{F}$ can be represented as a linear subspace through any orthogonalisation procedure like singular value decomposition (SVD) [19]. Let $\mathcal{F} = \boldsymbol{U}\boldsymbol{D}\boldsymbol{V}^{\top}$ be the SVD of $\mathcal{F}$. The first m columns of $\boldsymbol{U}$ represent an optimised subspace of order m. The Grassmann manifold $\mathcal{G}_{d,m}$ is the set of m-dimensional linear subspaces of $\mathbb{R}^d$. An element of $\mathcal{G}_{d,m}$ can be represented by an orthonormal matrix $\boldsymbol{Y}$ of size $d \times m$ such that $\boldsymbol{Y}^{\top}\boldsymbol{Y} = \boldsymbol{I}_m$, where $\boldsymbol{I}_m$ is the $m \times m$ identity matrix.

3   Classification on Riemannian Manifolds

3.1   Nearest-Neighbour Classifier

The Nearest Neighbour (NN) approach classifies a query data based on the most similar observation in the annotated training set [20]. To decide whether two observations are similar we will employ two metrics: the log-Euclidean distance for SPD matrices [17] and the Projection Metric for LS [21].

The log-Euclidean distance (d_{spd}) is one of the most popular metrics for SPD matrices due to its accuracy and low computational complexity [22]; it is defined as:

$$d_{\mathrm{spd}}(C_1, C_2) = ||\log(C_1) - \log(C_2)||_F \tag{5}$$

where $\log(\cdot)$ is the matrix-logarithm and $||\cdot||_F$ denotes the Frobenius norm on matrices.

As for LS, a common metric to measure the similarity between two subspaces is via principal angles [21]. The metric can include the smallest principal angle, the largest principal angle, or a combination of all principal angles [21,23]. In this work we have selected the Projection Metric which uses all the principal angles [21]:

$$d_{\mathrm{ls}}(Y_1, Y_2) = \left(m - \sum_{i=1}^{m} \cos^2 \theta_i \right)^{1/2} \tag{6}$$

where m is the size of the subspace.

The principal angles can be easily computed from the SVD of $Y_1^\top Y_2 = U(\cos\Theta)V^\top$, where $U = [u_1 \cdots u_m]$, $V = [v_1 \cdots v_m]$, and $\cos\Theta = \mathrm{diag}(\cos\theta_1, \cdots, \cos\theta_m)$.

3.2 Kernel Approach

Manifolds can be mapped to Euclidean spaces using Mercer kernels [23–25]. This transformation allows us to employ algorithms originally formulated for $\mathbb{R}^n$ with manifold value data. Several kernels for the set of SPD matrices have been proposed in the literature [24–26]. One kernel based on the log-Euclidean distance is derived in [27] and various kernels can be generated, including [23]:

$$K_{\mathrm{spd}}^{\mathrm{rbf}}(C_1, C_2) = \exp\left(-\gamma_r \cdot ||\log(C_1) - \log(C_2)||_F^2 \right) \tag{7}$$

$$K_{\mathrm{spd}}^{\mathrm{poly}}(C_1, C_2) = \left(\gamma_p \cdot \mathrm{tr}\left[\log(C_1)^\top \log(C_2)\right]\right)^d \tag{8}$$

Similar to SPD kernels, many kernels have been proposed for LS [19,28]. Various kernels can be generated from the projection metric, such as [23]:

$$K_{\mathrm{ls}}^{\mathrm{rbf}}(Y_1, Y_2) = \exp\left(-\gamma_r \cdot ||Y_1 Y_1^\top - Y_2 Y_2^\top||_F^2 \right) \tag{9}$$

$$K_{\mathrm{ls}}^{\mathrm{poly}}(Y_1, Y_2) = \left(\gamma_p \cdot ||Y_1^\top Y_2||_F^2 \right)^m \tag{10}$$

The parameters γ_r and γ_p are defined in Sect. 5. The kernels are used in combination with Support Vector Machines (SVMs) [4].

3.3 Kernelised Sparse Representation

Recently, several works show the efficacy of sparse representation methods for addressing manifold feature classification problems [29,30]. Here, each manifold point is represented by its sparse coefficients. Let $\mathcal{X} = \{X_j\}_{j=1}^{J}$ be a population of Riemannian points (where X_j is either a SPD matrix or a LS) and $\mathcal{D} = \{D_i\}_{i=1}^{K}$ be the Riemannian dictionary of size K, where each element represents an atom. Given a kernel $k(\cdot, \cdot)$, induced by the feature mapping function $\phi : \mathbb{R}^d \to \mathbb{H}$, we seek to learn a dictionary and corresponding sparse code $s \in \mathbb{R}^K$ such that $\phi(X)$ can be well approximated by the dictionary $\phi(\mathcal{D})$. The kernelised dictionary learning in Riemannian manifolds optimises the following objective function [29,30]:

$$\min_{s} \left(\left\| \phi(X) - \sum_{i=1}^{K} s_i \phi(D_i) \right\|_{F}^{2} + \lambda \|s\|_1 \right) \tag{11}$$

over the dictionary and the sparse codes $\mathcal{S} = \{s_j\}_{j=1}^{J}$. After initialising the dictionary $\mathcal{D}$, the objective function is solved by repeating two steps (sparse coding and dictionary update). In the sparse coding step, $\mathcal{D}$ is fixed and $\mathcal{S}$ is computed. In the dictionary update step, $\mathcal{S}$ is fixed while $\mathcal{D}$ is updated, with each dictionary atom updated independently.

For the sparse representation on SPD matrices, each atom $D_i \in \mathbb{R}^{d \times d}$ and each element $X \in \mathbb{R}^{d \times d}$ are SPD matrices. The dictionary is learnt following [24], where the dictionary is initialised using the Karcher mean [31]. For the sparse representation on LS, the dictionary $D_i \in \mathbb{R}^{d \times m}$ and each element $X \in \mathbb{R}^{d \times m}$ are elements of $\mathcal{G}_{d,m}$ and need to be determined by the Kernelised Grassmann Dictionary Learning algorithm proposed in [30]. We refer to the kernelised sparse representation (KSR) for SPD matrices and LS as KSR$_{\text{spd}}$ and KSR$_{\text{ls}}$, respectively.

4 Classification via Gaussian Mixture Models and Fisher Vectors

A **Gaussian Mixture Model** (GMM) is a weighted sum of K component Gaussian densities [4]:

$$p(f|\lambda) = \sum_{k=1}^{K} w_k \mathcal{N}(f|\mu_k, \Sigma_k) \tag{12}$$

where f is a d-dimensional feature vector, w_k is the weight of the k-th Gaussian (with constraints $0 \leq w_k \leq 1$ and $\sum_{k=1}^{K} w_k = 1$), and $\mathcal{N}(f|\mu_k, \Sigma_k)$ is the component Gaussian density with mean μ and covariance matrix Σ, given by:

$$\mathcal{N}(f|\mu, \Sigma) = \frac{1}{(2\pi)^{\frac{d}{2}}|\Sigma|^{\frac{1}{2}}} \exp\left\{ -\frac{1}{2}(f - \mu)^\top \Sigma^{-1}(f - \mu) \right\} \tag{13}$$

The complete Gaussian mixture model is parameterised by the mean vectors, covariance matrices and weights of all component densities. These parameters are collectively represented by the notation $\lambda = \{w_k, \boldsymbol{\mu}_k, \boldsymbol{\Sigma}_k\}_{k=1}^{K}$. For the GMM, we learn one model per action. This results in a set of GMM models that we will express as $\{\lambda_a\}_{a=1}^{A}$, where A is the total number of actions. For each testing video $\mathcal{V}$, the feature vectors in set $\mathcal{F}$ are assumed independent, so the average log-likelihood of a model λ_a is computed as:

$$\log p(\mathcal{F}|\lambda_a) = \frac{1}{N} \sum_{n=1}^{N} \log p(\boldsymbol{f}_n|\lambda_a) \tag{14}$$

We classify each video to the model a which has the highest average log-likelihood.

The **Fisher Vector** (FV) approach encodes the deviations from a probabilistic visual dictionary, which is typically a GMM with diagonal covariance matrices [32]. The parameters of a GMM with K components can be expressed as $\lambda = \{w_k, \boldsymbol{\mu}_k, \boldsymbol{\sigma}_k\}_{k=1}^{K}$, where, w_k is the weight, $\boldsymbol{\mu}_k$ is the mean vector, and $\boldsymbol{\sigma}_k$ is the diagonal covariance matrix for the k-th Gaussian. The parameters are learned using the Expectation Maximisation algorithm [4] on training data. Given the pooled set of features $\mathcal{F}$ from video $\mathcal{V}$, the deviations from the GMM are then accumulated using [32]:

$$\mathcal{G}_{\boldsymbol{\mu}_k}^{\mathcal{F}} = \frac{1}{N\sqrt{w_k}} \sum_{n=1}^{N} \gamma_n(k) \left(\frac{\boldsymbol{f}_n - \boldsymbol{\mu}_k}{\boldsymbol{\sigma}_k}\right) \tag{15}$$

$$\mathcal{G}_{\boldsymbol{\sigma}_k}^{\mathcal{F}} = \frac{1}{N\sqrt{2w_k}} \sum_{n=1}^{N} \gamma_n(k) \left[\frac{(\boldsymbol{f}_n - \boldsymbol{\mu}_k)^2}{\boldsymbol{\sigma}_k^2} - 1\right] \tag{16}$$

where vector division indicates element-wise division and $\gamma_n(k)$ is the posterior probability of $\boldsymbol{f}_n$ for the k-th component: $\gamma_n(k) = w_k \mathcal{N}(\boldsymbol{f}_n|\boldsymbol{\mu}_k, \boldsymbol{\sigma}_k) / \left(\sum_{i=1}^{K} w_i \mathcal{N}(\boldsymbol{f}_n|\boldsymbol{\mu}_i, \boldsymbol{\sigma}_i)\right)$.

The Fisher vector for each video $\mathcal{V}$ is represented as the concatenation of $\mathcal{G}_{\boldsymbol{\mu}_k}^{\mathcal{F}}$ and $\mathcal{G}_{\boldsymbol{\sigma}_k}^{\mathcal{F}}$ (for $k = 1, \ldots, K$) into vector $\mathcal{G}_{\lambda}^{\mathcal{F}}$. As $\mathcal{G}_{\boldsymbol{\mu}_k}^{\mathcal{F}}$ and $\mathcal{G}_{\boldsymbol{\sigma}_k}^{\mathcal{F}}$ are d-dimensional, $\mathcal{G}_{\lambda}^{\mathcal{F}}$ has the dimensionality of $2dK$. Power normalisation is then applied to each dimension in $\mathcal{G}_{\lambda}^{\mathcal{F}}$. The power normalisation to improve the FV for classification was proposed in [33] of the form $z \leftarrow \text{sign}(z)|z|^{\rho}$, where z corresponds to each dimension and the power coefficient $\rho = 1/2$. Finally, l_2-normalisation is applied. Note that we have omitted the deviations for the weights as they add little information [32]. The FVs are fed to a linear SVM for classification, where the similarity between vectors is measured using dot-products [32].

5   Datasets and Setup

For our experiments, we use three datasets: KTH [13], UCF-Sports [14], and UT-Tower [15]. See Fig. 1 for examples of actions. In the following sections, we describe how each of the datasets is employed, and we provide a description of the setup used for the experiments.

Datasets. The KTH dataset [13] contains 25 subjects performing 6 types of human actions and 4 scenarios. The actions included in this dataset are: boxing, handclapping, handwaving, jogging, running, and walking. The scenarios include indoor, outdoor, scale variations, and varying clothes. Each original video of the KTH dataset contains an individual performing the same action. The image size is 160×120 pixels, and temporal resolution is 25 frames per second. For our experiments we only use scenario 1.

The UCF-Sports dataset [14] is a collections of 150 sport videos or sequences. This datasets consists of 10 actions: diving, golf swinging, kicking a ball, lifting weights, riding horse, running, skate boarding, pommel horse, high bar, and walking. The number of videos per action varies from 6 to 22. The videos presented in this dataset have varying backgrounds. We use the bounding box enclosing the person of interest provided with the dataset where available. We create the corresponding 10 bounding boxes not provided with the dataset. The bounding box size is 250×400 pixels. The UT-Tower dataset [15] contains 9 actions performed 12 times. In total, there are 108 low-resolution videos. The actions include: pointing, standing, digging, walking, carrying, running, wave1, wave2, and jumping. The videos were recorded in two scenes (concrete square and lawn). As the provided bounding boxes have variable sizes, we resize the resulting boxes to 32×32.

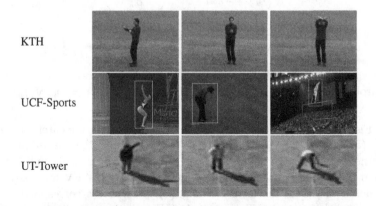

Fig. 1. Examples from the three datasets.

Setup. We use the Leave-One-Out (LOO) protocol suggested by each dataset. We leave one sample video out for testing on a rotating basis for UT-Tower and UCF-Sports. For KTH we leave one person out. For each video we extract a set of $d = 14$ dimensional features vectors as explained in Sect. 2. We only use feature vectors with a gradient magnitude greater that a threshold τ. The threshold τ used for selecting low-level feature vectors was set to 40 as per [2].

For each video, we obtain one SPD matrix and one LS. In order to obtain the optimised linear subspace $\mathcal{G}_{d,m}$ in the the manifold representation, we vary

$m = 1, \cdots, d$. We test with manifolds kernels using various parameters. The set of parameters was used as proposed in [23]. Polynomial kernels $K_{\text{spd}}^{\text{poly}}$ and $K_{\text{ls}}^{\text{rbf}}$ are generated by taking $\gamma_p = 1/d_p$ and $d_p = \{1, 2, \cdots, d\}$. Projection RBF kernels are generated with $\gamma_r = \frac{1}{d}2^\delta$ and $\delta = \{-10, -9, \cdots, 9\}$ for $K_{\text{spd}}^{\text{rbf}}$, and $\delta = \{-14, -12, \cdots, 20\}$ for $K_{\text{ls}}^{\text{rbf}}$. For the sparse representation of SPD matrices and LS we have used the code provided by [24,30]. Kernels are used in combination with SVM for final classification. We report the best accuracy performance after iterating with various parameters.

For the FV representation, we use the same set-up as in [6]. We randomly sampled 256,000 features from training videos and then the visual dictionary is learnt with 256 Gaussians. Each video is represented by a FV. The FVs are fed to a linear SVM for classification. For the GMM modelling, we learn a model for each action using all the feature vectors belonging to the same action. For each action a GMM is trained with $K = 256$ components.

6   Comparative Evaluation

We perform two sets of experiments: (i) in ideal conditions, where the classification is carried out using each original dataset, and (ii) in realistic and challenging conditions where testing videos are modified by scale changes and translations.

6.1   Ideal Conditions

We start our experiments using the NN classifier for both Riemannian representations: SPD matrices and LS. For LS we employ the projection metric as per Eq. (6) and for SPD matrices we employ the log-Euclidean distance as per Eq. (5). We tune the parameter m (subspace order) for each dataset. The kernels selected for SPD matrices and LS are described in Eqs. (7), (8), (9), (10) and their parameters are selected as per Sect. 5.

We present a summary of the best performance obtained for the manifold representations using the optimal subspace for LS and also the optimal kernel parameters for both representations. Similarly, we report the best accuracy performance for the kernelised sparse representations KSR_{spd} and KSR_{ls}. Moreover, we include the performance for the GMM and FV representations.

The results are presented in Table 1. First of all, we observe that using a SVM for action recognition usually leads to a better accuracy than NN. In particular, we notice that the NN approach performs quite poorly. The NN classifier may not be effective enough to capture the complexity of the human actions when there is insufficient representation of the actions (one video is represented by one SPD matrix or one LS). Secondly, we observe that among the manifold techniques, SPD based approaches perform better than LS based approaches. While LS capture only the dominant eigenvectors [34], SPD matrices capture both the eigenvectors and eigenvalues [35]. The eigenvalues of a covariance matrix typify the variance captured in the direction of each eigenvector [35].

Table 1. Accuracy of action recognition in ideal conditions.

	KTH	UCF-Sports	UT-Tower	average
d_{spd} + NN	76.0 %	76.5 %	73.1 %	75.2 %
d_{ls} + NN	67.3 %	65.7 %	76.8 %	69.9 %
$K_{\mathrm{spd}}^{\mathrm{poly}}$ + SVM	92.0 %	75.2 %	87.9 %	85.0 %
$K_{\mathrm{spd}}^{\mathrm{rbf}}$ + SVM	84.0 %	79.2 %	81.5 %	81.6 %
$K_{\mathrm{ls}}^{\mathrm{poly}}$ + SVM	56.0 %	50.3 %	42.6 %	49.6 %
$K_{\mathrm{ls}}^{\mathrm{rbf}}$ + SVM	76.0 %	61.7 %	79.6 %	72.4 %
KSR$_{\mathrm{spd}}$ + SVM	80.0 %	76.5 %	81.5 %	79.3 %
KSR$_{\mathrm{ls}}$ + SVM	74.0 %	72.5 %	83.3 %	77.3 %
GMM	86.7 %	80.5 %	87.9 %	85.0 %
FV + SVM	**96.7 %**	**88.6 %**	**92.5 %**	**92.6%**

Despite KSR$_{\mathrm{spd}}$ showing superior performance in other computer vision tasks [24], it is not the case for the action recognition problem. We conjecture this is due to the lack of labelled training data (each video is represented by only one SPD matrix), which may yield a dictionary with bad generalisation power. Moreover, sparse representations can be over-pruned, being caused by discarding several representative points that may be potentially useful for prediction [36].

Although kernel approaches map the data into higher spaces to allow linear separability, K_{spd}^{poly} exhibits on average a similar accuracy to GMM which does not transform the data. GMM is a weighted sum of Gaussian probability densities, which in addition to the covariance matrices, it uses the means and weights to determine the average log-likelihood of a set of feature vectors from a video to belong to a specific action. While SPD kernels only use covariance matrices, GMMs use both covariance matrices and means. The combination of both statistics has proved to increase the accuracy performance in other classification tasks [32,37]. FV outperforms all the classification methods with an average accuracy of 92.6 %, which is 7.6 points higher than both GMM and K_{spd}^{poly}. Similarly to GMM, FV also incorporates first and second order statistics (means and covariances), but it has additional processing in the form of power normalisation. It is shown in [33] that when the number of Gaussians increases, the FV turns into a sparser representation and it negatively affects the linear SVM which measures the similarity using dot-products. The power normalisation unsparsifies the FV making it more suitable for linear SVMs. The additional information provided by the means and the power normalisation explains the superior accuracy performance of FV.

6.2 Challenging Conditions

In this section, we evaluate the performance on all datasets under consideration when the testing videos have translations and scale variations. We have selected the following approaches for this evaluation: d_{spd}, $K_{\text{spd}}^{\text{poly}}$, $K_{\text{ls}}^{\text{rbf}}$, and FV. We discard d_{ls}, as its performance is too low and presents similar behaviour to d_{spd}. We do not include experiments on KSR_{spd} and KSR_{ls}, as we found that they show similar trends as $K_{\text{spd}}^{\text{poly}}$ and $K_{\text{ls}}^{\text{rbf}}$, respectively. Alike, GMM exhibits similar behaviour as FV.

For this set of experiments, the training is carried out using the original datasets. For the analysis of translations, we have translated (shifted) each testing video vertically and horizontally. For the evaluation under scale variations, each testing video is shrunk or magnified. For both cases, we replace the missing pixels simply by copying the nearest rows or columns. See Fig. 2 for examples of videos under challenging conditions.

The results for scale variations and translations are shown in Figs. 3 and 4, respectively. These results reveal that all the analysed approaches are susceptible to translation and scale variations. Both kernel based methods, $K_{\text{spd}}^{\text{poly}}$ and $K_{\text{ls}}^{\text{rbf}}$, exhibit sharp performance degradation even when the scale is only magnified or compressed by a factor of 0.05 %. Similarly, for both kernels the accuracy rapidly decreases with a small translation. The NN classification using the log-Euclidean distance (d_{spd}) is less sensitive to both variations. It can be explained by the fact that log-Euclidean metrics are by definition invariant by any translation and scaling in the domain of logarithms [22]. FV presents the best behaviour under moderate variations in both scale and translation. We attribute this to the loss of explicit spatial relations between object parts.

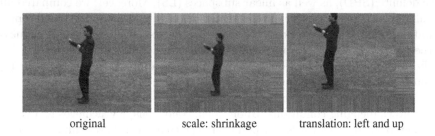

original   scale: shrinkage   translation: left and up

Fig. 2. Examples of challenging conditions.

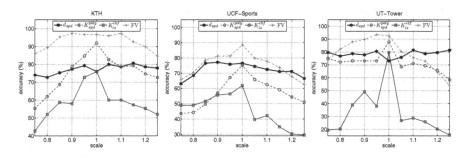

Fig. 3. Results for scale variation; scale >1 means magnification, while <1 means shrinkage.

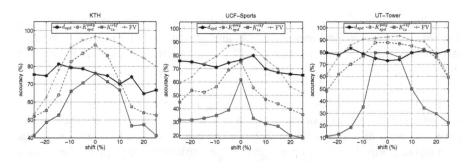

Fig. 4. Results for translation experiments. Each testing video is translated vertically and horizontally at the same time. A positive percentage indicates the video has been translated to the right and bottom while a negative percentage indicates the video has been translated to the left and up.

7   Main Findings

In this paper, we have presented an extensive empirical comparison among existing techniques for the human action recognition problem. We have carried out our experiments using three popular datasets: KTH, UCF-Sports and UT-Tower. We have analysed Riemannian representations including nearest-neighbour classification, kernel methods, and kernelised sparse representations. For Riemannian representation we used covariance matrices of features, which are symmetric positive definite (SPD), as well as linear subspaces (LS). Moreover, we compared all the aforementioned Riemannian representations with GMM and FV based representations, using the same extracted features. We also evaluated the robustness of the most representative approaches to translation and scale variations.

For manifold representations, all SPD matrices approaches surpass their LS counterpart, as a result of the use of not only the dominant eigenvectors but also the eigenvalues. The FV representation outperforms all the techniques under ideal and challenging conditions. Under ideal conditions, FV achieves an overall accuracy of 92.6%, which is 7.6 points higher than both GMM and the polynomial kernel using SPD matrices (K_{spd}^{poly}). FV encodes more information than Riemmannian based methods, as it characterises the deviation from a probabilistic visual dictionary (a GMM) using means and covariance matrices. Moreover, FV is less sensitive under moderate variations in both scale and translation.

Acknowledgements. NICTA is funded by the Australian Government via the Department of Communications, and the Australian Research Council via the ICT Centre of Excellence program.

References

1. Turaga, P., Veeraraghavan, A., Srivastava, A., Chellappa, R.: Statistical computations on Grassmann and Stiefel manifolds for image and video-based recognition. IEEE Trans. Pattern Anal. Mach. Intell. **33**, 2273–2286 (2011)

2. Carvajal, J., Sanderson, C., McCool, C., Lovell, B.C.: Multi-action recognition via stochastic modelling of optical flow and gradients. In: Workshop on Machine Learning for Sensory Data Analysis (MLSDA), pp. 19–24 (2014)
3. Lin, W., Sun, M.T., Poovandran, R., Zhang, Z.: Human activity recognition for video surveillance. In: International Symposium on Circuits and Systems (ISCAS), pp. 2737–2740 (2008)
4. Bishop, C.M.: Pattern Recognition and Machine Learning. Springer, New York (2006)
5. Csurka, G., Perronnin, F.: Fisher vectors: beyond bag-of-visual-words image representations. In: Richard, P., Braz, J. (eds.) VISIGRAPP 2010. CCIS, vol. 229, pp. 28–42. Springer, Heidelberg (2011)
6. Wang, H., Schmid, C.: Action recognition with improved trajectories. In: International Conference on Computer Vision (ICCV) (2013)
7. Aggarwal, J., Ryoo, M.: Human activity analysis: a review. ACM Comput. Surv. **43**, 16:1–16: 43 (2011)
8. Ke, S.R., Thuc, H.L.U., Lee, Y.J., Hwang, J.N., Yoo, J.H., Choi, K.H.: A review on video-based human activity recognition. Computers **2**, 88 (2013)
9. Poppe, R.: A survey on vision-based human action recognition. Image Vis. Comput. **28**, 976–990 (2010)
10. Weinland, D., Ronfard, R., Boyer, E.: A survey of vision-based methods for action representation, segmentation and recognition. Comput. Vis. Image Underst. **115**, 224–241 (2011)
11. Hassner, T.: A critical review of action recognition benchmarks. In: Computer Vision and Pattern Recognition Workshops (CVPRW), pp. 245–250 (2013)
12. Pérez, Ó., Piccardi, M., García, J., Molina, J.M.: Comparison of classifiers for human activity recognition. In: Mira, J., Álvarez, J.R. (eds.) IWINAC 2007. LNCS, vol. 4528, pp. 192–201. Springer, Heidelberg (2007)
13. Schuldt, C., Laptev, I., Caputo, B.: Recognizing human actions: a local SVM approach. In: International Conference on Pattern Recognition (ICPR), vol. 3, pp. 32–36 (2004)
14. Rodriguez, M., Ahmed, J., Shah, M.: Action MACH a spatio-temporal maximum average correlation height filter for action recognition. In: Conference on Computer Vision and Pattern Recognition (CVPR), pp. 1–8 (2008)
15. Chen, C.C., Ryoo, M.S., Aggarwal, J.K.: UT-Tower Dataset: Aerial View Activity Classification Challenge (2010)
16. Ali, S., Shah, M.: Human action recognition in videos using kinematic features and multiple instance learning. Pattern Anal. Mach. Intell. **32**, 288–303 (2010)
17. Guo, K., Ishwar, P., Konrad, J.: Action recognition from video using feature covariance matrices. IEEE Trans. Image Process. **22**, 2479–2494 (2013)
18. Sanin, A., Sanderson, C., Harandi, M., Lovell, B.: Spatio-temporal covariance descriptors for action and gesture recognition. In: Workshop on Applications of Computer Vision (WACV), pp. 103–110 (2013)
19. Harandi, M.T., Sanderson, C., Shirazi, S., Lovell, B.C.: Kernel analysis on Grassmann manifolds for action recognition. Pattern Recogn. Lett. **34**, 1906–1915 (2013)
20. Narasimha Murty, M., Susheela Devi, V.: Nearest neighbour based classifiers. In: Pattern Recognition: An Algorithmic Approach. Undergraduate Topics in Computer Science, pp. 48–85. Springer, London (2011). doi:10.1007/978-0-85729-495-1_3
21. Hamm, J., Lee, D.D.: Grassmann discriminant analysis: a unifying view on subspace-based learning. In: International Conference on Machine Learning (ICML), pp. 376–383 (2008)

22. Arsigny, V., Fillard, P., Pennec, X., Ayache, N.: Log-Euclidean metrics for fast and simple calculus on diffusion tensors. Magn. Reson. Med. **56**, 411–421 (2006)
23. Vemulapalli, R., Pillai, J., Chellappa, R.: Kernel learning for extrinsic classification of manifold features. In: Conference on Computer Vision and Pattern Recognition (CVPR), pp. 1782–1789 (2013)
24. Harandi, M.T., Sanderson, C., Hartley, R., Lovell, B.C.: Sparse coding and dictionary learning for symmetric positive definite matrices: a kernel approach. In: Fitzgibbon, A., Lazebnik, S., Perona, P., Sato, Y., Schmid, C. (eds.) ECCV 2012, Part II. LNCS, vol. 7573, pp. 216–229. Springer, Heidelberg (2012)
25. Jayasumana, S., Hartley, R., Salzmann, M., Li, H., Harandi, M.: Kernel methods on the Riemannian manifold of symmetric positive definite matrices. In: Conference on Computer Vision and Pattern Recognition (CVPR), pp. 73–80 (2013)
26. Zhang, J., Wang, L., Zhou, L., Li, W.: Learning discriminative Stein kernel for SPD matrices and its applications. IEEE Trans. Neural Netw. Learn. Syst. (in press)
27. Wang, R., Guo, H., Davis, L., Dai, Q.: Covariance discriminative learning: a natural and efficient approach to image set classification. In: Conference on Computer Vision and Pattern Recognition (CVPR), pp. 2496–2503 (2012)
28. Shirazi, S., Harandi, M., Sanderson, C., Alavi, A., Lovell, B.: Clustering on Grassmann manifolds via kernel embedding with application to action analysis. In: International Conference on Image Processing (ICIP), pp. 781–784 (2012)
29. Wu, Y., Jia, Y., Li, P., Zhang, J., Yuan, J.: Manifold kernel sparse representation of symmetric positive-definite matrices and its applications. IEEE Trans. Image Process. **24**, 3729–3741 (2015)
30. Harandi, M., Sanderson, C., Shen, C., Lovell, B.: Dictionary learning and sparse coding on Grassmann manifolds: an extrinsic solution. In: International Conference on Computer Vision (ICCV), pp. 3120–3127 (2013)
31. Bini, D.A., Iannazzo, B.: Computing the Karcher mean of symmetric positive definite matrices. Linear Algebra Appl. **438**, 1700–1710 (2013)
32. Sánchez, J., Perronnin, F., Mensink, T., Verbeek, J.: Image classification with the Fisher vector: theory and practice. Int. J. Comput. Vision **105**, 222–245 (2013)
33. Perronnin, F., Sánchez, J., Mensink, T.: Improving the Fisher kernel for large-scale image classification. In: Daniilidis, K., Maragos, P., Paragios, N. (eds.) ECCV 2010, Part IV. LNCS, vol. 6314, pp. 143–156. Springer, Heidelberg (2010)
34. Shirazi, S., Sanderson, C., McCool, C., Harandi, M.T.: Bags of affine subspaces for robust object tracking. In: IEEE International Conference on Digital Image Computing: Techniques and Applications (2015). http://dx.org/10.1109/DICTA.2015.7371239
35. Traore, I., Ahmed, A.A.E.: Continuous Authentication Using Biometrics: Data, Models, and Metrics, 1st edn. IGI Global, Hershey (2011)
36. Hirose, S., Nambu, I., Naito, E.: An empirical solution for over-pruning with a novel ensemble-learning method for fMRI decoding. J. Neurosci. Methods **239**, 238–245 (2015)
37. Aggarwal, N., Agrawal, R.: First and second order statistics features for classification of magnetic resonance brain images. J. Signal Inf. Process. **3**, 146–153 (2012)

Rigidly Self-Expressive Sparse Subspace Clustering

Linbo Qiao[1,2(✉)], Bofeng Zhang[1], Yipin Sun[1], and Jinshu Su[1,2]

[1] College of Computer, National University of Defense Technology,
Changsha 410073, China
[2] National Laboratory for Parallel and Distributed Processing,
National University of Defense Technology,
Changsha 410073, China
{qiao.linbo,bfzhang,yipinsun,sjs}@nudt.edu.cn

Abstract. Sparse subspace clustering is a well-known algorithm, and it is widely used in many research field nowadays, and a lot effort has been contributed to improve it. In this paper, we propose a novel approach to obtain the coefficient matrix. Compared with traditional sparse subspace clustering (SSC) approaches, the key advantage of our approach is that it provides a new perspective of the self-expressive property. We call it rigidly self-expressive (RSE) property. This new formulation captures the rigidly self-expressive property of the data points in the same subspace, and provides a new formulation for sparse subspace clustering. Extensions to traditional SSC could also be cooperating with this new formulation. We present a first-order algorithm to solve the nonconvex optimization, and further prove that it converges to a KKT point of the nonconvex problem under certain standard assumptions. Extensive experiments on the Extended Yale B dataset, the USPS digital images dataset, and the Columbia Object Image Library shows that for images with up to 30 % missing pixels the clustering quality achieved by our approach outperforms the original SSC.

Keywords: Sparse subspace clustering · Rigidly self-expressive · Optimization method

1 Introduction

Subspace clustering naturally arises with the emergence of high-dimensional data. It refers to the problem of finding multiple low-dimensional subspaces underlying a collection of data points sampled from a high-dimensional space and simultaneously partitioning these data into subspaces. Making use of the low intrinsic dimension of input data and the assumption of data lying in a union of linear or affine subspaces, subspace clustering assigns each data point to a subspace, in which data points residing in the same subspace belong to the same cluster. Subspace clustering has been applied to various areas such as computer vision [11],

L. Qiao—The work was partially supported by the National Natural Science Foundation of China under Grant No. 61303264 and Grant No. 61202482.

H. Cao et al. (Eds.): PAKDD 2016 Workshops, LNAI 9794, pp. 101–114, 2016.
DOI: 10.1007/978-3-319-42996-0_9

signal processing [16], and bioinformatics [13]. In the past two decades, numerous algorithms to subspace clustering have been proposed, including K-plane [3], GPCA [24], Spectral Curvature Clustering [4], Low Rank Representation (LRR) [15], Sparse Subspace Clustering (SSC) [7], *etc.* Among these algorithms, the recent work of Sparse Subspace Clustering (SSC) has been recognized to enjoy promising empirical performance.

In this paper, we propose a novel approach beyond SSC to obtain the coefficient matrix. Compared with the approaches mentioned above, the key advantage of our approach is that it provides a new perspective of the self-expressive property. We call it rigidly self-expressive (RSE) property. The model that we build for subspace clustering incorporates rigidly self-expressive property to obtain the coefficient matrix. This formulation generalizes traditional SSC, and captures the expressive property of the data points in the same subspace. We present a first-order algorithm to solve the nonconvex optimization, and further prove that it converges to a KKT point of the nonconvex problem under certain standard assumptions. Extensive experiments on the Extended Yale B dataset [14], the USPS digital images dataset [12], and the Columbia Object Image Library (COIL20) [17] show that for images with up to 30 % missing pixels the clustering quality achieved by our approach outperforms the original SSC.

2   Sparse Subspace Clustering

Assume there are N data points $y_i \in \mathbb{R}^{d_i}, i = 1, \cdots, N$ lying in the union of the linear or affine subspaces $S_i, i = 1, ..., n$, each of dimension $d_i \leq M$ for $i = 1, \cdots, n$. The observed data is reshaped as an matrix with each data point as one column in it

$$Y = [y_1 \cdots y_N] = [Y_1 \cdots Y_N]\Gamma \tag{1}$$

where $Y \in \mathbb{R}^{M \times N}$ with each data point as one column of the matrix and $\Gamma \in \mathbb{R}^{N \times N}$ is an unknown permutation matrix. The subspace clustering focus on the number of subspaces and the membership of each data point to its corresponding subspace.

The SSC algorithm [8] assumes the data can be sparsely represented by the data in a union of subspaces, which is called *self-expressive*. Based on the observation, we can write each data point as

$$y_i = Yc_i, \quad c_{ii} = 0, \tag{2}$$

where $c_i = [c_{i1} \; c_{i2} \; \cdots \; c_{iN}]$ and the constraint $c_{ii} = 0$ eliminates the trivial solution of writing a point as a linear combination of itself. When the data points are well distributed inside each subspace, the relationship among the data points is theoretically analyzed in [9], which formulate the problem as

$$\min_C \|C\|_1$$
$$s.t. \; Y = YC, \quad \text{diag}(C) = 0. \tag{3}$$

where $C = [c_1 \; c_2 \; \cdots \; c_N] \in \mathbb{R}^{N \times N}$ is the matrix whose i-th column corresponds to the sparse representation of y_i, c_i, and $\text{diag}(C) \in \mathbb{R}^N$ is the vector of the diagonal elements of C.

Considering there are outliers and noise in real world data, the model is extended as a more practical one

$$Y = YC + E + Z,$$
$$\text{diag}(C) = 0. \tag{4}$$

where E denotes the matrix form of outlying entries which has only a few large non-zero elements, and Z denotes the matrix form of noise,the formulation (3) is extended to handle the real-world problems with considering

$$\min_{(C,E,Z)} \; \|C\|_1 + \lambda_e \|E\|_1 + \tfrac{\lambda_z}{2} \|Z\|_F^2$$
$$s.t. \quad Y = YC + E + Z, \tag{5}$$
$$\text{diag}(C) = 0.$$

In the formulation, $Y \in R^{M \times N}$ is the original data set without any noise and outliers, Z and E correspond to noise and sparse outliers respectively, $\lambda_e > 0$, $\lambda_z > 0$ are two trade-off parameters balancing the three terms in the objective function, and the $\text{diag}(C)$ is a vector whose elements are the diagonal entries of the matrix C.

For the case that the data corrupted by outliers, Candes *et al.* [22,23] give geometric insights which show that the method would succeed when the dataset is corrupted with possibly overwhelmingly many outliers. For the case that the data is corrupted by noise Z Wang and Xu [25] show that when the amount of noise is small enough, the subspaces are sufficiently separated, and the data are well distributed, the matrix of coefficients gives the correct clustering with high probability.

3   Rigidly Self-Expressive SSC

The sparse subspace clustering algorithm mainly takes advantage of the *self-expressiveness* property of the data. Specifically speaking, each data point in a union of subspaces can be efficiently expressed as a combination of other points in the same dataset.

However, in many real-world problems, data are always corrupted by noise and sparse outlying entries at the same time due to measurement noise or data collection techniques. For instance, in clustering of human faces, images can be corrupted by errors due to speculation, cast shadow, and occlusion [26]. Similarly, in the motion segmentation problem, because of the malfunctioning of the tracker, feature trajectories can be corrupted by noise or can have entries with large errors [28]. In such cases, the data do not lie perfectly in a union of subspaces, which means that *the noise and outlier free data* $\hat{Y}$ *does not exactly lie in the union of the subspaces of observed data* Y, and the observed data points Y lie in a space contaminated with outlier E and noise Z. Considering the self-expressiveness in the formulation (5), it is not appropriate to use the linear combination YC to represent the data points $\hat{Y}$.

In this paper we improve the SSC formulation in [9], and present a rigidly self-expressive formulation, named Rigidly Self-Expressive Sparse Subspace Clustering (RSE-SSC), using a sparse linear combination $\hat{Y}C$ of the original subspaces to represent the original data points $\hat{Y}$ without noise and outliers, and the observed data set is expressed as the sum of the original data set and noise and outliers. Here we consider the optimization problem with the same objective value function with the original SSC, but totally different constraints on data points. Letting $\hat{Y}$ the data points lie in the original subspaces without outliers nor noise, and the constraints

$$
\begin{aligned}
Y &= \hat{Y} + E + Z, \\
\hat{Y} &= \hat{Y}C, \\
\mathrm{diag}(C) &= 0.
\end{aligned} \tag{6}
$$

are used to express the sparse representation. The observed data Y is naturally expressed as the sum of the exactly original data set and noise and outliers. And the appropriate sparse subspace clustering (RSE-SSC) is formulated as (7)

$$
\begin{aligned}
\min_{(\hat{Y},C,E,Z)} \quad & \|C\|_1 + \lambda_e\|E\|_1 + \tfrac{\lambda_z}{2}\|Z\|_F^2 \\
\mathrm{s.t.} \quad & Y = \hat{Y} + E + Z, \\
& \hat{Y} = \hat{Y}C, \\
& \mathrm{diag}(C) = 0.
\end{aligned} \tag{7}
$$

In the formulation, $\hat{Y} \in R^{M \times N}$ is the original data set without any noise and outliers, Z and E correspond to noise and sparse outliers respectively, $\lambda_e > 0$, $\lambda_z > 0$ are two trade-off parameters balancing the three terms in the objective function, and the $\mathrm{diag}(C)$ is a vector whose elements are the diagonal entries of the matrix C.

The sparse coefficients again encode information about memberships of data to subspaces, which are used in a spectral clustering framework, as before. The algorithm for RSE-SSC is shown in the following section.

4   Solving the Sparse Optimization Problem

The proposed convex programs can be solved via generic convex solvers. However, the computational costs of generic solvers typically is high and these solvers do not scale well with the dimension and the number of data points. In this section, we study efficient implementations of the proposed sparse optimizations using an Alternating Direction Method of Multipliers (ADMM) method [1,2]. We first consider the most general optimization problem

$$
\begin{aligned}
\min_{(\hat{Y},C,E,Z)} \quad & \|C\|_1 + \lambda_e\|E\|_1 + \tfrac{\lambda_z}{2}\|Z\|_F^2 \\
\mathrm{s.t.} \quad & \hat{Y} = \hat{Y}C, \\
& Y = \hat{Y} + E + Z, \\
& \mathrm{diag}(C) = 0.
\end{aligned} \tag{8}
$$

Utilizing the equality constraint $Y = \hat{Y} + E + Z$, we can eliminate Z from the optimization problem (7) to generate a concise formulation without Z which is equivalent to solve the original optimization problem. The optimization problem is formulated as

$$\min_{(\hat{Y}, C, E)} \quad \|C\|_1 + \lambda_e \|E\|_1 + \tfrac{\lambda_z}{2} \|Y - \hat{Y} - E\|_F^2$$
$$\text{s.t.} \quad \hat{Y} = \hat{Y}C, \tag{9}$$
$$\text{diag}(C) = 0.$$

where Z is eliminated from the optimization program, and there are fewer variables and this will cut down the computational cost in each iteration as each variable shall be updates in each iteration of ADMM.

However there is no simple way to update C in each iteration, in order to obtain efficient updates on the optimization variables, we introduce an auxiliary matrix $A \in \mathbb{R}^{N \times N}$, and equivalently transform the optimization problem (9) to the optimization problem

$$\min_{(\hat{Y}, C, E, A)} \quad \|C\|_1 + \lambda_e \|E\|_1 + \tfrac{\lambda_z}{2} \|Y - \hat{Y} - E\|_F^2$$
$$\text{s.t.} \quad \hat{Y} = \hat{Y}A, \tag{10}$$
$$A = C - \text{diag}(C).$$

It should be noted that the solution $(\hat{Y}; C; E)$ of optimization problem (10) concides with the solution of optimization problem (9), also concides with the solution of optimization problem (7). As shown in the Algorithm 1, the updating of variable C is much simpler in each iteration. Following the ADMM framework, we add those two constraints $\hat{Y} = \hat{Y}A$ and $A = C - \text{diag}(C)$ of (10) as two penalty terms with parameter $\rho > 0$ to the objective function, and also introduce Lagrange multipliers for the two equality constraints, then we can write the augmented Lagrangian function of (10) as

$$\mathcal{L}(\hat{Y}, C, E, A; \Delta_1, \Delta_2)$$
$$:= \|C\|_1 + \lambda_e \|E\|_1 + \tfrac{\lambda_z}{2} \|Y - \hat{Y} - E\|_F^2$$
$$+ \tfrac{\rho}{2} \|\hat{Y}A - \hat{Y}\|_F^2 + \tfrac{\rho}{2} \|A - C + \text{diag}(C)\|_F^2 \tag{11}$$
$$+ \text{tr}(\Delta_1^\top (\hat{Y}A - Y)) + \text{tr}(\Delta_2^\top (A - C + \text{diag}(C))).$$

where the matrix $\Delta_1, \Delta_2 \in \mathbb{R}^{N \times N}$ is the Lagrange multipliers for the two equality constraints in (10), $\text{tr}(\cdot)$ denotes the trace operator of a given matrix. The algorithm then iteratively updates the variables $A, C, E, \hat{Y}$ and the Lagrange multipliers Δ_1, Δ_2.

In the k-th iteration, we denote the variables by A^k, C^k, E^k, $\hat{Y}^k$, and the Lagrange multipliers by Δ_1^k, Δ_2^k. Given A^k, C^k, E^k, $\hat{Y}^k$, Δ_1^k, Δ_2^k, ADMM iterates as follows

---

Algorithm 1.   ADMM algorithm for solving program (10)

Input: $\hat{Y}^0, A^0, C^0, E^0, \Delta_1^0, \Delta_2^0$
Output: $\hat{Y}, A, C, E, \Delta_1, \Delta_2$
1: **Initialization:** Set $maxIter = 10^4$, $k = 0$, $Terminate = False$
2: **while**(Terminate == False) **do**
3:     Update A^{k+1} by solving the following system of linear equations

$$\rho((\hat{Y}^k)^\top \hat{Y}^k + I)A = \rho((\hat{Y}^k)^\top \hat{Y}^k + C^k) + \rho\text{diag}(C^k) + (\hat{Y}^k)^\top \Delta_1^k - \Delta_2^k,$$

4:     Update C^{k+1} as $C^{k+1} = J^{k+1} - \text{diag}(J^{k+1})$, where $J^{k+1} = T_{\frac{1}{\rho}}(A^{k+1} + \Delta_2^k/\rho)$,
5:     Update E^{k+1} as $E^{k+1} = T_{\frac{\lambda_e}{\lambda_z}}(\hat{Y}^k - Y)$,
6:     Update $\hat{Y}^{k+1}$ by the solving system of linear equations

$$\hat{Y}(\lambda_z I + \rho(A^{k+1} - I)(A^{k+1} - I)^\top) = \lambda_z(Y - E^{k+1}) - \Delta_1(A^{k+1} - I)^\top,$$

7:     Update Δ_1^{k+1} as $\Delta_1^{k+1} := \Delta_1^k + \rho(\hat{Y}^{k+1}A^{k+1} - \hat{Y}k + 1)$,
8:     Update Δ_2^{k+1} as $\Delta_2^{k+1} := \Delta_2^k + \rho(A^{k+1} - C^{k+1})$,
9:     $k = k + 1$,
10:    **if** $k \geq maxIter$ or $\|\hat{Y}A^k - \hat{Y}\|_F^2 \leq \epsilon$ or $\|A^k - C^k\|_F^2 \leq \epsilon$ or $\|A^k - A^{k-1}\| \leq \epsilon$ or $\|C^k - C^{k-1}\| \leq \epsilon$ or $\|E^k - E^{k-1}\| \leq \epsilon$ or $\|\hat{Y}^k - \hat{Y}^{k-1}\| \leq \epsilon$
       then
       $Terminate = True$
11:    **end if**
12: **end while**

$$\hat{Y}^{k+1} := \underset{\hat{Y}}{\text{argmin}}\, \mathcal{L}(\hat{Y}, A^{k+1}, C^{k+1}, E^{k+1}; \Delta_1^k, \Delta_2^k), \tag{12a}$$

$$A^{k+1} := \underset{A}{\text{argmin}}\, \mathcal{L}(\hat{Y}^k, A, C^k, E^k; \Delta_1^k, \Delta_2^k), \tag{12b}$$

$$C^{k+1} := \underset{C}{\text{argmin}}\, \mathcal{L}(\hat{Y}^k, A^{k+1}, C, E^k; \Delta_1^k, \Delta_2^k), \tag{12c}$$

$$E^{k+1} := \underset{E}{\text{argmin}}\, \mathcal{L}(\hat{Y}^k, A^{k+1}, C^{k+1}, E; \Delta_1^k, \Delta_2^k), \tag{12d}$$

$$\Delta_1^{k+1} := \Delta_1^k + \rho(\hat{Y}A - \hat{Y}), \tag{12e}$$

$$\Delta_2^{k+1} := \Delta_2^k + \rho(A - C). \tag{12f}$$

Then we show how to solve the six subproblems in (12a), (12b), (12c), (12d), (12e) and (12f) in the ADMM algorithm. After all these subproblems solved, we will give the framework of the algorithm that summarize our ADMM algorithm for solving (10) in Algorithm 1.

These three steps are repeated until convergence is achieved or the number of iterations exceeds a maximum iteration number. The algorithm will stop when these conditions satisfied $\|\hat{Y}A^k - \hat{Y}\|_F^2 \leq \epsilon, \|A^k - C^k\|_F^2 \leq \epsilon, \|A^k - A^{k-1}\| \leq \epsilon, \|C^k - C^{k-1}\| \leq \epsilon, \|E^k - E^{k-1}\| \leq \epsilon, \|\hat{Y}^k - \hat{Y}^{k-1}\| \leq \epsilon$, where ϵ denotes the error tolerance for the primal and dual residuals. In practice, the choice of $= 10^4$ works well in real experiments. In summary, Algorithm 1 shows the updates for the ADMM implementation of the optimization problem (10).

5   Convergence Analysis

Similar to [21,27], in this section, we provide a convergence analysis for the proposed ADMM algorithm showing that under certain standard conditions, any limit point of the iteration sequence generated by Algorithm 1 is a KKT point of (10).

Theorem 1. *Let* $X := (\hat{Y}, C, W, E)$ *and* $\{X^k\}_{k=1}^{\infty}$ *be generated by Algorithm 1. Assume that* $\{X^k\}_{k=1}^{\infty}$ *is bounded and* $\lim_{k\to\infty}(X^{k+1} - X^k) = 0$. *Then any accumulation point of* $\{X^k\}_{k=1}^{\infty}$ *is a KKT point of problem* (10).

For ease of presentation, we define $S_1 := \{C | \text{diag}(C) = 0\}$, and use $\mathcal{P}_S(\cdot)$ to denote the projection operator onto set S. It is easy to verify that the KKT conditions for (10) are:

$$\partial \mathcal{L}_Y(\hat{Y}, A, C, E; \Delta_1, \Delta_2) = 0, \tag{13a}$$

$$\partial \mathcal{L}_A(\hat{Y}, A, C, E; \Delta_1, \Delta_2) = 0, \tag{13b}$$

$$\partial \mathcal{L}_C(\hat{Y}, A, C, E; \Delta_1, \Delta_2) = 0, \tag{13c}$$

$$\partial \mathcal{L}_E(\hat{Y}, A, C, E; \Delta_1, \Delta_2) = 0, \tag{13d}$$

$$\hat{Y} - \hat{Y}A = 0, \tag{13e}$$

$$\mathcal{P}_S(A) = A, \tag{13f}$$

where $\partial f(x)$ is the subdifferential of function f at x.

Proof. Assume $\hat{X} := (\hat{Y}, \hat{C}, \hat{W}, \hat{E})$ is a limit point of $\{X^k\}_{k=1}^{\infty}$. We will show that $\hat{X}$ satisfies the KKT conditions in (13). As (12a) and (12b) are guaranteed by the algorithm construction, it directly implies that $\hat{X}$ satisfies (13a) and (13b). We rewrite the updating rules 12e and 12f in Algorithm 1 as

$$E^{k+1} - E^k = \mathcal{T}_{\frac{\lambda_e}{\lambda_z}}(\hat{Y}^k - Y) - \mathcal{T}_{\frac{\lambda_e}{\lambda_z}}(\hat{Y}^{k-1} - Y) \tag{14a}$$

$$C^{k+1} - C^k = J^{k+1} - \text{diag}(J^{k+1}) - (J^k - \text{diag}(J^k)) \tag{14b}$$

$$\Delta_1^{k+1} - \Delta_1^k = \rho(\hat{Y}A - \hat{Y}), \tag{14c}$$

$$\Delta_2^{k+1} - \Delta_2^k = \rho(A - C). \tag{14d}$$

The assumption $\lim_{k\to\infty}(X^{k+1} - X^k) = 0$ implies that the left hand sides in (15) all go to zero. Therefore,

$$\rho(\hat{Y}A - \hat{Y}) \to 0 \tag{15a}$$

$$\rho(A - C) \to 0 \tag{15b}$$

Hence, we only need to verify that $\hat{X}$ satisfies the other two conditions in (13).

For convenience, let us first ignore the projection in (13e). Then for $\tau_2 > 0$, (13e) is equivalent to

$$\tau_2 \rho Y^T(Y - YC) + C \in \tau_2 \partial \|C\|_1 + C \triangleq \mathcal{Q}_{\tau_2}(C) \tag{16}$$

with the scalar function $\mathcal{Q}_{\tau_2}(t) := \tau_2 \partial(|t|_1) + t$ applied element-wise to C. It is easy to verify that $\mathcal{Q}_{\tau_2}(t)$ is monotone and $\mathcal{Q}_{\tau_2}^{-1}(t) = \mathrm{shrink}_1(t, \tau_2)$. By applying $\mathcal{Q}_{\tau_2}^{-1}(\cdot)$ to both sides of (16), we get

$$C = \mathrm{shrink}_1(\tau_2 \rho Y^T(Y - YC) + C, \tau_2). \tag{17}$$

By invoking the definition of g_C^k leads to

$$\hat{C} = \mathcal{P}_{S_2}(\mathrm{shrink}_1(\tau_2 \rho \hat{Y}^T(\hat{Y} - \hat{Y}\hat{C}) + \hat{C}, \tau_2)),$$

which implies that $\hat{X}$ satisfies (13c) and (13d) when the projection function is considered.

In summary, $\hat{X}$ satisfies the KKT conditions (13). Thus, any accumulation point of $\{X^k\}_{k=1}^{\infty}$ is a KKT point of problem (10).

6   Experiments

In this section, we apply our RSE-SSC approach to three different data sets. We will mainly focus on the comparison of our approach with SSC proposed in [9]. The MATLAB codes of SSC were downloaded from http://www.cis.jhu.edu/~ehsan/code.htme.

6.1   The Dataset

We applied our Algorithm 2 to three public datasets: the Extended Yale B dataset[1], the USPS digital images dataset[2], and the COIL20 dataset[3].

The Extended Yale B dataset is a well-known dataset for face clustering, which consists of images taken from 38 human subjects, and 64 frontal images for each subject were acquired under different illumination conditions and a fixed pose. To reduce the computational cost and memory requirements of the algorithms, we downsample the raw images into the size of 48×42. Thus, each image is in dimension of $2,016$.

The USPS dataset is relatively difficult to handle, in which there are $7,291$ labeled observations and each observation is a digit of 16×16 grayscale image and of different orientations. The number of each digit varies from 542 to $1,194$. To reduce the time and memory cost of the expriement, we randomly chose 100 images of each digit in our experiment.

The COIL20 dataset is a database consisting of $1,440$ grayscale images of 20 objects. Images of the 20 objects were taken to pose intervals of 5 degrees, which results in 72 images per object. All $1,440$ normalized images of 20 objects are used in our experiment.

---

[1]   http://vision.ucsd.edu/~leekc/ExtYaleDatabase/ExtYaleB.html.
[2]   http://statweb.stanford.edu/~tibs/ElemStatLearn/data.html.
[3]   http://www.cs.columbia.edu/CAVE/software/softlib/coil-20.php.

Algorithm 2.   Algorithm for RSE-SSC

Input: A set of points $\{M_i\}_{i=1}^N$ (with missing entries and outlying entries) lying in a union of L linear subspaces $\{S_\ell\}_{\ell=1}^L$

Output: Clustering results of the data points

1: Normalization: normalize the data points.
2: RSE-SSC solve the RSE-SSC optimization problem (7) by algorithm introduced in Sect. 4.
3: Post-processing: for each C_i, keep its largest T coefficients in absolute magnitude, and set the remaining coefficients to zeros.
4: Similarity graph: form a similarity graph with N nodes representing the data points, and set the weights of the edges between the nodes by $W = |C| + |C|^T$.
5: Clustering: apply the normalized spectral clustering approach in [18] to the similarity graph.

6.2 Post-Processing and Spectral Clustering

After solving optimization problem (7), we obtain the clustered images and the sparse coefficient matrix C. Similar to [6], we perform some post-processing procedure on C. For each coefficient vector C_i, we keep its largest T coefficients in absolute magnitude and set the remaining coefficients to zeros. The affinity matrix W associated with the weighted graph $\mathcal{G}$ is then constructed as $W = |C| + |C|^T$. To obtain the final clustering result, we apply the normalized spectral clustering approach proposed by Ng *et al.* [18]. Thus, the whole procedure of our RSE-SSC based clustering approach can be described as in Algorithm 2.

For SSC [7], we find that it performs better without the normalization of data and post-processing of the coefficient matrix C. As a result, we ran the codes provided by the authors directly. Note that the same spectral clustering algorithm was applied to the coefficient matrix obtained by SSC.

6.3 Implementation Details

Considering that the number of subspaces affects the clustering and recovery performance of algorithms, we applied algorithms under cases of $L = 3, 5, 8$, where L denotes the number of subspaces, i.e., the number of different subjects. To shorten the testing time, L subjects were chosen in the following way. In the Extended Yale B dataset, all the 38 subjects were divided into four groups, where the four groups correspond to subjects 1 to 10, 11 to 20, 21 to 30, and 31 to 38, respectively. L subjects were chosen from the same group. For example, when $L = 5$, the number of possible 5 subjects is $3\binom{10}{5} + \binom{8}{5} = 812$. Among these 812 possible choices, 20 trials were randomly chosen to test the proposed algorithms under the condition of L subspaces. To study the effect of the fraction of missing entries in clustering and recovery performance of algorithms, we artificially corrupted images into 3 missing rate levels 10 %, 20 % to 30 %. To make the comparison of different algorithms as fair as possible, we randomly generated the missing images first, and then all algorithms were applied to the same randomly corrupted images to cluster the images and recover the missing pixels.

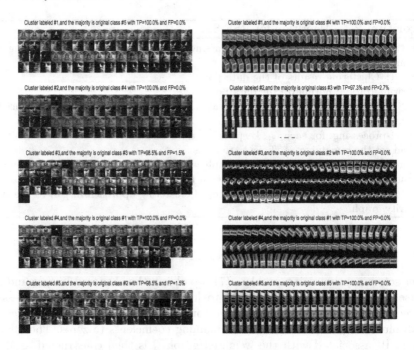

(a) Clustered images from Extended Yale (b) Clustered images from Columbia objects

Fig. 1. Clustered images from Extended Yale B face images and Columbia objects images within 5 subspaces with 10 % entries missing

To generate corrupted images with a specified missing fraction range from, we randomly removed squares whose size is no larger than 10×10, repeatedly until the total fraction of missing pixels is no less than the specified fraction.

In Algorithm 2 (RSE-SSC), we initialise Y by filling in each missing pixel with the average value of corresponding pixels in other images with known pixel value. We implement SSC proposed in [7] in two different ways. In Algorithm "SSC-AVE", we fill in the missing entries in the same way as "RSE-SSC", and in Algorithm "SSC-0", we fill in the missing entries by 0. We use the subspace clustering error (SCE), which is defined as

$$SCE := (\# \text{ of misclassified images})/(\text{total } \# \text{ of images}),$$

to demonstrate the clustering quality. For each set of L with different percentage of missing pixels, the averaged SCE over 20 random trials are calculated.

In Algorithm 1, we choose $\lambda_e = \lambda_z = 5 \times 10^{-2}$, total loss threshold $tol = 5 \times 10^{-6}$, maximum iterations $maxIter = 5 \times 10^3$ in all experiments. We set $\rho = 1000/\mu$, where $\mu := \min_i \max_{j \neq i} |Y_i^T Y_j|$ to avoid trivial solutions. It should be noted that ρ actually changes in each iteration, because matrix Y is updated in each iteration. To accelerate the convergence of Algorithm 1, we adopt the following stopping criterion to terminate the algorithm $\|\hat{Y}A^k - \hat{Y}\|_F^2 + \|A^k - C^k\|_F^2 + \|A^k - A^{k-1}\| + \|C^k - C^{k-1}\| + \|E^k - E^{k-1}\| + \|\hat{Y}^k - \hat{Y}^{k-1}\| < tol$ or the iteration number exceeds the $maxIter$.

Table 1. SCE-Mean of RSE-SSC and SSC with different fraction of missing entries for different datasets

Missing rate=10%			Missing rate=20%			Missing rate=30%		
SSC-0	SSC-AVE	RSE-SSC	SSC-0	SSC-AVE	RSE-SSC	SSC-0	SSC-AVE	RSE-SSC
Yale B dataset: 3 subjects								
5.83	5.20	3.78	27.00	7.57	6.12	51.84	14.68	8.24
Yale B dataset: 5 subjects								
5.62	4.76	5.25	40.32	17.23	8.29	54.28	32.23	13.75
Yale B dataset: 8 subjects								
7.81	6.45	5.72	42.18	40.37	15.42	60.62	46.57	18.19
USPS dataset: 3 subjects								
0.07	0.07	0.07	9.07	9.33	7.43	10.52	9.97	8.34
USPS dataset: 5 subjects								
8.76	7.68	3.74	23.51	21.69	18.54	24.55	21.06	20.74
USPS dataset: 8 subjects								
12.50	10.11	7.86	36.81	34.59	21.35	46.93	29.08	26.53
COIL20 dataset: 3 subjects								
6.99	6.74	5.87	38.47	19.75	7.63	45.74	19.72	8.94
COIL20 dataset: 5 subjects								
7.79	9.17	7.13	41.76	18.60	9.36	46.74	26.36	11.82
COIL20 dataset: 8 subjects								
11.55	9.44	9.56	41.94	28.32	15.27	48.51	35.54	18.62

6.4   Results

We report the experimental results in Table 1. It shows the SCE of three algorithms, where "SCE-mean" represent the mean of the SCE in percentage over 20 random trials. From Table 1, we can see that when the images are incomplete, for example when $L = 3$, the mean of SCE is usually smaller than 7%. This means that the percentage of misclassified images is smaller than 7%. It can been seen that our Algorithm 2 gives better results on clustering errors in most situations. Especially, when $spa = 20\%$ and 30%, the mean clustering errors are much smaller than the ones given by SSC-AVE and SSC-0, this phenomena is more obvious with the increase of number of subjects. These comparison results show that our RSE-SSC model can cluster images very robustly and greatly outperforms SSC.

The subfigures (a) and (b) of Fig. 1 show the clustering results of one instance of $L = 5$ using Algorithm 2 for the Extended Yale B dataset and the COIL dataset. After applying our algorithm, each image is labled with a class ID, and comparing to the original class ID we could calculate the True Positive Rate and False Positive Rate of each original individual. The misclassified images in each cluster are labeled with colored rectangles and the true positive rate (TP) and false positive rate are also given as the title of the subfigures. Most of the misclassified images, as we can see, are not in good illumination conditions and they are thus difficult to be classified. Removing these illumination conditions will improve the experimental results a lot. We only show the results of one instance of $L = 5$ for the Extended Yale B dataset and the COIL20 dataset. The results on all datasets will be fully displayed in a longer version.

It should be noted that, due to the limited space, we just present results on the Extended Yale B dataset and the COIL dataset with 10% entries missing, the other two missing rate level will be provided in a longer version or in the form of supplementary material. In the supplementary material, Fig. 1, Fig. 2 and Fig. 3 show the results for the Extended Yale B dataset, the COIL dataset and the USPS dataset with $L = 5$ using Algorithm 2. Figure 4, Fig. 5 and Fig. 6 show the accordingly clustering results of $L = 8$ using Algorithm 2 for these datasets.

7   Conclusions

Sparse subspace clustering is a well-known algorithm, and it is widely used in many research field nowadays, and a lot effort has been contributed to improve it. In this paper, we propose a novel approach to obtain the coefficient matrix. Compared with traditional sparse subspace clustering (SSC) approaches, the key advantage of our approach is that it provides a new perspective of the self-expressive property. We call it rigidly self-expressive (RSE) property. This new formulation captures the rigidly self-expressive property of the data points in the same subspace, and provides a new formulation for sparse subspace clustering. Extensions to traditional SSC could also be cooperate with this new formulation, and this could lead to a serial of approaches based on rigidly self-expressive property. We present a first-order algorithm to solve the nonconvex optimization, and further prove that it converges to a KKT point of the nonconvex problem under certain standard assumptions. Extensive experiments on the Extended Yale B dataset, the USPS digital images dataset, and the Columbia Object Image Library show that for images with up to 30% missing pixels the clustering quality achieved by our approach outperforms the original SSC.

References

1. Boyd, S., Parikh, N., Chu, E., Peleato, B., Eckstein, J.: Distributed optimization and statistical learning via the alternating direction method of multipliers. Found. Trends in Mach. Learn. **3**(1), 1–122 (2011)
2. Boyd, S.P., Vandenberghe, L.: Convex Optimization. Cambridge University Press, Cambridge (2004)
3. Bradley, P.S., Mangasarian, O.L.: K-plane clustering. J. Global Optim. **16**(1), 23–32 (2000)
4. Chen, G.L., Lerman, G.: Spectral curvature clustering (SCC). Int. J. Comput. Vis. **81**(3), 317–330 (2009)
5. Daubechies, I., Defrise, M., De Mol, C.: An iterative thresholding algorithm for linear inverse problems with a sparsity constraint. Commun. Pure Appl. Math. **57**(11), 1413–1457 (2004)

6. Dyer, E.L., Sankaranarayanan, A.C., Baraniuk, R.G.: Greedy feature selection for subspace clustering. J. Mach. Learn. Res. **14**(1), 2487–2517 (2013)
7. Elhamifar, E.: Sparse modeling for high-dimensional multi-manifold data analysis. Ph.D. thesis, The Johns Hopkins University (2012)
8. Elhamifar, E., Vidal, R.: Sparse subspace clustering. In: Proceedings of CVPR, vol. 1–4, pp. 2782–2789 (2009)
9. Elhamifar, E., Vidal, R.: Sparse subspace clustering: algorithm, theory, and applications. IEEE Trans. Pattern Anal. Mach. Intell. **35**(11), 2765–2781 (2013)
10. Grant, M., Boyd, S., Ye, Y.: CVX: matlab software for disciplined convex programming (2008)
11. Ho, J., Yang, M.-H., Lim, J., Lee, K.-C., Kriegman, D.: Clustering appearances of objects under varying illumination conditions. In: Proceedings 2003 IEEE Computer Society Conference on Computer Vision and Pattern Recognition, vol. 1, pp. I-11–I-18. IEEE (2003)
12. Hull, J.J.: A database for handwritten text recognition research. IEEE Trans. Pattern Anal. Mach. Intell. **16**(5), 550–554 (1994)
13. Kriegel, H.-P., Krger, P., Zimek, A.: Clustering high-dimensional data: a survey on subspace clustering, pattern-based clustering, and correlation clustering. ACM Trans. Knowl. Discov. Data (TKDD) **3**(1), 1 (2009)
14. Lee, K.-C., Ho, J., Kriegman, D.J.: Acquiring linear subspaces for face recognition under variable lighting. IEEE Trans. Pattern Anal. Mach. Intell. **27**(5), 684–698 (2005)
15. Liu, G., Xu, H., Yan, S.: Exact subspace segmentation and outlier detection by low-rank representation. In: Proceedings of AISTATS, pp. 703–711 (2012)
16. Lu, Y.M., Do, M.N.: Sampling signals from a union of subspaces. IEEE Sig. Proc. Mag. **25**(2), 41–47 (2008)
17. Nene, S.A., Nayar, S.K., Murase, H.: Columbia object image library (coil-20). Technical report CUCS-005-96 (1996)
18. Ng, A.Y., Jordan, M.I., Weiss, Y.: On spectral clustering: analysis and an algorithm. Proc. NIPS **14**, 849–856 (2002)
19. Ramamoorthi, R.: Analytic PCA construction for theoretical analysis of lighting variability in images of a lambertian object. IEEE Trans. Pattern Anal. Mach. Intell. **24**(10), 1322–1333 (2002)
20. Rao, S.R., Tron, R., Vidal, R., Ma, Y.: Motion segmentation via robust subspace separation in the presence of outlying, incomplete, or corrupted trajectories. In: IEEE Conference on Computer Vision and Pattern Recognition, CVPR 2008, pp. 1–8. IEEE (2008)
21. Shen, Y., Wen, Z., Zhang, Y.: Augmented lagrangian alternating direction method for matrix separation based on low-rank factorization. Optim. Methods Softw. **29**(2), 239–263 (2014)
22. Soltanolkotabi, M., Candes, E.J.: A geometric analysis of subspace clustering with outliers. Ann. Stat. **40**(4), 2195–2238 (2012)
23. Soltanolkotabi, M., Elhamifar, E., Candes, E.J.: Robust subspace clustering. Ann. Stat. **42**(2), 669–699 (2014)
24. Vidal, R.E.: Generalized principal component analysis (GPCA): an algebraic geometric approach to subspace clustering and motion segmentation. Ph.D. thesis, University of California at Berkeley (2003)
25. Wang, Y.-X., Xu, H.: Noisy sparse subspace clustering. In: Proceedings of ICML, pp. 89–97 (2013)

26. Wright, J., Ganesh, A., Rao, S., Peng, Y., Ma, Y.: Robust principal component analysis: exact recovery of corrupted low-rank matrices via convex optimization. In: Proceedings of NIPS, pp. 2080–2088 (2009)
27. Xu, Y., Yin, W., Wen, Z., Zhang, Y.: An alternating direction algorithm for matrix completion with nonnegative factors. Front. Math. China **7**(2), 365–384 (2012)
28. Zappella, L., Llado, X., Salvi, J.: Motion segmentation: a review. Artif. Intell. Res. Dev. **184**, 398–407 (2008)

Joint Recognition and Segmentation of Actions via Probabilistic Integration of Spatio-Temporal Fisher Vectors

Johanna Carvajal[1,3], Chris McCool[2], Brian Lovell[1], and Conrad Sanderson[1,3,4(✉)]

[1] University of Queensland, Brisbane, Australia
[2] Queensland University of Technology, Brisbane, Australia
[3] NICTA, Brisbane, Australia
[4] Data61, CSIRO, Brisbane, Australia
conrad.sanderson@nicta.com.au

Abstract. We propose a hierarchical approach to multi-action recognition that performs joint classification and segmentation. A given video (containing several consecutive actions) is processed via a sequence of overlapping temporal windows. Each frame in a temporal window is represented through selective low-level spatio-temporal features which efficiently capture relevant local dynamics. Features from each window are represented as a Fisher vector, which captures first and second order statistics. Instead of directly classifying each Fisher vector, it is converted into a vector of class probabilities. The final classification decision for each frame is then obtained by integrating the class probabilities at the frame level, which exploits the overlapping of the temporal windows. Experiments were performed on two datasets: s-KTH (a stitched version of the KTH dataset to simulate multi-actions), and the challenging CMU-MMAC dataset. On s-KTH, the proposed approach achieves an accuracy of 85.0 %, significantly outperforming two recent approaches based on GMMs and HMMs which obtained 78.3 % and 71.2 %, respectively. On CMU-MMAC, the proposed approach achieves an accuracy of 40.9 %, outperforming the GMM and HMM approaches which obtained 33.7 % and 38.4 %, respectively. Furthermore, the proposed system is on average 40 times faster than the GMM based approach.

1   Introduction

Research on human action recognition can be divided into two areas: (i) single-action recognition, and (ii) multi-action recognition. In most computer vision literature, action recognition approaches have concentrated on single actions, where each video to be classified contains only one action. However, when observing realistic human behaviour in natural settings, the fundamental problem is segmenting and recognising actions from a *multi-action* sequence [1]. It is challenging due to the high variability of appearances, shapes, possible occlusions, large variability in the temporal scale and periodicity of human actions, the complexity of articulated motion, the exponential nature of all possible movement combinations, as well as the prevalence of irrelevant background [2,3].

H. Cao et al. (Eds.): PAKDD 2016 Workshops, LNAI 9794, pp. 115–127, 2016.
DOI: 10.1007/978-3-319-42996-0_10

Hoai et al. [2] address joint segmentation and classification by classifying temporal regions using a multi-class Support Vector Machine (SVM) and performing segmentation using dynamic programming. A similar approach is presented in [4], where the temporal relationship between actions is considered. Borzeshi et al. [5] proposed the use of hidden Markov models (HMMs) with irregular observations (termed HMM-MIO) to perform multi-action recognition. More recently, Carvajal et al. [6] proposed to model each action using a Gaussian mixture model (GMM) approach where classification decisions are made using overlapping temporal windows. A drawback of [2,4,5] is that they have a large number of parameters to optimise. Furthermore, [5] requires an extra stage to reduce dimensionality due to use of very high dimensional feature vectors, while [2,4] require fully labelled annotations for training. One downside of [6] is that for each action and scenario, a model with a large number of Gaussians is required, making the system computationally expensive.

Typically, the aforementioned approaches used for the multi-action recognition task can be classified as either generative or discriminative models. The approaches presented in [5,6] are generative models, while those presented in [2,4] are discriminative models. Generative and discriminative models have complementary strengths. Generative models can easily deal with variable length sequences and missing data, while also being easier to design and implement [7,8]. In contrast, discriminative models often achieve superior classification and generalisation performance [7,8]. An ideal recognition system would hence combine these two separate but complementary approaches.

The Fisher vector (FV) approach [7,9,10] allows for the fusion of both generative and discriminative models. In contrast to the popular Bag of Words (BoW) approach [11] which describes images by histograms of visual words, the FV approach describes images by deviations from a probabilistic visual vocabulary model. The resulting vectors can then be used by an SVM for final classification. Recently, FV has been successfully applied to the single-action recognition problem [12,13].

A reliable low-level feature descriptor is a crucial stage for the success of an action recognition system. One popular descriptor for action recognition is Spatio-Temporal Interest Points (STIPs) [14]. However, STIP based descriptors have several drawbacks [15,16]: they are computationally expensive, unstable, imprecise and can result in unnecessarily sparse detections. See Fig. 1 for a demonstration of STIP based detection. Other feature extraction techniques used for action recognition include gradients [6] and optical flow [16,17]. Each pixel in the gradient image helps extract relevant information, eg. edges (see Fig. 1). Since the task of action recognition is based on a sequence of frames, optical flow provides an efficient way of capturing the local dynamics [16].

Contributions. In this paper we propose a novel hierarchical system to perform multi-action segmentation and recognition. A given video is processed as a sequence of overlapping temporal windows. Each frame in a temporal window is represented through selective low-level spatio-temporal features, based on a combination of gradients with optical flow. Interesting features from each

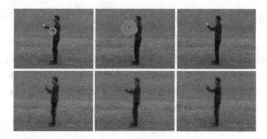

Fig. 1. Top row: feature extraction based on Spatio-Temporal Interest Points (STIPs) is often unstable, imprecise and overly sparse. Bottom row: interest pixels (marked in red) obtained using magnitude of gradient. (Color figure online)

temporal window are then pooled and processed to form a Fisher vector. Instead of directly classifying each Fisher vector, a multi-class SVM is employed to generate a vector of probabilities, with one probability per class. The final classification decision (action label) for each frame is then obtained by integrating the class probabilities at the frame level, which exploits the overlapping of the temporal windows. The proposed system hence combines the benefits of generative and discriminative models.

To the best of our knowledge, the combination of probabilistic integration with Fisher vectors is novel for the *multi-action* segmentation and recognition problem. In contrast to [2,4,5], the proposed system requires fewer parameters to be optimised. We also avoid the need for a custom dynamic programming definition as in [2,4]. Lastly, unlike the GMM approach proposed in [6] the proposed method requires only one GMM for all actions, making it considerably more efficient.

2   Proposed Method

The proposed system has a hierarchical nature, stemming from progressive reduction and transformation of information, starting at the pixel level. The system is comprised of four main components:

1. Division of a given video into overlapping multi-frame temporal windows, followed by extracting interesting low-level spatio-temporal features from each frame in each window.
2. Pooling of the interesting features from each temporal window to generate a sequence of Fisher vectors.
3. Conversion of each Fisher vector into a vector of class probabilities with the aid of a multi-class SVM.
4. Integration of the class probabilities at the frame level, leading to the final classification decision (action label) for each frame.

Each of the components is explained in more detail in the following subsections.

2.1   Overlapping and Selective Feature Extraction

A video $\mathcal{V} = (I_t)_{t=1}^T$ is an ordered set of T frames. We divide $\mathcal{V}$ into a set of overlapping temporal windows $(\mathcal{W}_s)_{s=1}^S$, with each window having a length of L frames. To achieve overlapping, the start of each window is one frame after the start of the preceding window. Each temporal window is hence defined as a set of frame identifiers: $\mathcal{W}_s = (t_{\text{start}}, \ldots, t_{\text{start}-1+L})$.

Each frame $I_t \in \mathbb{R}^{r \times c}$ can be represented by a set of feature vectors $F_t = \{f_p\}_{p=1}^{N_t}$ (with $N_t < r \cdot c$) corresponding to interesting pixels. Following [6], we first extract the following $D = 14$ dimensional feature vector for each pixel in a given frame t:

$$f = [\, x, \ y, \ g, \ o \,] \tag{1}$$

where x and y are the pixel coordinates, while g and o are defined as:

$$g = \left[\, |J_x|, \ |J_y|, \ |J_{yy}|, \ |J_{xx}|, \ \sqrt{J_x^2 + J_y^2}, \ \text{atan}\frac{|J_y|}{|J_x|} \,\right] \tag{2}$$

$$o = \left[\, u, \ v, \ \frac{\partial u}{\partial t}, \ \frac{\partial v}{\partial t}, \ \left(\frac{\partial u}{\partial x} + \frac{\partial v}{\partial y}\right), \ \left(\frac{\partial v}{\partial x} - \frac{\partial u}{\partial y}\right) \,\right] \tag{3}$$

The first four gradient-based features in Eq. (2) represent the first and second order intensity gradients at pixel location (x, y). The last two gradient features represent gradient magnitude and gradient orientation. The optical flow based features in Eq. (3) represent in order: the horizontal and vertical components of the flow vector, the first order derivatives with respect to time, the divergence and vorticity of optical flow [17].

Typically only a subset of the pixels in a frame correspond to the object of interest. As such, we are only interested in pixels with a gradient magnitude greater than a threshold τ [18]. We discard feature vectors from locations with a small magnitude. In other words, only feature vectors corresponding to interesting pixels are kept. This typically results in a variable number of feature vectors per frame. See the bottom part in Fig. 1 for an example of the retained pixels.

2.2   Representing Windows as Fisher Vectors

Given a set of feature vectors, the Fisher Vector approach encodes the deviations from a probabilistic visual dictionary, which is typically a diagonal GMM. The parameters of a GMM with K components can be expressed as $\{w_k, \mu_k, \sigma_k\}_{k=1}^K$, where, w_k is the weight, μ_k is the mean vector, and σ_k is the diagonal covariance matrix for the k-th Gaussian. The parameters are learned via the Expectation Maximisation algorithm [19] on training data.

For each temporal window $\mathcal{W}_s$, the feature vectors are pooled into set X containing $N = \sum_{t \in \mathcal{W}_s} N_t$ vectors. The deviations from the GMM are then accumulated via [10]:

$$\mathcal{G}_{\mu_k}^X = \frac{1}{N\sqrt{w_k}} \sum_{n=1}^N \gamma_n(k) \left(\frac{f_n - \mu_k}{\sigma_k}\right) \tag{4}$$

$$\mathcal{G}_{\sigma_k}^X = \frac{1}{N\sqrt{2w_k}} \sum_{n=1}^N \gamma_n(k) \left[\frac{(f_n - \mu_k)^2}{\sigma_k^2} - 1\right] \tag{5}$$

where vector division indicates element-wise division and $\gamma_n(k)$ is the posterior probability of f_n for the k-th component: $\gamma_n(k) = w_k \mathcal{N}(f_n|\mu_k, \sigma_k)/$ $\left(\sum_{i=1}^{K} w_i \mathcal{N}(f_n|\mu_i, \sigma_i)\right)$.

The Fisher vector for window $\mathcal{W}_s$ is represented as the concatenation of $\mathcal{G}_{\mu_k}^X$ and $\mathcal{G}_{\sigma_k}^X$ (for $k = 1, \ldots, K$) into vector $\boldsymbol{\Phi}_s$. As $\mathcal{G}_{\mu_k}^X$ and $\mathcal{G}_{\sigma_k}^X$ are D-dimensional, $\boldsymbol{\Phi}_s$ has the dimensionality of $2DK$. Note that we have omitted the deviations for the weights as they add little information [10].

2.3 Generation of Probability Vectors

For each Fisher vector we generate a vector of probabilities, with one probability per action class. First, a multi-class SVM [20] is used to predict class labels, outputting a set of raw scores. The scores are then transformed into a probability distribution over classes by applying Platt scaling [21]. The final probability vector derived from Fisher vector $\boldsymbol{\Phi}_s$ is expressed as:

$$q_s = [P(l = 1|\boldsymbol{\Phi}_s), \; \cdots, \; P(l = A|\boldsymbol{\Phi}_s)] \tag{6}$$

where l indicates an action class label and A is the number of action classes. The parameters for the multi-class SVM are learned using Fisher vectors obtained from pre-segmented actions in training data.

2.4 Integrating Probability Vectors to Label Frames

As the temporal windows are overlapping, each frame is present in several temporal windows. We exploit the overlapping to integrate the class probabilities at the frame level. The total contribution of the probability vectors to each frame t is calculated by:

$$Q_t = \sum_{s=1}^{S} \mathbf{1}_{\mathcal{W}_s}(t) \cdot q_s \tag{7}$$

where $\mathbf{1}_{\mathcal{W}_s}(t)$ is an indicator function, resulting in 1 if $t \in \mathcal{W}_s$, and 0 otherwise. The estimated action label for frame t is then calculated as:

$$\widehat{l}_t = \arg\max_{l=1,\ldots,A} Q_t^{[l]} \tag{8}$$

where $Q_t^{[l]}$ indicates the l-th element of Q_t.

3 Experiments

We evaluated our proposed method for joint action segmentation and recognition on two datasets: **(i)** a stitched version of the KTH dataset [22], and **(ii)** the challenging Carnegie Mellon University Multi-Modal Activity Dataset (CMU-MMAC) [23]. The results are reported in terms of frame-level accuracy as the ratio between the number of matched frames over the total number of frames.

The s-KTH (stitched KTH) dataset is obtained by simply concatenating existing single-action instances into sequences [5]. The KTH dataset contains 25 subjects performing 6 types of human actions and 4 scenarios. The scenarios vary from indoor, outdoor, scale variations, and different clothes. Each original video of the KTH dataset [22] contains an individual performing the same action. This action is performed four times and each subdivision or action-instance (in terms of start-frame and end-frame) is provided as part of the dataset. This dataset contains 2391 action-instances, with a length between 1 and 14 s [24]. The image size is 160×120 pixels, and temporal resolution is 25 frames per second.

The action-instances (each video contains four instances of the action) were picked randomly, alternating between the two groups of {boxing, hand-waving, hand-clapping} and {walking, jogging, running} to accentuate action boundaries. See Fig. 2 for an example. The dataset was divided into two sets as in [5,6]: one for training and one for testing. In total, 64 and 36 multi-action videos were used for training and testing, respectively. We used 3-fold cross-validation.

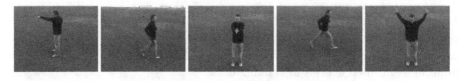

Fig. 2. Example of a multi-action sequence in the stitched version of the KTH dataset (s-KTH): boxing, jogging, hand clapping, running, hand waving and walking.

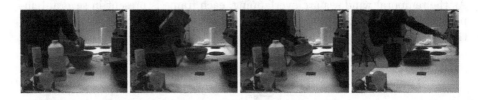

Fig. 3. Example of a challenging multi-action sequence in the CMU-MMAC kitchen dataset: crack, read, stir, and switch-on.

The CMU-MMAC dataset is considerably more challenging as it contains realistic multi-action videos [23]. A kitchen was built to record subjects preparing and cooking food according to five recipes. This dataset has occlusions, a cluttered background, and many distractors such as objects being deliberately moved. For our experiments we have used the same subset as per [5], which contains 12 subjects making brownies. The subjects were asked to make brownies in a natural way (no instructions were given). Each subject making the brownie is partially seen, as shown in Fig. 3.

The videos have a high resolution and are longer than in s-KTH. The image size is 1024×768 pixels, and temporal resolution is 30 frames per second. The average duration of a video is approximately 15,000 frames and the average length of an action instance is approximately 230 frames (7.7 s), with a minimum length of 3 frames (0.1 s) and a maximum length of 3,269 frames (108 s) [5]. The dataset was annotated using 14 labels, including the actions *close, crack, open, pour, put, read, spray, stir, switch-on, take, twist-off, twist-on, walk*, and the remaining actions (eg. frames in between two distinct actions) were grouped under the label *none* [25]. We used 12-fold cross-validation, using one subject for testing on a rotating basis.

All videos were converted into gray-scale. Additionally, the videos from the CMU-MMAC dataset were re-scaled to 128×96 to reduce computational requirements. Based on [6] and preliminary experiments on both datasets, we used $\tau = 40$, where τ is the threshold used for selection of interesting low-level feature vectors (Sect. 2.1). Although the interesting feature vectors are calculated in all frames, we only use the feature vectors extracted from every second frame in order to speed up processing.

Parameters for the visual vocabulary (GMM) were learned using a large set of descriptors obtained from training videos. Specifically, we randomly sampled 100,000 feature vectors for each action and then pooled all the resultant feature vectors from all actions for training. Experiments were performed with three separate GMMs with varying number of components: $K = \{64, 128, 256\}$. We have not evaluated larger values of K due to increased computational complexity and hence the exorbitant amount of time required to process the large CMU-MMAC dataset.

To learn the parameters of the multi-class SVM, we used video segments containing single actions. For s-KTH this process is straightforward as the videos have been previously segmented. The CMU-MMAC dataset contains continuous multi-actions. For this reason, to train our system we obtain one Fisher vector per action in each video, using the low-level feature vectors belonging to that specific action.

3.1 Effect of Window Length and Dictionary Size

We have evaluated the performance of two variants of the proposed system: **(1)** probabilistic integration with Fisher vectors (**PI-FV**), and **(2)** probabilistic integration with BoW histograms (**PI-BoW**), where the Fisher vector representation is replaced with BoW representation. We start our experiments by studying the influence of the segment length L, expressed in terms of seconds. The results are reported in Figs. 4 and 5, in terms of average accuracy over the folds.

Using the PI-FV variant (Fig. 4), we found that using $L = 1s$ and $K = 256$ leads to the best performance on the s-KTH dataset. For the CMU-MMAC dataset, the best performance is obtained with $L = 2.5\,s$ and $K = 64$. Note that using larger values of K (128 and 256) leads to worse performance. We attribute this to the large variability of appearance in the dataset, where the training data may not be a good representative of test data. As such, using a large value of K may lead to overfitting to the training data.

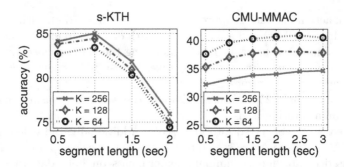

Fig. 4. Performance of the proposed **PI-FV** approach for varying the segment length on the s-KTH and CMU-MMAC datasets, in terms of average frame-level accuracy over the folds.

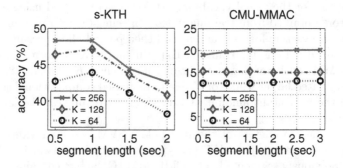

Fig. 5. As per Fig. 4, but showing the performance of the **PI-BoW** variant (where the Fisher vector representation is replaced with BoW representation).

The optimal segment length for each dataset is different. We attribute this to the s-KTH dataset containing short videos whose duration is between $1s$ and $7s$, while CMU-MMAC has a large range of action durations between $0.1s$ and $108s$. While the optimal values of L and K differ across the datasets, the results also show that relatively good overall performance across both datasets can be obtained with $L = 1s$ and $K = 64$.

The results for the PI-BoW variant are shown in Fig. 5. The best performance for the PI-BoW variant on the s-KTH dataset is obtained using $L = 1s$ and $K = 256$, while on the CMU-MMAC dataset it is obtained with $L = 2.5s$ and $K = 256$. These are the same values of L and K as for the PI-FV variant. However, the performance of the PI-BoW variant is consistently worse than the PI-FV variant on both datasets. This can be attributed to the better representation power of FV. Note that the visual dictionary size K for BoW is usually higher in order to achieve performance similar to FV. However, due to the large size of the CMU-MMAC dataset, and for direct comparison purposes, we have used the same range of K values throughout the experiments.

3.2   Confusion Matrices

Figures 6 and 7 show the confusion matrices for the PI-FV and PI-BoW variants on the CMU-MMAC dataset. The confusion matrices show that in 50 % of the cases (actions), the PI-BoW variant is unable to recognise the correct action. Furthermore, the PI-FV variant on average obtains better action segmentation than PI-BoW.

For five actions (*crack, open, read, spray, twist-on*), PI-FV has accuracies of 0.5 % or lower. Action *crack* implies crack and pour eggs into a bowl, but it's annotated only as *crack*, leading to confusion between *crack* and *pour*. We suspect that actions *read* and *spray* are poorly modelled due to lack of training data; they are performed by a reduced number of subjects. Action *twist-on* is confused with *twist-off* which are essentially the same action.

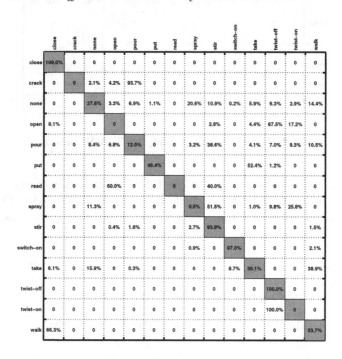

Fig. 6. Confusion matrix for the PI-FV variant on the CMU-MMAC dataset.

3.3   Comparison with GMM and HMM-MIO

We have compared the performance of the PI-FV and PI-BoW variants against the HMM-MIO [5] and stochastic modelling [6] approaches previously used for multi-action recognition. The comparative results are shown in Table 1.

The proposed PI-FV method obtains the highest accuracy of 85.0 % and 40.9 % for the s-KTH and CMU-MMAC datasets, respectively. In addition to higher accuracy, the proposed method has other advantages over previous techniques. There is just one global GMM (representing the visual vocabulary).

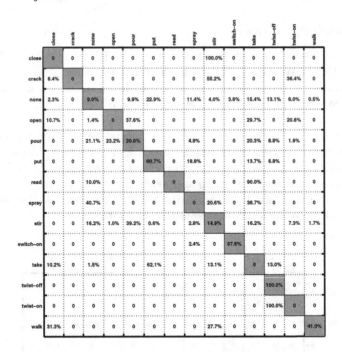

Fig. 7. As per Fig. 6, but using the PI-BoW variant.

This is in contrast to [6] which uses one GMM (with a large number of components) for each action, leading to high computational complexity. The HMM-MIO method in [5] requires the search for many optimal parameters, whereas the proposed method has just two parameters (L and K).

Table 1. Comparison of the proposed methods (PI-FV and PI-BoW) against several recent approaches on the stitched version of the KTH dataset (s-KTH) and the challenging CMU-MMAC dataset.

Method	s-KTH	CMU-MMAC
HMM-MIO [5]	71.2%	38.4%
Stochastic modelling [6]	78.3%	33.7%
PI-FV	**85.0%**	**40.9%**
PI-BoW	48.0%	20.1%

3.4 Wall-Clock Time

Lastly, we provide an analysis of the computational cost (in terms of wall-clock time) of our system and the stochastic modelling approach. The wall-clock time is measured under optimal configuration for each system, using a Linux machine with an Intel Core processor running at 2.83 GHz.

On the s-KTH dataset, the stochastic modelling system takes on average 228.4 min to segment and recognise a multi-action video. In comparison, the proposed system takes 5.6 min, which is approximately 40 times faster.

4 Conclusions and Future Work

In this paper we have proposed a hierarchical approach to multi-action recognition that performs joint segmentation and classification in videos. Videos are processed through overlapping temporal windows. Each frame in a temporal window is represented using selective low-level spatio-temporal features which efficiently capture relevant local dynamics and do not suffer from the instability and imprecision exhibited by STIP descriptors [14]. Features from each window are represented as a Fisher vector, which captures the first and second order statistics. Rather than directly classifying each Fisher vector, it is converted into a vector of class probabilities. The final classification decision for each frame (action label) is then obtained by integrating the class probabilities at the frame level, which exploits the overlapping of the temporal windows.

The proposed approach has a lower number of free parameters than previous methods which use dynamic programming or HMMs [5]. It is also considerably less computationally demanding compared to modelling each action directly with a GMM [6].

Experiments were done on two datasets: s-KTH (a stitched version of the KTH dataset to simulate multi-actions), and the more challenging CMU-MMAC dataset (containing realistic multi-action videos of food preparation). On s-KTH, the proposed approach achieves an accuracy of 85.0 %, considerably outperforming two recent approaches based on GMMs and HMMs which obtained 78.3 % and 71.2 %, respectively. On CMU-MMAC, the proposed approach achieves an accuracy of 40.9 %, outperforming the GMM and HMM approaches which obtained 33.7 % and 38.4 %, respectively. Furthermore, the proposed system is on average 40 times faster than the GMM based approach.

Possible future areas of exploration include the use of the fast Fisher vector variant proposed in [26], where for each sample the deviations for only one Gaussian are calculated. This can deliver a large speed up in computation, at the cost of a small drop in accuracy [27].

Acknowledgements. NICTA is funded by the Australian Government through the Department of Communications, as well as the Australian Research Council through the ICT Centre of Excellence program.

References

1. Buchsbaum, D., Canini, K.R., Griffiths, T.: Segmenting and recognizing human action using low-level video features. In: Annual Conference of the Cognitive Science Society (2011)

2. Hoai, M., Lan, Z.Z., De la Torre, F.: Joint segmentation and classification of human actions in video. In: IEEE Conference on Computer Vision and Pattern Recognition (CVPR), pp. 3265–3272 (2011)
3. Shi, Q., Wang, L., Cheng, L., Smola, A.: Discriminative human action segmentation and recognition using semi-Markov model. In: IEEE Conference on Computer Vision and Pattern Recognition (CVPR), pp. 1–8 (2008)
4. Cheng, Y., Fan, Q., Pankanti, S., Choudhary, A.: Temporal sequence modeling for video event detection. In: Conference on Computer Vision and Pattern Recognition (CVPR), pp. 2235–2242 (2014)
5. Borzeshi, E., Perez Concha, O., Xu, R., Piccardi, M.: Joint action segmentation and classification by an extended hidden Markov model. IEEE Sig. Process. Lett. **20**, 1207–1210 (2013)
6. Carvajal, J., Sanderson, C., McCool, C., Lovell, B.C.: Multi-action recognition via stochastic modelling of optical flow and gradients. In: Workshop on Machine Learning for Sensory Data Analysis (MLSDA), pp. 19–24. ACM (2014). http://dx.doi.org/10.1145/2689746.2689748
7. Jaakkola, T., Haussler, D.: Exploiting generative models in discriminative classifiers. Adv. Neural Inf. Process. Syst. **11**, 487–493 (1998)
8. Lasserre, J., Bishop, C.M.: Generative or discriminative? Getting the best of both worlds. In: Bernardo, J., Bayarri, M., Berger, J., Dawid, A., Heckerman, D., Smith, A., West, M. (eds.) Bayesian Statistics, vol. 8, pp. 3–24. Oxford University Press, Oxford (2007)
9. Csurka, G., Perronnin, F.: Fisher vectors: beyond bag-of-visual-words image representations. In: Richard, P., Braz, J. (eds.) VISIGRAPP 2010. CCIS, vol. 229, pp. 28–42. Springer, Heidelberg (2011)
10. Sánchez, J., Perronnin, F., Mensink, T., Verbeek, J.: Image classification with the Fisher vector: theory and practice. Int. J. Comput. Vis. **105**, 222–245 (2013)
11. Wang, H., Ullah, M.M., Klaser, A., Laptev, I., Schmid, C.: Evaluation of local spatio-temporal features for action recognition. Br. Mach. Vis. Conf. (BMVC) **124**(1–124), 11 (2009)
12. Oneata, D., Verbeek, J., Schmid, C.: Action and event recognition with Fisher vectors on a compact feature set. In: International Conference on Computer Vision (ICCV), pp. 1817–1824 (2013)
13. Wang, H., Schmid, C.: Action recognition with improved trajectories. In: International Conference on Computer Vision (ICCV) (2013)
14. Laptev, I.: On space-time interest points. Int. J. Comput. Vis. **64**, 107–123 (2005)
15. Cao, L., Tian, Y., Liu, Z., Yao, B., Zhang, Z., Huang, T.: Action detection using multiple spatial-temporal interest point features. In: International Conference on Multimedia and Expo (ICME), pp. 340–345 (2010)
16. Kliper-Gross, O., Gurovich, Y., Hassner, T., Wolf, L.: Motion interchange patterns for action recognition in unconstrained videos. In: Fitzgibbon, A., Lazebnik, S., Perona, P., Sato, Y., Schmid, C. (eds.) ECCV 2012, Part VI. LNCS, vol. 7577, pp. 256–269. Springer, Heidelberg (2012)
17. Ali, S., Shah, M.: Human action recognition in videos using kinematic features and multiple instance learning. IEEE Trans. Pattern Anal. Mach. Intell. **32**, 288–303 (2010)
18. Guo, K., Ishwar, P., Konrad, J.: Action recognition from video using feature covariance matrices. IEEE Trans. Image Process. **22**, 2479–2494 (2013)
19. Bishop, C.M.: Pattern Recognition and Machine Learning. Springer, New York (2006)

20. Crammer, K., Singer, Y.: On the algorithmic implementation of multiclass kernel-based vector machines. J. Mach. Learn. Res. **2**, 265–292 (2001)
21. Platt, J.C.: Probabilistic outputs for support vector machines and comparisons to regularized likelihood methods. Adv. Large Margin Classifiers **10**, 61–74 (1999)
22. Schuldt, C., Laptev, I., Caputo, B.: Recognizing human actions: a local SVM approach. Int. Conf. Pattern Recogn. (ICPR) **3**, 32–36 (2004)
23. De la Torre, F., Hodgins, J.K., Montano, J., Valcarcel, S.: Detailed human data acquisition of kitchen activities: the CMU-multimodal activity database (CMU-MMAC). In: CHI Workshop on Developing Shared Home Behavior Datasets to Advance HCI and Ubiquitous Computing Research (2009)
24. Baccouche, M., Mamalet, F., Wolf, C., Garcia, C., Baskurt, A.: Sequential deep learning for human action recognition. In: Salah, A.A., Lepri, B. (eds.) HBU 2011. LNCS, vol. 7065, pp. 29–39. Springer, Heidelberg (2011)
25. Spriggs, E.H., Torre, F.D.L., Hebert, M.: Temporal segmentation and activity classification from first-person sensing. In: IEEE Workshop on Egocentric Vision, CVPR (2009)
26. Simonyan, K., Vedaldi, A., Zisserman, A.: Deep Fisher networks for large-scale image classification. In: Burges, C., Bottou, L., Welling, M., Ghahramani, Z., Weinberger, K. (eds.) Advances in Neural Information Processing Systems, vol. 26, pp. 163–171 (2013)
27. Parkhi, O.M., Simonyan, K., Vedaldi, A., Zisserman, A.: A compact and discriminative face track descriptor. In: Conference on Computer Vision and Pattern Recognition (CVPR) (2014)

Learning Multi-faceted Activities from Heterogeneous Data with the Product Space Hierarchical Dirichlet Processes

Thanh-Binh Nguyen$^{(\boxtimes)}$, Vu Nguyen, Svetha Venkatesh, and Dinh Phung

Centre for Pattern Recognition and Data Analytics,
Deakin University, Geelong, Australia
thanhbi@deakin.edu.au

Abstract. Hierarchical Dirichlet processes (HDP) was originally designed and experimented for a single data channel. In this paper we enhanced its ability to model heterogeneous data using a richer structure for the base measure being a product-space. The enhanced model, called Product Space HDP (PS-HDP), can (1) simultaneously model heterogeneous data from multiple sources in a Bayesian nonparametric framework and (2) discover multilevel latent structures from data to result in different types of topics/latent structures that can be explained jointly. We experimented with the MDC dataset, a large and real-world data collected from mobile phones. Our goal was to discover *identity–location–time* (a.k.a *who-where-when*) patterns at different levels (globally for all groups and locally for each group). We provided analysis on the activities and patterns learned from our model, visualized, compared and contrasted with the ground-truth to demonstrate the merit of the proposed framework. We further quantitatively evaluated and reported its performance using standard metrics including F1-score, NMI, RI, and purity. We also compared the performance of the PS-HDP model with those of popular existing clustering methods (including K-Means, NNMF, GMM, DP-Means, and AP). Lastly, we demonstrate the ability of the model in learning activities with missing data, a common problem encountered in pervasive and ubiquitous computing applications.

1 Introduction

Big data is providing us with data not only large in the amount but also multiform: text, image, graphic, video, speech, and so forth. Besides, data are often disrupted, irregular and disparate, resulting in missing data which is difficult to deal with. For example, while a post on Facebook may have texts and emotion tags but not a photo, another post may have texts, a video, but without any emotion tag. This diversity, heterogeneity and incompleteness of data cause trouble to data scientists as machine learning methods are typically designed to work with only one data type and/or not designed to work with missing elements.

Usually, useful patterns in heterogeneous data, such as daily life activities from mobile data, are not appearing in form of raw data, but have to be learned

© Springer International Publishing Switzerland 2016
H. Cao et al. (Eds.): PAKDD 2016 Workshops, LNAI 9794, pp. 128–140, 2016.
DOI: 10.1007/978-3-319-42996-0_11

or inferred by exploiting the rich dependency between multiple channels of data. Extracting these hidden patterns has been challenging the data mining and machine learning fields for the last few decades – a field known as latent variable modelling.

A recent tremendously successful latent model is the Latent Dirichlet Allocation (LDA) [1] and its Bayesian nonparametric version, the Hierarchical Dirichlet Processes (HDP) [22]. These are Bayesian topic models, which extract the latent patterns in form of probability distributions. However, although the statistical foundation is generic, these models were originally developed to deal with a single data channel, often to model words in document corpus. In this paper, we extend the machinery of HDP to extract richer, high-order latent patterns from heterogeneous data through the use of a richer base measure distribution being the product-space. This method allows heterogeneous data from multiples sources can be exploited simultaneously and take their correlated information into account of the learning process. We term our model the Product Space HDP (PS-HDP) model. Although the model has all advantages of hierarchical nonparametric modeling which automatically discover the space of latent patterns and activities from the data, its major strength lies in the product-space approach which can deal with multiple heterogeneous data sources and with missing elements.

We experiment our proposed PS-HDP model on the Nokia Mobile Data Challenge (MDC) dataset [9] to discover interesting *identity–location–time* (a.k.a *who-where-when*) patterns, which are known to be useful for mobile context-aware applications [21], or for human dynamics understanding [18]. First, we extract only the Bluetooth and WiFi-related data along with their timestamps from the MDC dataset. After that, we feed these data into our PS-HDP model to discover *identity–location–time* patterns at multiple levels including (1) global level (i.e. patterns occur across all participants) and (2) local level (i.e. patterns occurs for a specific participant). Those patterns are then visualized and analyzed against the ground truth to show that the model can automatically discover interesting patterns from data. Next, we evaluate quantitatively the performance of the proposed model over the standard metrics including F1-score, normalized mutual information (NMI), rand index (RI) and purity. These metrics are then compared with those from popular clustering methods, including K-Means, Nonnegative Matrix Factorization (NNMF) [10], Gaussian Mixture Model (GMM) [13], DP-Means [8], and Affinity Propagation (AP) [6]. Finally, we demonstrate the ability of the PS-HDP model in dealing with missing data. The experimental results show that when more data is observed (i.e. less missing data), the F1-score and purity increase consistently.

In short, our main contributions in this paper include: (1) a novel Bayesian nonparametric model which can simultaneously model heterogeneous data from multiple sources to discover multilevel latent structures from data that can be explained jointly; (2) an application of learning hidden activities from heterogeneous data collected from multiple sensors, which is important in the area of pervasive and ubiquitous computing, using the proposed model on MDC dataset, a large and real world dataset collected from mobile phones.

2 Related Works

2.1 Pattern Discovery from Heterogeneous Data

Discovery of hidden patterns from heterogeneous data has been a challenge in machine learning and data mining. As machine learning algorithms are typically designed to work with only one specific data type (e.g. continuous, discrete), most of the previous works treat each data channel separately. For example, in the combined mining method [2], K different miners has been applied on K data sources to get K corresponding sets of patterns. After that, a merger is used to combine these sets to get global patterns (i.e. patterns from all data sources). Unfortunately, this approach is usually time-consuming, and more importantly, unable to exploit the correlating information between these data sources during the learning process to create better patterns.

Recently, researchers have been trying to leverage the advances of Bayesian nonparametric approach to propose unifying models to learn and discover patterns from multiple data sources. One common strategy is to model one data source as the primary data (called *content*), while treating other data sources as secondary data (called *contexts*). Contexts are viewed as distributions over some index space and both contents and contexts are modelled jointly. For example, Phung et al. [19] proposed an integration of the HDP and the nested Dirichlet process (nDP) with shared mixture components to jointly model contexts and contents respectively, where mixture components could be integrated out under a suitable parameterization. The authors showed that their model achieved good results in the field of computer vision. In another topic modelling work, Nguyen et al. [16] used documents as primary data, and used other information (e.g. time, authors) as contexts. In this model, secondary data channels should be collected in group-level, called group-level contexts [17]. More recently, Huynh et al. [7] have developed a full Bayesian nonparametric approach to model correlation structures among multiple and heterogeneous data sources. Choosing a data source as the primary data (*content*), they induce a mixture distribution over the data using HDP. Other data sources, also generated from HDP, are treated as *context(s)* and are assumed to be mutually independent given the *content*. However, in some applications, choosing one data source to be the primary data is not an easy task. To our best knowledge, this work is the most similar to our work. However, our approach differs from this one as it treats all data channels equally and hence does not require to specify *contexts* and *content*.

2.2 Discovery of Interaction and Mobility Patterns from Bluetooth and WiFi Data

Bluetooth data is widely used in the proximity detection problems. In particular, mobile Bluetooth data is usually used to detect surrounding people to discover interaction patterns of a person. Do and Gatica-Perez [3] used a large daily life Bluetooth data captured by smartphones to create a dynamic social network. Then, by using their proposed probabilistic model, they discovered different social contexts (such as group meeting or dinner with family) and interaction types (e.g. office interaction, personal interaction). In another approach,

Nguyen et al. [14] used HDP to discover interaction types from Bluetooth data from honest social signals captured by sociometric badges. Then, they clustered mixtures proportions from HDP using Affinity Propagation algorithm to extract contexts and communities.

While Bluetooth data is useful for discover surrounding people, WiFi data is usually used to infer locations. A smartphone is able to scan for surrounding WiFi hotspots. Each WiFi hotspot has a unique identified fingerprint (i.e. its MAC address). Assuming that the location of a WiFi hotspot is never changed, one can use its fingerprint as an indicator of the location where a person is at. From the raw WiFi scans, different approaches are used to discover locations. Dousse et al. [4] used the OPTICS clustering to group similar scans to a cluster representing a place. However, using OPTICS algorithm, the number of clusters must be provided beforehand. Nguyen et al. [15], in contrast, using the AP algorithm to discover interesting locations without the need of specifying the number of clusters. Furthermore, from interesting locations, they can also learn daily routines and mobility patterns of mobile phone users.

3   Framework

3.1   Hierarchical Dirichlet Processes (HDP)

Let J be the number of groups and $\{x_{j1}, \ldots, x_{jN_j}\}$ be N_j observations associated with group j which are assumed to be exchangeable within the group. Under HDP framework, each group j is endowed with a random group-specific mixture distribution G_j which is statistically connected with other mixture distributions via another Dirichlet Process (DP) sharing the same base probability measure G_0:

$$G_j \mid \alpha, G_0 \stackrel{\text{iid}}{\sim} \text{DP}\,(\alpha, G_0) \qquad (j = 1, \ldots, J) \qquad (1)$$

$$G_0 \mid \gamma, H \sim \text{DP}\,(\gamma, H)\,. \qquad (2)$$

This generative process further indicates that G_j (s) are exchangeable at the group level and conditionally independent given the base measure G_0, which is also a random probability measure distributed according to another DP.

It is clear from the definition of the HDP that G_j's, G_0 and H share the same support Θ. Then the local atoms in group j is draw as $\theta_{ji} \stackrel{\text{iid}}{\sim} G_j$ and the observation is generated following $x_{ji} \sim F\,(\theta_{ji})$.

We present the stick-breaking representation of HDP for posterior inference which can be summarized following. We draw a global mixing weight $\beta \sim \text{GEM}(\gamma)$, then generate the topics $\phi_k \stackrel{\text{iid}}{\sim} H(\lambda)$. The global atom G_0 in Eq. 2 can be characterized as $G_0 = \sum_{k=1}^{\infty} \delta_{\phi_k} \times \beta_m$. We next sample the mixing proportion for each document j such that $\pi_j \stackrel{\text{iid}}{\sim} \text{DP}\,(\alpha\beta)$. The local atom in each document is represented as $G_j = \sum_{k=1}^{\infty} \pi_{j,k} \times \delta_{\phi_k}$. Finally, we draw the latent assignment $z_{ji} \stackrel{\text{iid}}{\sim} \text{Mult}(\pi_j)$ and observation $x_{ji} \stackrel{\text{iid}}{\sim} F(\phi_{z_{ji}})$ accordingly.

HDP is originally applied for nonparametric text modelling, but it is also applied in the field of natural language processing to detect how many grammar symbols exist in a particular set of sentences [11]. Another extension of HDP as Dynamic HDP [20] is for modelling time series documents. Evolutionary HDP (EvoHDP) [23] is for multiple correlated time-varying corpora by adding time dependencies to the adjacent epochs. In EvoHDP, each HDP is built for multiple corpora at each time epoch, and the time dependencies are incorporated into adjacent epochs under the Markovian assumption. Specifically, the dependency is formulated by mixing two distinct Dirichlet processes (DPs) (one is the DP model for the previous epoch, and the other is an updating DP model). The model inference is implemented by a cascaded Gibbs sampling scheme.

3.2   Product-Space HDP (PS-HDP)

HDP is a powerful topic model to learn latent topics and patterns; however, although the statistical background is generic, it was originally designed and experimented for a single data channel. The Product Space HDP (PS-HDP) is an extension of the HDP model using a richer structure for the base measure being a product-space. It can be described as follow. The data consist of J groups, each of which contain N_j data points. Each data point i (in group j) is a collection of observations, denoted as $\{x_{ji}^1, x_{ji}^2, ..., x_{ji}^C\}$ from C data sources which can be heterogeneous. To have matters concrete, we assume a group is a user and a data point is an interaction between users. Each interaction includes three channels of information such that x_{ji}^1 is a timestamp (Gaussian distribution), x_{ji}^2 and x_{ji}^3 are a Bluetooth and a WiFi signal respectively (Multinomial distribution).

Stochastic Representation. Let $H_1, H_2, ..., H_C$ be the base measure (for each data sources) generating the global atom G_0 from Dirichlet Process with concentration parameter γ as $G_0 = \langle G_0^1 G_0^2 ... G_0^C \rangle \sim \mathrm{DP}\,(\gamma, H_1 \times H_2 \times ... H_C)$ where $H_1 \times H_2 \times ... H_C$ is the product of base measure. Then, each group j will have a local atom G_j drawn from DP with the concentration parameter α and the global atom G_0 as $G_j = \langle G_j^1 G_j^2 ... G_j^C \rangle \sim \mathrm{DP}\,(\alpha, G_0)$. In other words, each random group-specific mixture distribution G_j sharing the same base probability measure G_0. Next, the atom for each data point i in group j at channel c is iid drawn as $\theta_{ji}^c \overset{\text{iid}}{\sim} G_j^c$ and the observation is generated subsequently $x_{ji}^c \sim F^c\left(\theta_{ji}^c\right)$.

Stick-Breaking Representation. For posterior inference, we characterize the above stochastic view using stick-breaking representation. We draw the global weight $\beta \sim \mathrm{GEM}\,(\gamma)$ and the topics (or patterns) $\phi_k^c \overset{\text{iid}}{\sim} H_c, \forall k = 1, ..., \infty, \forall c = 1...C$ such that the global atom $G_0 = \sum_{k=1}^{\infty} \beta_k \delta_{\langle \phi_k^1, ..., \phi_k^C \rangle}$. For each group j, the local weight $\pi_j \overset{\text{iid}}{\sim} \mathrm{DP}\,(\alpha, \beta)$ such that $G_j = \sum_{k=1}^{\infty} \pi_{jk} \delta_{\langle \phi_k^1, ..., \phi_k^C \rangle}$. Then, the data point label $z_{ji} \sim \mathrm{Mult}\,(\pi_j)$. Finally, the observation is generated using the corresponding topic $\phi_{z_{ji}}^c$ as $x_{ji}^c \sim F^c\left(\phi_{z_{ji}}^c\right)$, $\forall j = 1, 2..., J$, $\forall i = 1..N_j$, $\forall c = 1...C$. Figure 1 shows the graphical models of the PS-HDP from the stochastic view and the stick-breaking view.

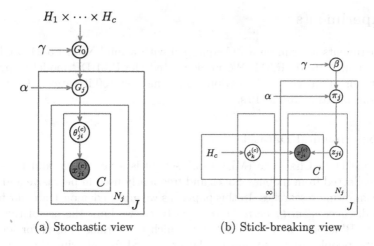

Fig. 1. The stochastic view and stick-breaking view of the Product Space HDP.

Posterior Inference. Our framework is a Bayesian model. For posterior inference, we utilize collapsed Gibbs sampling [12]. To integrate out π_j and ϕ_k due to conjugacy property, the two latent variables z_{ji} and β need to be sampled.

Sampling z_{ji}. We assign a data point x_{ji} to its component ϕ_k. The conditional distribution for z_{ji} is influenced by a collection of words associated with topic k across documents:

$$p\left(z_{ji} = k \mid \boldsymbol{x}, \boldsymbol{z}_{-ji}, \alpha, \beta, H\right) = p\left(z_{ji} = k \mid \boldsymbol{z}_{-j}, \alpha, \beta\right) \times$$
$$p\left(x_{ji} \mid z_{ji} = k, \{x_{j'i'} \mid z_{j'i'} = k, \forall (j'i' \neq ji)\}, H\right)$$
$$= \begin{cases} \left(n_{jk}^{-ji} + \alpha\beta_k\right) \times f_k^{-x_{ji}}\left(x_{ji}\right) & \text{used } k \\ \alpha \times \beta_{\text{new}} \times f_{k^{\text{new}}}^{-x_{ji}}\left(x_{ji}\right) & \text{new } k. \end{cases}$$

The first term is recognized as the Chinese Restaurant Franchise (number of data points in group j follows topic k) while the second term is the predictive likelihood $f_k^{-x_{ji}}\left(x_{ji}\right)$.

Sampling β. We sample the global mixing weight follow the approach presented in [22] that we sample β jointly with the auxiliary variable $\boldsymbol{m}$ $(0 \leq m \leq n_{jk})$:

$$p\left(m_{jk} = m \mid \boldsymbol{z}, \boldsymbol{m}_{-jk}, \beta\right) \propto \text{Stirl}\left(n_{ij}, m_{jk}\right)\left(\alpha\beta_k\right)^m$$
$$p\left(\boldsymbol{\beta} \mid \boldsymbol{m}, \boldsymbol{z}, \alpha, \gamma\right) \propto \beta_{\text{new}}^{\gamma-1} \prod_{k=1}^{K} \beta_k^{\sum_j m_{jk}-1}$$

Sampling Hyperparameters α and γ. To make the model robust in identifying the unknown number of clusters, we resample hyperparameters in each Gibbs iteration. The lower concentration parameter α is described in [22]. The upper concentration parameter γ is followed the techniques of [5].

4 Experiments

Our experiments are run on a PC equipped with a Intel Xeon E5-2460 CPU (8 cores, 2.6 Ghz), 16 GB RAM. We implemented the PS-HDP model using C#. For posterior inference, we do a Gibbs sampling over 500 iterations. In average, each iteration costs around 19 s.

4.1 Experimental Dataset

The Mobile Data Challenge (MDC) dataset [9] is a very large and real-world dataset collected from mobile phones and frequently used in pervasive and ubiquitous computing researches. In this paper, as we aim to demonstrate our framework to discover *identity–location–time* patterns, we limit the use of the MDC dataset to Bluetooth and WiFi data, in which the former is used for identifying nearby people (*identity*) and the latter is used for inferring the significant locations of users (*location*). All data have also associated with timestamps that can be used to infer the change of patterns over *time*. The dataset also includes information about places where a user stayed at least 20 min, which can be used to extract the location ground-truth of each Bluetooth/WiFi scan, and the IMEI number of the phones, which are used to extract the identity ground-truth. The data were extracted as described below.

Bluetooth Data. For the convenience of the evaluation step, we keep only scans that include at least one identifiable device from the ground truth. Thus, only scans that capture one (or more) of participants' phones are retained.

WiFi Data. For WiFi data, we eliminate access points that has been scanned less than 10 times as they are not statistically meaningful and do not affect the location discovery. Empty scans after this elimination are also removed.

Matching Bluetooth and WiFi Scans. The Bluetooth and WiFi scans have sometimes different timestamps due to the design of the data collecting application. In our experiments, a Bluetooth and a WiFi scan is considered to be from the same scan if they have exactly the same timestamp.

Timestamp Data. As we aim to discover context patterns during a day, we only use the hour, minute and second information of timestamps. We also convert them to a real number of hour (e.g. 10 h and 30 min to 10.5 h).

The MDC dataset has millions of scans. As we aim to demonstrate the ability to deal with multiple sources of the PS-HDP model, we want to keep the experimental dataset in an appropriate size. Thus, we select a month (Feb 2011 in our experiments), and then extract all scans in this month. Moreover, the MDC dataset is imbalanced as some users have much higher number of scans than others. To keep it balanced, we randomly choose at most 200 scans for each user. The final dataset includes 98 users with 16,950 scans (data points) in total, including 107 unique Bluetooth IDs and 1385 unique WiFi hotspot IDs.

4.2 Discovery of Joint *Identity–Location–Time* Patterns with Complete Data

We feed the extracted experimental dataset in Sect. 4.1 to our PS-HDP model, where the Bluetooth and WiFi data are modelled by multinomial distributions, whilst the Time data is modelled by a Gaussian distribution. At the end, there were totally 46 patterns (clusters) discovered. Each pattern has information of the time (represented by a mean and a variance) at which the pattern occurs; the probability of each Bluetooth ID presenting in the pattern; and the probability of each WiFi hotspot presenting in the pattern.

We display each pattern by three plots. The top plot displays the mean and the variance of the time. The middle plot display the top ten Bluetooth IDs. The bottom plot display the place ID at which the top 10 WiFi hotspot IDs are located. Both Bluetooth ID and place ID are displayed using tag cloud technique, where the size of each number reflects the contribution of the corresponding ID to the cluster. As a result, there could be some IDs with very small probability cannot be seen on the plot. This situation occurs frequently for the Bluetooth IDs. Figure 2 shows an example pattern, where users who are corresponding to Bluetooth ID 24, 77, 22, 78, 84, and 94 often meet each other around 19:00 at a location where the WiFi hotspot is located.

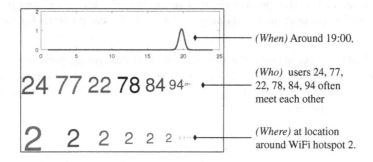

Fig. 2. Representation of *Who-When-Where* pattern.

Among 46 discovered patterns, we can find some interesting ones. For example, Fig. 3 shows two patterns 23 and 25 in which the Bluetooth ID 48 and 30 (which are corresponding to two specific participants) are usually co-exist at the place ID number 1, but at different time. The pattern 23 shows that they are usually at the place ID 1 at around 4:00, whereas the pattern 25 shows that they also meet each other at the same place at around 21:00. Furthermore, we can see that at 4:00 the person corresponding to the Bluetooth ID 48 (person 48) is more likely at the place ID 1 than the person corresponding to the Bluetooth ID 30 (person 30). The situation change at 21:00, where the person 30 presents at the place ID 1 more frequent than the person 48. These two patterns would not be discovered if one treat each data channel (i.e. Bluetooth and WiFi) independently. It shows the advantage of our model over traditional approaches.

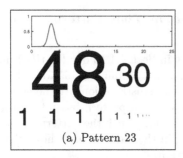

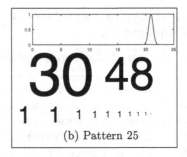

Fig. 3. Two patterns with the same Bluetooth IDs and place, but different time.

4.3 Multilevel Pattern Analysis

We further analyze multilevel patterns at global (for all participants) and local (for each participant) levels. We aim to discover which patterns are regular for all users (e.g., what users often interact with each other, where the locations are, and when they meet). Similarly, we learn the local regular pattern for individuals (e.g., who are this user often interacting with, at what locations, and when). We will ask similar questions for infrequent patterns at multilevel. To answer these questions, we utilize the global weight β to analyze the level of global patterns and the mixing proportion π_j to analyze the level of local patterns for user j.

Global Pattern Analysis. We rely on β to find interesting patterns globally. Figure 5 shows the pattern that has the largest β_k value (pattern number 6) and the pattern that has a smallest β_k value (pattern number 12), as well as the β_k values of all 46 patterns.

Local Pattern Analysis. After running the PS-HDP model, we got a mixing proportion vector for each participant and cluster assignment for each data point. Using these information, we can rebuild patterns for each participant using only data points scanned by his phone. To help finding interesting patterns for each participant, we built a small application which let user choose a user (represented by a Bluetooth ID) and the application visualizes the two most interesting patterns (i.e. one has the largest and one has the smallest π_{ji} value) inferred from the data of that participant. Figure 4 shows the 2 most interesting patterns for the user corresponding to the Bluetooth ID 77.

Furthermore, we compute a similarity matrix between 98 users using the Euclidian distance of user's mixture proportions. After that, we feed this similarity matrix into the Affinity Propagation clustering algorithm [6] to automatically group users together. We also compute the linear correlation coefficients from the users' mixture proportions as shown in the Fig. 6. We can see that users with similar correlation coefficients have been grouped together, showing that the mixture proportions produced by our PS-HDP model are meaningful.

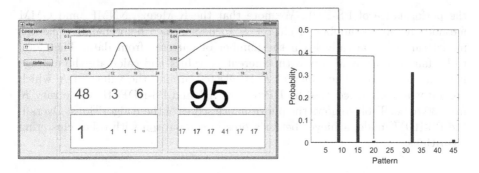

Fig. 4. Local patterns corresponding to the largest *(left)* and the smallest *(right)* π_{ji} values of the participant 77.

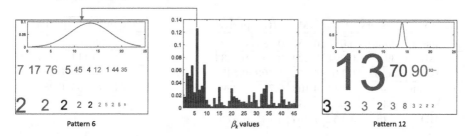

Fig. 5. Global patterns. *Left* and *Right*: the pattern corresponding to the largest and smallest β_k values respectively. *Middle*: β_k values of all patterns.

4.4   Evaluation of Performance

After running the PS-HDP model, each data point will be assigned to a cluster through the indicator z_{ji}. Besides that, from the ground truth, the location of each data point could be known. We rely on this information to evaluate the clustering performance of our approach. To get the baselines, we run some quantitative clustering algorithms including K-Means, Non-negative Matrix Factorization (NNMF), Gaussian Mixture Model (GMM), DP-Means, and Affinity Propagation (AP) on the same dataset and use their performance results to compare with

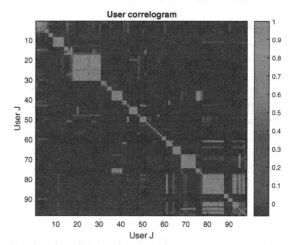

Fig. 6. Correlogram of users' mixture proportions.

the performance of PS-HDP. We note that the K-Means, NNMF, and GMM methods require a number of cluster K to be specified beforehand, while our model can automatically learn the number of patterns from data. Therefore, to be fair, we run K-Means with different K values and calculate the average performance scores. The range of K is selected around the values of K which are automatically discovered by DP-means, AP, and PS-HDP. Here, we vary K from 30 to 60. Table 1 shows the performance scores of these algorithms. Overall, the PS-HDM model achieves better scores in comparison with other clustering algorithms.

Table 1. Performance of different clustering algorithms on the MDC dataset (note that F1-scores are usually low on pervasive data).

Algo.	Clusters	F1	NMI	RI	purity
K-Means	30-60	0.081	0.155	0.780	0.439
NNMF	30-60	0.094	0.320	0.790	0.543
GMM	30-60	0.116	0.345	**0.793**	0.545
DP-Means	48	0.122	0.103	0.757	0.399
AP	37	0.069	0.143	0.785	0.417
PS-HDP	46	**0.154**	**0.367**	0.781	**0.573**

Table 2. F1-score and purity w.r.t. different amount of missing data.

Amount	F1	purity
70%	0.109	0.253
50%	0.114	0.259
30%	0.134	0.288
10%	0.155	0.289

4.5 Discovery of Joint *Identity–Location–Time* Patterns with Missing Data

To demonstrate the pattern discovery ability of our framework on data with missing values, we create 4 settings with different amount of missing data. More specifically, from the complete dataset in Sect. 4.1, we randomly choose m data points (with m repeatedly set to 70%, 50%, 30% and 10% of total data points) and set their Bluetooth data as missing values. Each of these generated datasets is then inputted to the PS-HDP model and performance metrics are calculated (similar to the complete data settings). The experimental results show that F1-score and the purity increase when less missing data occurs (as shown in Table 2). In other words, the more data is observed, the better patterns are. It means that the PS-HDP model can deal well with data even if they have missing values.

5   Conclusion

We presented a full Bayesian nonparametric model, called the Product Space HDP, which is extended from the HDP model by using a richer structure for the base measure being a product-space. Its major strengths and advantages firstly inherited from the Bayesian nonparametric approach including the ability to automatically grow the model complexity, hence does not require to know number of clusters beforehand; and secondly lie in the product-space approach which can deal with multiple heterogeneous data sources and with missing elements. The difference of our approach over existing ones is that it treats data from all sources equally, therefore does not require to specify the *content* and *contexts* channels. We apply the proposed model to one of the most fundamental problems in pervasive and ubiquitous computing: learning hidden activities from heterogeneous data collected from multiple sensors. Experimental results showed advantages of the PS-HDP model, including the ability of learning complex hidden patterns with good performance over popular existing clustering methods.

References

1. Blei, D., Ng, A., Jordan, M.: Latent Dirichlet allocation. J. Mach. Learn. Res. **3**, 993–1022 (2003)
2. Cao, L., Zhang, H., Zhao, Y., Luo, D., Zhang, C.: Combined mining: discovering informative knowledge in complex data. Trans. SMC **41**(3), 699–712 (2011)
3. Do, T.M.T., Gatica-Perez, D.: Human interaction discovery in smartphone proximity networks. Pers. Ubiquit. Comput. **17**(3), 413–431 (2013)
4. Dousse, O., Eberle, J., Mertens, M.: Place learning via direct wifi fingerprint clustering. In: Mobile Data Management (MDM), pp. 282–287. IEEE (2012)
5. Escobar, M., West, M.: Bayesian density estimation and inference using mixtures. J. Am. Stat. Assoc. **90**(430), 577–588 (1995)
6. Frey, B.J., Dueck, D.: Clustering by passing messages between data points. Science **315**(5814), 972–976 (2007). http://www.sciencemag.org/content/315/5814/972
7. Huynh, V., Phung, D., Nguyen, L., Venkatesh, S., Bui, H.H.: Learning conditional latent structures from multiple data sources. In: Cao, T., Lim, E.-P., Zhou, Z.-H., Ho, T.-B., Cheung, D., Motoda, H. (eds.) PAKDD 2015. LNCS, vol. 9077, pp. 343–354. Springer, Heidelberg (2015)
8. Kulis, B., Jordan, M.I.: Revisiting k-means: new algorithms via bayesian nonparametrics. In: Proceedings of the ICML (2012)
9. Laurila, J.K., Gatica-Perez, D., Aad, I., Bornet, O., Do, T.M.T., Dousse, O., Eberle, J., Miettinen, M., et al.: The mobile data challenge: big data for mobile computing research. In: Pervasive Computing (2012)
10. Lee, D.D., Seung, H., et al.: Learning the parts of objects by non-negative matrix factorization. Nature **401**(6755), 788–791 (1999)
11. Liang, P., Petrov, S., Jordan, M.I., Klein, D.: The infinite PCFG using hierarchical dirichlet processes. In: EMNLP 2007, pp. 688–697 (2007)
12. Liu, J.: The collapsed Gibbs sampler in Bayesian computations with applications to a gene regulation problem. Am. Stat. Assoc. **89**, 958–966 (1994)
13. McLachlan, G., Peel, D.: Finite Mixture Models. Wiley, New York (2004)
14. Nguyen, T.C., Phung, D., Gupta, S., Venkatesh, S.: Extraction of latent patterns and contexts from social honest signals using hierarchical Dirichlet processes. In: PERCOM, pp. 47–55 (2013)
15. Nguyen, T.B., Nguyen, T.C., Luo, W., Venkatesh, S., Phung, D.: Unsupervised inference of significant locations from wifi data for understanding human dynamics. In: Proceedings of MUM 2014, pp. 232–235 (2014)

16. Nguyen, T., Phung, D., Venkatesh, S., Nguyen, X., Bui, H.: Bayesian nonparametric multilevel clustering with group-level contexts. In: ICML, pp. 288–296 (2014)
17. Nguyen, V., Phung, D., Venkatesh, S., Bui, H.H.: A Bayesian nonparametric approach to multilevel regression. In: Cao, T., Lim, E.-P., Zhou, Z.-H., Ho, T.-B., Cheung, D., Motoda, H. (eds.) PAKDD 2015. LNCS, vol. 9077, pp. 330–342. Springer, Heidelberg (2015)
18. Pentland, A.: Automatic mapping and modeling of human networks. Phys. A: Stat. Mech. Appl. **378**(1), 59–67 (2007)
19. Phung, D., Nguyen, X., Bui, H., Nguyen, T., Venkatesh, S.: Conditionally dependent Dirichlet processes for modelling naturally correlated data sources. Technical report, Pattern Recognition and Data Analytics, Deakin University (2012)
20. Ren, L., Dunson, D.B., Carin, L.: The dynamic hierarchical Dirichlet process. In: Proceedings of the 25th ICML 2008, pp. 824–831. ACM, New York (2008)
21. Schilit, B.N., Theimer, M.M.: Disseminating active map information to mobile hosts. IEEE Netw. **8**(5), 22–32 (1994)
22. Teh, Y., Jordan, M., Beal, M., Blei, D.: Hierarchical Dirichlet processes. J. Am. Stat. Assoc. **101**(476), 1566–1581 (2006)
23. Zhang, J., Song, Y., Zhang, C., Liu, S.: Evolutionary hierarchical dirichlet processes for multiple correlated time-varying corpora. In: SIGKDD, pp. 1079–1088 (2010)

Phishing Detection on Twitter Streams

Se Yeong Jeong, Yun Sing Koh$^{(\boxtimes)}$, and Gillian Dobbie

Department of Computer Science, The University of Auckland,
Auckland, New Zealand
sjeo017@aucklanduni.ac.nz,{ykoh,gill}@cs.auckland.ac.nz

Abstract. With the prevalence of cutting-edge technology, the social media network is gaining popularity and is becoming a worldwide phenomenon. Twitter is one of the most widely used social media sites, with over 500 million users all around the world. Along with its rapidly growing number of users, it has also attracted unwanted users such as scammers, spammers and phishers. Research has already been conducted to prevent such issues using network or contextual features with supervised learning. However, these methods are not robust to changes, such as temporal changes or changes in phishing trends. Current techniques also use additional network information. However, these techniques cannot be used before spammers form a particular number of user relationships. We propose an unsupervised technique that detects phishing in Twitter using a 2-phase unsupervised learning algorithm called PDT (Phishing Detector for Twitter). From the experiments we show that our technique has high accuracy ranging between 0.88 and 0.99.

Keywords: Phishing Detector · Twitter stream · DBSCAN

1 Introduction

As the user base of Twitter steadily grows into the millions, real time search systems and different types of mining tools are emerging to enable people to track events and news on Twitter. These services are appealing mechanisms to ease the spread of news and allow users to discuss events and post their status, but opens up opportunities for new forms of spam and cybercrime. Twitter has become a target for spammers to disseminate their target messages. Spammers post tweets containing typical words of a trending topic and URLs, usually obfuscated by URL shorteners that lead users to completely unrelated websites.

Phishing is the fraudulent attempt to obtain sensitive information such as usernames, passwords, personal details and banking details often for malicious reasons under the disguise of a trustworthy entity in an electronic community. Traditionally, phishing emails contain links that take advantage of a user's trust. Phishing sites are usually almost identical imitations of genuine ones, taking advantage of average users to obtain private information, generally financial details. With an increased popularity in social media networks, links to phishing sites are commonly found on these platforms. These links are often masked in

© Springer International Publishing Switzerland 2016
H. Cao et al. (Eds.): PAKDD 2016 Workshops, LNAI 9794, pp. 141–153, 2016.
DOI: 10.1007/978-3-319-42996-0_12

shortened URLs to hide true URLs. This category of spam can jeopardise and de-value real time search services unless an efficient and accurate automated mechanism to detect phishers is found.

Although the research community and industry have been developing techniques to identify phishing attacks through other media [6,8–10] such as email and instant messaging, there is very little research that provides a deeper understanding of phishing in online social media. Moreover these phishers are sophisticated and adaptable to game the system with fast evolving content and network patterns. Phishers continually change their phishing behaviour patterns to avoid being detected. It is challenging for existing anti-phishing systems to quickly respond to newly emerging patterns for effective phishing detection. Moreover relying on the network connection information means that the phishers would have to have been active over a period to build up the connections. A good anti-phishing detection algorithm should be able to detect phishing as efficiently and early as possible.

We proposed a two phase approach called Phishing Detector for Twitter (PDT), that combines a density based clustering algorithm, DBSCAN, with DerTIA algorithm used in detecting attacks on recommender systems. We adapted both these approaches to detect phishing on Twitter. The main contributions of this paper are outlined as follows: (1) Introduced a phishing detection algorithm, PDT, an unsupervised learning approach, which does not rely on social influence (social network connections); (2) Described a systematic feature selection and analysis process.

The remainder of this paper is structured as follows. Section 2 discusses various methods researchers have designed to confront this problem of detecting phishing or spam in Twitter and other media. Then in Sect. 3, we review the outline of our technique. Section 4 details the data collection methodology of our research. Section 5 discusses selected features, performs analysis on features from collected samples. Section 3 details our unsupervised technique to detect phishing in Twitter. In Sect. 7, we review experimental setups and results on several data sets. Lastly, Sect. 8 concludes the paper.

2   Related Work

Phishing has been found in various traditional web applications such as emails, websites, blogs, forums and social media networks. Numerous preventative methods have been developed to fight against phishing.

List-Based Techniques. The list-based anti-phishing mechanism is a technique commonly used at low cost. Its strength comes from speed and simplicity. Classifying requires a simple lookup on the maintained database. Blacklists [14] are built into modern web browsers. A major drawback of the list-based mechanisms is that the accuracy is highly dependent on the completeness of the list. It takes time and effort to maintain the lists. Google uses automated proprietary algorithms to maintain a list of fraud websites whereas PhishTank [1] relies on contributions from online communities.

Machine Learning Based Techniques. With increases in computing power, phishing detections involving machine learning has emerged [2]. These approaches utilise one or more characteristics found on a site and build rules to detect phishing. Pre-labelled samples have a pivotal role in buiding a classifier. Garera *et al.* [9] proposed a technique that uses structure of URL in conjunction with logistic regression classification and Google PageRank in order to determine if a URL is legitimate or phishing.

The following two techniques employ a visual cue in detection. GoldPhish by Dunlop *et al.* [7] implements an unusual classification approach that takes a screenshot of a target website and comparies it with a genuine one to find any discrete differences. In addition to the visual comparison, the classifier considers the extracted text from optical character recognition on the screenshot in the judgement. Zhang *et al.* [18] handled visual content differently. The system first takes a screenshot of the page in question and generates a unique signature from the captured image then the image is labelled by Visual Similarity Assessment (Earth Mover's Distance). At the same time, the system extracts textual information from processed content. The textual features are then classified using Naïve Bayes' Rule and combined with labelled image features. The classifications are evaluated by a statistical model to determine the final label. Cantina+ [16] is another feature based approach that detects phishing. It makes use of features found in DOM, search engines and third party services with machine learning techniques. The accompanying two novel filters are used to help reduce incorrectly labelled data and accomplish runtime speedup.

Phishing Detection Techniques for Twitter. There is no denying that social media networks have become the main target for spammers due to their increase in popularity in today's world. Yardi *et al.* [17] studied spam in Twitter using network and temporal properties. Machine learning algorithms are incorporated in these techniques in order to uncover patterns exploited by spammers. In [15], the authors proposed a method that utilises graph-based and content-based features for Naïve Bayesian classifiers to distinguish the suspicious behaviors from normal Tweets. CAT [4] and the proposed method in [5] also use classification techniques to detect spammers. While the previously mentioned studies see spam detection as a classification problem, Miller *et al.* [13] viewed it as an anomaly detection problem. Two data stream algorithms, DenStream and StreamKM++, were used to facilitate spam identification. As opposed to spam detection on Twitter, there are a few studies carried out on phishing detection on Twitter. PhishAri [3] is a system that detects malicious URLs in tweets using URL-based, WHOIS-based, user-based and network-based features using a random forest classification algorithm. Warningbird [11] is another detection system by Lee *et al.* Unlike other conventional classifiers which are built on Twitter-based and URL-based features, Warningbird relies on the correlations of URL redirect chains that share the same redirection servers.

Current techniques suffer from similar limitations which include (1) difficulty in detecting phishers before they are sufficient inter-user relationships (or network information); (2) lack of robustness to changes within phishing trends; (3) timeliness and a significant effort to maintain the completeness in List-based techniques.

3   Overview: Phishing Detector for Twitter (PDT)

Given the ever-changing nature of the Twitter stream and behaviour of phishers, we postulate that unsupervised learning techniques could be a better way to detect phishing. This section details unsupervised learning algorithms and the cluster classifier that are used to identify phishing tweets. We propose a new technique called Phishing Detector for Twitter (PDT). Our approach has two phases. In Phase 1 we used DBSCAN to determine legitimate and phishing tweets. However as DBSCAN is a strict approach there are clusters with data points that are difficult to classify as legitimate or phishing. These indeterminate tweets (data points) are then passed into Phase 2. By using this two phase approach we are able to increase the accuracy of phishing detection significantly.

In the following sections we will discuss the data collection methodology, along side feature selection and the analysis we carried out. We then discuss our PDT approach in detail.

4   Data Collection Methodology

In this section, we describe the method of data collection and how each sample was labelled for this research.

Crawling Tweets. For this study, tweets were collected using the Twitter Public Streaming API. The API offers samples of public data flowing through Twitter around the world in real time. After a sample dataset was completed, tweets that did not contain URLs were removed from the dataset since they are irrelevant to the study. On October 4th, 2014, we collected 25, 350 tweets and of those, 5, 151 with URLs were used in this research as the initial experimental set. We later crawled additional tweets as validation sets.

Labeling Samples as Phishing or Legitimate. Despite having an unsupervised learning approach it was necessary to have suitable ground truth datasets to validate our results. Thus we annotated the collected tweets as phishing or legitimate by utilising two phishing blacklists from Google Safe Browsing API and Twitter. If a user is suspended, we have labelled this user as a spammer, therefore all of the URLs in his tweets were marked as phishing sites. Due to delays in Twitters phishing detection algorithm, we have waited for seven days and checked URLs against the databases to label the collected messages.

5   Feature Selection and Analysis

Previous studies on email phishing show that some features of URLs and email can be used to determine if a URL is malicious. In terms of Twitter, it lacks some of the features that emails hold, however, they may be substituted by other metadata that only a tweet embeds.

User Features. Each Twitter user has extra information that can be utilised to identify phishing tweets along with other features. We identified seven user features and they are shown in Table 1.

Table 1. Identified User Features

Feature	Type	Description
Follower count	numeric	Number of Twitter users who follows the user
Following count	numeric	Number of Twitter users who are followed by the user
Age of account	numeric	Number of days since creation of account
Favourites count	numeric	Number of tweets that the user marked as favourite
Lists count	numeric	Number of lists that the user was subscribed to
Presence of description	nominal	Existence of profile description
Verified user flag	nominal	Whether the user's account was verified by Twitter. Verification is used to establish authenticity of identities of key individuals and brands on Twitter

Tweet Features. Malicious tweets change their attributes over time to get higher visibility in the global ecosystem. Such tweets try to gain attraction by including keywords of trending topics (often by using hashtags), mentioning popular users (denoted by @) and following other active users. They include such tokens to increase their visibility to users who use Twitter's search facility or external search engines. By mentioning genuine users randomly, phishing tweets can make themselves visible to those users. Additional metadata of a tweet can be retrieved via a Twitter API. This includes, but is not limited to, retweet counts, favourite counts and a Boolean flag a user may set to indicate presence of possible sensitive information. We identified eight tweet features shown in Table 2.

Table 2. Identified Tweet Features

Feature	Type	Description
Message length	numeric	Number of characters in a tweet
Retweet count	numeric	Number of times a tweet was retweeted by other users
Favourites count	numeric	Number of times a tweet was marked as favourite by other users
URL count	numeric	Number of URLs found in a tweet
Hashtag count	numeric	Number of hashtags (#keyword) found in a tweet
Mention count	numeric	Number of user mentions (@user) found in a tweet
Presence of geolocation	nominal	Existence of geolocation data in a tweet
Sensitive flag	nominal	Existence of user-set sensitive flag in the tweet's metadata

URL Features. A number of case studies on detecting phishing emails have already revealed that URL features contribute to the identification of phishing sites. Many phishing sites abuse browser redirection to bypass blacklists therefore the number of redirections between the initial URL and the final URL is another feature we collected. We have also identified extra features from WHOIS for our collected sample domains. We identified five URL features shown in Table 3.

Table 3. Identified URL Features

Feature	Type	Description
URL length	numeric	Number of characters found in a URL
Domain length	numeric	Number of characters found in the domain of a URL
Redirection count	numeric	Number of redirection hops between the initial URL and the final URL
Age of domain	numeric	Number of days since the registered date of the domain
Dot count	numeric	Number of dots (.) found in a URL. For example, www.auckland.ac.nz has 3 dots

Feature Analysis. Prior to designing our phishing detection technique, two analyses were executed to gain better insight into the feature set and eliminate any visible noise features in the early phase. In addition to the datasets we collected, we have also obtained datasets from a group of authors who have completed similar work in Miller *et al.* [13].

Table 4 presents the ranking of features based on $\overline{\chi^2}$ values from our sample set. It can be noted that the most important features are URL count, age of account and dot count. Research on Twitter spammers presented by Benevenuto et al. displays a similar behaviour [5].

Table 4. Results of χ^2 computation on the sample set

Feature	χ^2	$p-value$	Feature	χ^2	$p-value$
URL count	0.1092	0.8501	Listed count	19.3584	0.3060
Age of account	0.3190	0.7264	Url length	50.1056	0.0001
Dot count	0.3547	0.7114	Favourites count	1381.7993	0.1552
Redirection count	0.7762	0.4426	Following count	1526.8343	0.0392
Mention count	0.9181	0.4675	Age of domain	2558.3320	0.0404
Hashtag count	1.2330	0.3447	Follower count	3156.6372	0.0893
Domain length	10.4100	0.0101	Tweets count	26550.8693	0.0024

6   PDT Approach

In this section we describe our PDT approach in detail. In Sect. 6.1 we discuss the DBSCAN technique which was used in Phase 1, and in Sect. 6.2 we discuss the Der-TIA approach adapted for our technique.

6.1   Phase 1: DBSCAN

Density Based Spatial Clustering of Applications with Noise (DBSCAN) is a density based data clustering algorithm. The principal idea of this algorithm is that a set of points closely packed together forms a cluster and any data points in the low density region are labelled as outliers.

Cluster Classifier. DBSCAN can cluster data only and is unable to assign them into phishing or non-phishing categories. In order to carry out the assignment, Ordinary Least Squares (OLS) method was used, which computes the linear approximation for each pairwise feature. Distinctive linear regressions for the feature pairs were identified for all clusters. They were further analysed and patterns were observed as shown in Fig. 1 to draw four rules as described in Table 5. This was carried out on the initial set.

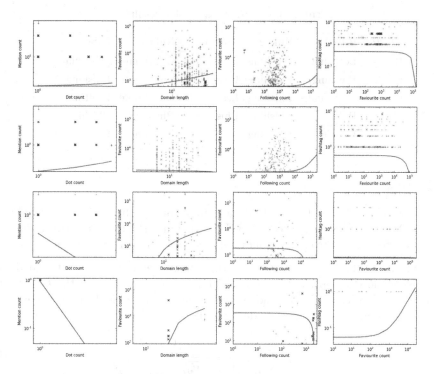

Fig. 1. Observed OLS patterns for pairwise features in clusters plotted on log-log charts. Red markers represent phishing samples and blue markers represent legitimate samples. The first two clusters are labelled as legitimate and the remaining clusters are labelled as phishing. (Color figure online)

Table 5. Cluster classification rules (β is the regression coefficient in OLS method)

Rule	Feature pair	Condition	Decision
Rule 1	Dot count vs. Mention count	$\beta < 0$	Phishing
Rule 2	Domain length vs. Favourites count	$\beta > 0$	Phishing
Rule 3	Following count vs. Favourites count	$\beta < 0$	Phishing
Rule 4	Hashtags count vs. Favourites count	$\beta > 0$	Phishing

The minimum requirement size of a cluster is 30 data points. If the size is less than 30, the cluster is considered as insufficient to comprise any one of the patterns we identified earlier. Such clusters are then indeterminate. The second phase is necessary to filter the phishing data point from the clusters that were indeterminate. Additionally, a cluster is determined by this procedure when at least 3 out of 4 labels are the same.

If the numbers of phishing and non-phishing labels are the same and the majority cannot be found from the results, then the cluster is also labelled as indeterministic as shown in Table 6. Data within clusters that were indeterminate were then pass through Phase 2.

Table 6. Cluster classification results

Cluster	Rule 1	Rule 2	Rule 3	Rule 4	Label
C1	Legitimate	Phishing	Legitimate	Legitimate	Legitimate
C2	Phishing	Phishing	Phishing	Legitimate	Phishing
C3	Legitimate	Phishing	Legitimate	Legitimate	Legitimate
C4	Phishing	Phishing	Phishing	Phishing	Phishing
C5	Legitimate	Phishing	Phishing	Legitimate	Indetermined

6.2   Phase 2: DeR-TIA

In order to classify indeterminate data points from the first phase, a technique called DeR-TIA by [19] is used. DeR-TIA combines the results of two different measures techniques to detect abnormalities in recommender systems.

DegSim. The first part of the algorithm finds the similarities between data sets using the Pearson correlation algorithm in conjunction with the k-Nearest Neighbour algorithm. The Pearson correlation algorithm yields a linear correlation (dependencies) between two data points.

$$W_{pq} = \frac{\sum_{f \in F}(V_{pf} - \overline{V_p})(V_{qf} - \overline{V_q})}{\sqrt{\sum_{f \in F}(V_{pf} - \overline{V_p})^2(V_{qf} - \overline{V_q})^2}} \tag{1}$$

where F is the set of all features, V_{pf} is the value of feature f in the data point p and $\overline{V_p}$ is the mean value of data point p. The outcomes from the above formula range between -1 and 1. A positive value indicates that the inputs have a positive correlation and vice versa. If there is no correlation found, the outcome will be 0 and the boundary values, -1 and 1, illustrate that there are very strong correlations. The closer the outcome value is to the boundary limits, the closer the data points to the line of best fit.

The DegSim attribute is defined as the average Pearson correlation value of the k-Nearest Neighbours (k-NN) over the k.

$$DegSim = \frac{\sum_{p=1}^{k} W_{pq}}{k} \qquad (2)$$

where W_{pq} is the Pearson correlation between data point p and q where k is the number of neighbours.

RDMA. The second part of the algorithm is Rating Deviation from Mean Agreement (RDMA) technique. This technique measures the deviation of agreement from other data points on the entire dataset. The RDMA measure is as follows:

$$RDMA_p = \frac{\sum_{f \in F} \frac{|V_{pf} - \overline{V_f}|}{NV_f}}{N_p} \qquad (3)$$

where N_p is the number of features data set p has, F is the set of all features, V_{pf} is the value of feature f in the data point p, $\overline{V_f}$ is the mean value of feature f in the entire sample set and NV_f is the overall number of feature f in the sample set.

Once values for RDMA and DegSim are computed, the dataset of each property is split into two clusters to find the legitimate and phishing groups using the k-means algorithm where the value of k fixed at 2. The labels of clusters are determined by the cluster size. As discussed earlier, the majority of the URLs in tweets are non-phishing, therefore the larger cluster is classified as legitimate. Then the phishing clusters from RDMA and DegSim are intersected to get the final set of phishing data points.

7   Experiments

To compare the performance of our technique, we anaylsed our technique against DBSCAN. The two major reasons we chose DBSCAN as our baseline algorithm were (1) DBSCAN is an unsupervised learning technique that does not require network data features [12], and (2) DBSCAN was used in Phase 1 of our technique, thus we are able to measure improvement rate of our second phase compared to using only DBSCAN.

7.1   Experimental Setup

The experimental environment is set up with a *t2.micro* compute instance running on Amazon Elastic Compute Cloud platform. *t2.micro* instances are configured with an Intel Xeon 2.5 GHz CPU and 1 G RAM. Public tweet stream crawler and analysis tools for this research are written in Python with scientific libraries such as numpy, scipy, mathplotlib and StatsModels. 15 distinct tweet sets (VS) were sampled. Table 7 summaries collected sample sets for this research.

Table 7. Samples information

Datasets	Collection time (UTC)	#tweets collected	#tweets with URLs	#legitimate tweets
VS 1	2015-04-30 04:06:01	28685	7459	7052
VS 2	2015-04-30 06:03:01	22553	7076	6381
VS 3	2015-04-30 10:02:01	26818	7900	7375
VS 4	2015-05-01 08:22:01	44216	12059	11164
VS 5	2015-05-01 22:47:01	55078	14213	13734
VS 6	2015-05-02 00:15:01	54100	13343	12648
VS 7	2015-05-02 06:51:01	45688	12819	12369
VS 8	2015-05-02 12:14:01	62837	14830	14346
VS 9	2015-05-02 16:41:02	68233	15907	15128
VS 10	2015-05-02 18:24:01	62074	14444	13809
VS 11	2015-05-03 00:46:01	55110	13991	13629
VS 12	2015-05-03 02:18:01	60620	13570	13093
VS 13	2015-05-03 06:55:01	51584	12727	12303
VS 14	2015-05-03 08:35:01	49417	12605	12206
VS 15	2015-05-03 10:03:01	53932	13623	12917

In order to evaluate the correctness of our experiment method based on the features set collected, the commonly accepted information retrieval metrics are used. Accuracy, precision, recall and f-measure are measures used to quantify the effectiveness of PDT.

7.2   Experimental Results

By using PDT we notice an average improvement of 63 % in accuracy and an average improvement of 47 % in f-measure compared against DBSCAN. We also note that although there were no increase in precision there was a 62 % increase in recall value when we compared DBSCAN to PDT. We do note that the original precision in DBSCAN was relatively high with an average pf 99.7 %. Any further improvements would have been marginal.

We discovered that the accuracy of the results from validation samples are noticeably higher than the initial experiment results. It can be speculated that with the underlying dynamic behaviour of social media, that either Twitter

Table 8. Obtained metrics from different samples

Datasets	DBSCAN				PDT			
	Accuracy	Precision	Recall	f-measure	Accuracy	Precision	Recall	f-measure
VS 1	0.4497	0.9975	0.4454	0.6158	0.9858	0.9989	0.9861	0.9924
VS 2	0.4624	0.9936	0.4595	0.6284	0.9816	0.9968	0.9828	0.9897
VS 3	0.3147	0.9920	0.3371	0.5032	0.9542	0.9949	0.9558	0.9750
VS 4	0.2212	0.9996	0.2247	0.3670	0.9671	0.9923	0.9720	0.9820
VS 5	0.2797	0.9982	0.2799	0.4372	0.9780	0.9971	0.9800	0.9885
VS 6	0.2674	0.9983	0.2717	0.4271	0.9684	0.9955	0.9711	0.9831
VS 7	0.3842	1.0000	0.3889	0.5600	0.9874	0.9998	0.9871	0.9934
VS 8	0.3481	1.0000	0.3518	0.5205	0.9873	0.9994	0.9874	0.9934
VS 9	0.3672	0.9986	0.3788	0.5493	0.9894	0.9991	0.9898	0.9944
VS 10	0.3853	0.9967	0.3948	0.5656	0.9851	0.9979	0.9865	0.9922
VS 11	0.3731	0.9969	0.3744	0.5444	0.9873	0.9987	0.9883	0.9935
VS 12	0.3943	0.9990	0.3975	0.5688	0.9892	0.9996	0.9892	0.9944
VS 13	0.3570	0.9991	0.3601	0.5294	0.9899	0.9996	0.9900	0.9948
VS 14	0.3397	0.9972	0.3501	0.5192	0.9793	0.9988	0.9798	0.9892
VS 15	0.3243	0.9991	0.3336	0.5002	0.9928	0.9994	0.9930	0.9962
StdDev	0.0645	0.0023	0.0626	0.0697	0.0107	0.0022	0.0098	0.0059

user's usages or phishing trend or both have been changed over the 208 day period since the time of the initial sample collection. We postulate that this is due to the adaptive nature of our unsupervised learning based technique, which can adapt to the continuously-changing Twitter ecosystem. The samples we collected over the three days show consistency in all metrics as supported by low standard deviation values. The Mann-Whitney test on the f-measures supports that PDT is significantly more accurate than DBSCAN with input parameters as $U = 16$, Z-ratio $= -4.2038$, $P \leq 0.05$ two-tailed (Table 8).

8   Conclusions

In this research we proposed a technique, called PDT, which is a two phase approach adapting both DBSCAN and DeR-TIA to improve the coverage. Our technique PDT shows promising outcomes. We showed that our technique produced high accuracy, precision, recall, and f-measure values compared to previous technique namely DBSCAN. Moreover PDT can adapt over time for phishing detection with behavioral changes in Twitter. We have shown that our technique worked over data collected from different periods of time. Using other traditional supervised methods we would not have been able to guarantee that it could adapt to the changing nature of the Twitter data.

For further development, phishing detection through a sliding window over the stream of new tweets would be useful. A fixed size window accepts new data from Twitter streams and eliminates obsolete data from the window pool. Thus ensuring recency of information evaluated and may increase the accuracy of the results produced.

References

1. Phishtank — join the fight against phishing, June 2015. https://phishtank.com
2. Abu-Nimeh, S., Nappa, D., Wang, X., Nair, S.: A comparison of machine learning techniques for phishing detection. In: Proceedings of the Anti-phishing Working Groups 2nd Annual eCrime Researchers Summit, pp. 60–69. ACM (2007)
3. Aggarwal, A., Rajadesingan, A., Kumaraguru, P.: Phishari: automatic realtime phishing detection on twitter. In: eCrime Researchers Summit (eCrime), 2012, pp. 1–12. IEEE (2012)
4. Amleshwaram, A.A., Reddy, N., Yadav, S., Gu, G., Yang, C.: Cats: characterizing automation of Twitter spammers. In: 2013 Fifth International Conference on Communication Systems and Networks (COMSNETS), pp. 1–10. IEEE (2013)
5. Benevenuto, F., Magno, G., Rodrigues, T., Almeida, V.: Detecting spammers on Twitter. In: Collaboration, Electronic Messaging, Anti-abuse and Spam Conference (CEAS), vol. 6, p. 12 (2010)
6. Chhabra, S., Aggarwal, A., Benevenuto, F., Kumaraguru, P.: Phi.sh/$ocial: the phishing landscape through short urls. In: Proceedings of the 8th Annual Collaboration, Electronic messaging, Anti-abuse and Spam Conference, pp. 92–101. ACM (2011)
7. Dunlop, M., Groat, S., Shelly, D.: Goldphish: using images for content-based phishing analysis. In: 2010 Fifth International Conference on Internet Monitoring and Protection (ICIMP), pp. 123–128. IEEE (2010)
8. Fette, I., Sadeh, N., Tomasic, A.: Learning to detect phishing emails. In: Proceedings of the 16th International Conference on World Wide Web, pp. 649–656. ACM (2007)
9. Garera, S., Provos, N., Chew, M., Rubin, A.D.: A framework for detection and measurement of phishing attacks. In: Proceedings of the 2007 ACM Workshop on Recurring Malcode, pp. 1–8. ACM (2007)
10. Klien, F., Strohmaier, M.: Short links under attack: geographical analysis of spam in a url shortener network. In: Proceedings of the 23rd ACM Conference on Hypertext and Social Media, pp. 83–88. ACM (2012)
11. Lee, S., Kim, J.: Warningbird: a near real-time detection system for suspicious urls in Twitter stream. IEEE Trans. Dependable Secure Comput. **3**, 183–195 (2013)
12. Liu, G., Qiu, B., Wenyin, L.: Automatic detection of phishing target from phishing webpage. In: 20th International Conference on Pattern Recognition (ICPR), pp. 4153–4156, August 2010
13. Miller, Z., Dickinson, B., Deitrick, W., Hu, W., Wang, A.H.: Twitter spammer detection using data stream clustering. Inf. Sci. **260**, 64–73 (2014)
14. Sheng, S., Wardman, B., Warner, G., Cranor, L., Hong, J., Zhang, C.: An empirical analysis of phishing blacklists. In: Sixth Conference on Email and Anti-Spam (CEAS), California, USA (2009)
15. Wang, A.H.: Don't follow me: spam detection in Twitter. In: Proceedings of the 2010 International Conference on Security and Cryptography (SECRYPT), pp. 1–10. IEEE (2010)

16. Xiang, G., Hong, J., Rose, C.P., Cranor, L.: Cantina+: a feature-rich machine learning framework for detecting phishing web sites. ACM Trans. Inf. Syst. Secur. (TISSEC) **14**(2), 21 (2011)
17. Yardi, S., Romero, D., Schoenebeck, G.: Detecting spam in a Twitter network. First Mon. **15**(1) (2010)
18. Zhang, H., Liu, G., Chow, T.W., Liu, W.: Textual and visual content-based anti-phishing: a Bayesian approach. IEEE Trans. Neural Netw. **22**(10), 1532–1546 (2011)
19. Zhou, W., Wen, J., Koh, Y.S., Alam, S., Dobbie, G.: Attack detection in recommender systems based on target item analysis. In: 2014 International Joint Conference on Neural Networks (IJCNN), pp. 332–339. IEEE (2014)

Image Segmentation with Superpixel Based Covariance Descriptor

Xianbin Gu$^{(\boxtimes)}$ and Martin Purvis

Department of Information Science, University of Otago, Dunedin, New Zealand
guxi0185@student.otago.ac.nz, martin.purvis@otago.ac.nz

Abstract. This paper investigates the problem of image segmentation using superpixels. We propose two approaches to enhance the discriminative ability of the superpixel's covariance descriptors. In the first one, we employ the Log-Euclidean distance as the metric on the covariance manifolds, and then use the RBF kernel to measure the similarities between covariance descriptors. The second method is focused on extracting the subspace structure of the set of covariance descriptors by extending a low rank representation algorithm on to the covariance manifolds. Experiments are carried out with the Berkly Segmentation Dataset, and compared with the state-of-the-art segmentation algorithms, both methods are competitive.

Keywords: Image segmentation · Superpixel · Low rank representation · Covariance matrix · Manifold

1 Introduction

Covariance matrix is widely used in image segmentation with whom those pixel-wise features, like color, gradient, etc., are assembled together into one symmetric positive definite matrix (Sym_d^+) named covariance descriptor. Research shows that such descriptor is a feature that highly discriminative for many image processing tasks, such as image classification, segmentation, and object recognition [11,13]

In image segmentation, the covariance descriptor is often built on some basic features of a group of pixels, like color, intensity, positions, or gradients, etc. And different combinations of basic features bring different covariance descriptors, which often influence the algorithms' performance. However, the research about how to construct covariance descriptors for a specific task is insufficient, and the relations between basic feature combinations and performance of the algorithms are still unclear.

Generally, researchers construct covariance descriptors by trying different basic feature combinations and taking the one that gives the best performance [12], i.e. by an empirical way. This may be handy for practice but lack of theory support.

Fortunately, there are some other options, which can enhance the discriminative ability of covariance descriptors without repeatedly testing the combinations of the features. These methods are based on two facts. First, in the view

© Springer International Publishing Switzerland 2016
H. Cao et al. (Eds.): PAKDD 2016 Workshops, LNAI 9794, pp. 154–165, 2016.
DOI: 10.1007/978-3-319-42996-0_13

of differential geometry, the covariance descriptors are symmetric positive definite matrices lying on a convex cone in the Euclidean space, i.e. they are the points on some Sym_d^+ manifolds. So, a proper defined metric on the Sym_d^+ will improve the performance of covariance descriptors. Secondly, there are always some correlations between the basic features that built up the covariance descriptor, which may bring noises. Thus, removing the noise in covariance descriptors is also beneficial.

To this end, we study the RBF kernel and Low Rank Representation algorithm on the Sym_d^+ manifolds and compare them with the state-of-the-art methods by experimenting on different covariance descriptors extracted from superpixels.

The rest of the paper is organized as follows. Section 2 presents a brief review of the algorithms and concepts that are necessary for this paper. Section 3 discusses different methods to measure the similarity of covariance descriptors. Section 4 is the comparison between the algorithms, and Sect. 5 gives the conclusion.

2   Background

2.1   Manifold, Covariance Descriptor and Multi-collinearity

A manifold $\mathcal{M}$ of dimension d is a topological space that is locally homeomorphic to open subset of the Euclidean space R^d [27]. For analysis on $\mathcal{M}$, there usually have two options. One is by embedding $\mathcal{M}$ into R^d so that to create a linear structure and the methods from Euclidean space can be directly applied. The alternative is concentrated on the intrinsic properties of $\mathcal{M}$, i.e. define a properly intrinsic metric of $\mathcal{M}$ and launch the analysis on the true structure of $\mathcal{M}$. The first method is more intuitive but less accurate because the extrinsic metric may not align with the intrinsic properties of the manifold. While the second method is able to represent the manifold structure precisely, but for analysis, it is not as friendly as in the Euclidean space.

Let $\mathbf{F} = (\mathbf{f}_1, ..., \mathbf{f}_n)^T$ be a feature array, where $\mathbf{f}_i$ is a vector whose entries are the observations of the i-th feature. A covariance descriptor is the covariance matrix of $\mathbf{F}$, which is defined as,

$$cov(\mathbf{F}) = \left[E((\mathbf{f}_i - \mu_i)^T (\mathbf{f}_j - \mu_j)) \right]_{n \times n}, \tag{1}$$

where, μ_i is the mean of the i-th feature $\mathbf{f}_i$, $[\cdot]_{n \times n}$ indicates an $n \times n$ matrix whose entry at position (i, j) is represented by the "·". Apparently, different sets of $\mathbf{f}_i$ generate different $cov(\mathbf{F})$, which makes the performance vary.

Collinearity (or multi-collinearity) is a term from statistics, which refers a linear association between two (or more) variables. Specifically, given a feature array $\mathbf{F}$, if there exists a set of not-all-zero scalar $\lambda_1, ..., \lambda_n$ that makes the following equation holds,

$$\lambda_1 \mathbf{f}_1 + \lambda_2 \mathbf{f}_2 + \cdots + \lambda_n \mathbf{f}_n + u = 0 \tag{2}$$

If $u = 0$, $\mathbf{F}$ is perfect multi-collinearity; while if $u \sim N(0, \sigma)$, $\mathbf{F}$ is nearly multi-collinearity. This multi-collinearity phenomenon is common in image segmentation because the variables in the feature array $\mathbf{F}$, like gradient, are computed from other containing variables (i.e. inclusion). If we consider Eq. (2) and Eq. (1) simultaneously, it is easy to see the inclusion may produce redundant entries and noises in $cov(\mathbf{F})$.

2.2 Segmentation with Superpixels

A cluster of pixels is called superpixel for whom its members are more similar between each other than those nonmembers. In [16], the authors have shown that image segmentation benefits from using superpixels. There are three advantages for superpixel based segmentation. Firstly, they dramatically reduce computation cost by representing pixels inside one superpixel as a whole. Secondly, regional features can be extracted from superpixels, which are more discriminative than pixel-wise features in many vision tasks. Thirdly, multi-scale techniques can be applied when considering different parameter settings (or, different algorithms) for superpixel generating as different scales.

In this paper, the segmentation is performed by a spectral clustering algorithm proposed in [16], which takes advantage of the superpixels. Briefly, this algorithm mainly contains three parts. The first one is superpixel generation. Similar to [11,16,25], we produce superpixels by Mean Shift algorithm [6] and Felzenszwalb-Huttenlocher algorithm [7] with a few sets of parameters. The second is graph construction. We construct a bipartite graph on the pixels and superpixels, and the superpixels are represented by covariance descriptors. We adopt different ways to measure the similarities of the superpixels, and the results are reported in Sect. 5. The third part is spectral clustering. We use T-cut [16] to reduce the computational cost. The framework is shown in Algorithm 1.

Algorithm 1. Superpixel-based Segmentation

Input: An image M and the number of segmentation k.
Output: A k-way segmentation of M.
 1: Create over segmentation of M by superpixel algorithms;
 2: Construct bipartite graph $G(X, Y, B)$ (refer to *Section* 3.1);
 3: Compute weights on the edges by some similarity measure (refer to Alg. 2 and Alg. 3);
 4: Partition G by T-cut.

---

3   Similarity Measurement

3.1   Construction of Bipartite Graph

Let $P = \{p_1, ..., p_n\}$ denotes the set of pixels of a given images and S be a collection $\{S_i\}$, where $S_i = \{s_t^{(i)}\}$ is a set of superpixels. A given bipartite graph

$G(X, Y, B)$ is built in this way: set $X = P \cup S$, $Y = S$ and let $B = E_1 \cup E_2$ be the edges, where E_1 and E_2 represent the edges in every vertex pair $(p_k, s_t^{(i)})$ and $(s_k^{(i)}, s_l^{(i)})$ respectively. A number of methods have been proposed to the similarities between superpixels (i.e., the weights on the edges in E_2). Some are based on geometry constrains [16], some are based on encoding techniques [25]. While in [11], a covariance descriptor based method was proposed, which employed color and a covariance matrix of the color value $[R, G, B]$ to assess the similarities in superpixels.

However, it is still necessary to explore the mechanism of making use of covariance descriptors. Our first thinking is to use the geodesics distance measuring the distance between the covariance descriptors. Secondly, we note that the multi-collinearity is almost inevitable when building the covariance descriptors, this encourages us to use the low rank representation algorithm.

3.2   The RBF Kernel

A dataset of $d \times d$ covariance matrices is lying on a manifold embedding in d^2-dimensional Euclidean space because the space of $d \times d$ covariance matrices is a convex cone in the d^2-dimensional Euclidean space.

It has been proofed that the geometry of the space Sym_d^+ can be well explained with a Riemannian metric which induced an infinite distance between an Sym_d^+ matrix and a non-Sym_d^+ matrix [2]. But different to [11], we use the Log-Euclidean distance, a geodesic distance, which makes it possible to embed the manifold into $\mathcal{RKHS}$ with RBF kernel [14].

The Log-Euclidean distance between covariance matrix X_i and X_j is defined as $d_{LE}(X_i, X_j) := \|Log(X_i) - Log(X_j)\|_F$. Respectively, the RBF kernel can be rewritten as,

$$k_{LE} : (X \times X) \to R : k_{LE}(X_i, X_j) := exp(-\sigma d_{LE}^2(X_i, X_j)) \qquad (3)$$

where, $\sigma > 0$ is a scale parameter. The similarity matrix is defined as $[B]_{ij} := (k_{LE}(X_i, X_j))$. Details are as Algorithm 2. Theoretically, the kernel method is more efficient, but it may not hold in our case. We give some possible explanation in Sect. 5.

Algorithm 2. Construct the Graph via RBF kernel

Input: The Graph $G(X, Y, B)$; parameter α and σ .
Output: A weighted Graph $G(X, Y, \tilde{B})$.
1: **for all** e in B **do**
2:   **if** $e \in E_2$ **then**
3:     $e = exp(-\sigma d_{LE}^2(s_k^{(i)}, s_l^{(i)}))$
4:   **else**
5:     $e = \alpha$
6:   **end if**
7: **end for**

3.3   Low Rank Representation for Sym_d^+

The low rank representation (LRR) algorithm [4,26] is proposed to remove the redundancy and noises in the dataset. For a given dataset X, the LRR algorithm finds a matrix Z, called low rank representation of X, such that $X = XZ + E$ holds, where E represents the noises. The performance of LRR is promising when X is a set of points in Euclidean space [5,10,19], and recently, it has been extended to data sets lying on manifolds [9,23,24].

Algorithm 3. Construct the Graph via LRR

Input: A collection of covariance matrix $\mathcal{S}$; parameter λ.
Output: A weighted similarity matrix $\tilde{B}$.
1: **for** $S_i = \{s_t^{(i)}\}_{t=1}^n$ in $\mathcal{S}$ **do**
2:    Compute Z_i of S_i:
3:    Initialize: $J = Z_i = 0$, $Y = 0$, $\mu = 10^{-6}$, $\mu_{max} = 10^{10}$, $\rho = 1.9$, $\epsilon = 10^{-8}$;
4:    **for** i=1:n **do**
5:       **for** j=1:n **do**
6:          $\Delta_{ij} = tr[(s_t^{(i)} s_t^{(j)})]$
7:       **end for**
8:    **end for**
9:    **while** not converged **do**
10:       Fix Z_i and update J by
             $J \leftarrow \Theta(Z_i + \frac{Y}{\mu})$;
11:       Fix J and update Z by
             $Z \leftarrow (\lambda\mu J - \lambda Y + 2\Delta)(2\Delta + \lambda\mu I)^{-1}$
12:       Check convergence,
13:       **if** $\|Z_i - J\|_F < \epsilon$ **then**
14:          break
15:       **else**
16:          Update Y and μ,
             $Y \leftarrow Y + \mu(Z_i - J)$
             $\mu \leftarrow min(\rho\mu, \mu_{max})$
17:       **end if**
18:    **end while**
19:    Compute Singular Value Decomposition of Z_i,
          $Z_i = U_i \Sigma_i V_i^T$
20:    Compute the weights on $e \in \{(s_k^{(i)}, s_l^{(i)})\}_{k,l=1}^n \subset B$ by
          $(\tilde{U}_i * \tilde{U}_i^t)^2$, where $\tilde{U}_i$ is the U_i normalized in rows.
21: **end for**

Let $\mathcal{X}$ be a 3-order tensor, which is stacked from covariance matrices $(X_i)_{d \times d}$, $i = 1, 2, ..., n$. By embedding $\mathcal{X}$ into the d^2-dimensional Euclidean space, our LRR model is set as follows,

$$\min_{E,Z} \|E\|_F^2 + \lambda\|Z\|_*,$$

$$s.t. \quad \mathcal{X} = \mathcal{X}_{\times_3} Z + E, \tag{4}$$

where, $\|\cdot\|_F$ is the *Frobenius* norm; $\|\cdot\|_*$ is the *nuclear* norm; λ is the balance parameter; $\times_3$ means mode-3 multiplication of a tensor and matrix [15]. Equation (4) can be solved via Augment Lagrangian Multiplier (ALM) [17]. Details are in Appendix.

Let Δ be a symmetric matrix, whose entries are $\Delta_{ij} = \Delta_{ji} = tr(X_i X_j)$, we can obtain a solution of Eq. (4) by iteratively updating the following variables,

$$J = \Theta(Z + \frac{Y}{\mu}), \tag{5}$$

and,

$$Z = (\lambda \mu J - \lambda Y + 2\Delta)(2\Delta + \lambda \mu I)^{-1}, \tag{6}$$

where, λ and μ are pre-setting parameters, Y is the Lagrange coefficient, $\Theta(\cdot)$ is the singular value thresholding operator [3].

Since the coefficient matrix Z contains the subspace information of the dataset, it is reasonable to define the similarity matrix as $[B]_{ij} := ([\widetilde{U}\widetilde{U}^T]_{ij})^2$ for spectral clustering, where, $\widetilde{U}$ is the row-normalized singular vector of Z [18]. Algorithm 3 gives the details.

4   Experiments

The experiments are set to compare the effects of different similarity measure algorithms of covariance descriptors. We construct the covariance descriptors with three different feature vectors named as CovI, CovII, CovIII respectively,

- $CovI : [R, G, B]$,
- $CovII : [R, G, B, I, \dfrac{\partial I}{\partial x}, \dfrac{\partial I}{\partial y}, \dfrac{\partial I}{\partial^2 x}, \dfrac{\partial I}{\partial^2 y}]$,
- $CovIII : [R, G, B, \dfrac{\partial R}{\partial x}, \dfrac{\partial R}{\partial y}, \dfrac{\partial G}{\partial x}, \dfrac{\partial G}{\partial y}, \dfrac{\partial B}{\partial x}, \dfrac{\partial B}{\partial y}, \dfrac{\partial R}{\partial^2 x}, \dfrac{\partial R}{\partial^2 y}, \dfrac{\partial G}{\partial^2 x}, \dfrac{\partial G}{\partial^2 y}, \dfrac{\partial B}{\partial^2 x}, \dfrac{\partial B}{\partial^2 y}]$.

From CovI to CovIII, the dimensionality of the covariance descriptor is increasing. For example, CovI contains the patterns in the R, G, B channels, while in CovIII, the patterns of their derivatives are also included. This means the covariance descriptors become more discriminative. But, since the partial derivatives are directly computed from other contained features, the tendencies of multi-collinearity are also growing.

The methods for similarity measurement include RBF kernel with Log-Euclidean distance (RBFLE) and Low Rank Representation (LRR).

All experiments are done with the Berkly Segmentation Dataset, a standard benchmark image segmentation dataset, which includes 300 natural images selected from diverse scene categories [1]. Besides, it also provide a number of human-annotated ground-truth descriptions for each image. In our experiments, every image is partitioned into K regions with $K \in [2, 40]$. And, the reported evaluation results are based on the K that provides the best performance of the algorithms.

4.1 The Settings

The same as in [11, 16, 25], the superpixels are generated by the Mean Shift algorithm with 3 different sets of parameters and the Felzenszwalb-Huttenlocher algorithm with 2 different sets of parameters; the weights on E_1 are fixed to 1×10^{-3}. For the RBF-LE, parameter σ is set as 20. In the LRR model, parameter λ is sensitive to noise level [18]. Since the BSDS contains images from different categories, which indicates the noise levels are different between images, we tuned λ for every image by a grid research in $\{1, 0.1, 0.01, 0.001\}$; a higher noise level is associated with a greater λ. In addition, we apply "k-nearest neighbor" to refine the similarity graph with $k = 1$.

4.2 The Evaluation

The performance of the algorithms is assessed by four popular segmentation evaluation methods, which includes the Probabilistic Rand Index (PRI) [22], the Variation of Information (VoI) [21], the Global Consistency Error (GCE) [20], and the Boundary Displacement Error (BDE) [8].

PRI is a nonparametric test, which measures the probability of an arbitrary pair of samples being labeled consistently in the two segmentations. A higher PRI value means better segmentation.

The VoI is a metric that relates to the conditional entropies between the class label distribution. It measures the sum of information loss and information gain between the two partitions, so it roughly measures the extent to which one clustering can explain the other. A lower VoI value indicates better segmentation result.

The GCE measures the difference between two regions that contain the same pixel in different segmentations. Particularly, this metric compensates for the difference in granularity. For GCE values, being close to 0 implies a good segmentation.

The BDE measures the average displacement error of boundary pixels between two segmentations. The error of one boundary pixel is defined as the distance between the pixel and the closest pixel in the other boundary image. A lower BDE value means less deviation between the segmentation and ground truth.

In addition, we rank the algorithms on each index and give the average rank (Avg.R, lower is better) of each algorithm, which gives a straightforward comparison between the methods.

4.3 Results

The evaluations of the algorithms are listed in the following tables. The results the state-of-art algorithms in [11, 16, 25] (i.e. SAS, ℓ_0-sparse, col+CovI) are also listed for reference.

Table 1 shows the best results of the algorithms proposed in this paper together with those reported in other papers. For CovII+LRR, the PRI is the

Table 1. Performance of different algorithms

Algorithms	PRI	VoI	GCE	BDE	Avg.R
SAS [16]	0.8319	1.6849	**0.1779**	11.2900	2.5
ℓ_0-sparse [25]	0.8355	1.9935	0.2297	**11.1955**	3.75
Col+CovI [11]	0.8495	**1.6260**	0.1785	12.3034	2.25
CovII+LRR	**0.8499**	1.7418	0.1915	12.7635	3
CovIII+RBFLE	0.8397	1.9026	0.2103	11.5557	3.5

Table 2. Performance of RBFLE and LRR with different covariance descriptors

Algorithms	PRI	VoI	GCE	BDE
CovI+RBFLE	0.8349	2.0148	0.2218	**12.5276**
CovI+LRR	**0.8454**	**1.7564**	**0.1885**	13.0427
CovII+RBFLE	0.8372	1.9466	0.2148	**11.6658**
CovII+LRR	**0.8499**	**1.7418**	**0.1915**	12.7635
CovIII+RBFLE	0.8397	1.9026	0.2103	**11.5557**
CovIII+LRR	**0.8451**	**1.7698**	**0.1932**	12.4837

highest and the rest index values are very close to the other algorithms. Table 2 demonstrates the results from RBFLE and LRR. The performance of LRR is overwhelming, which indicates noises reduction inside the covariance descriptor benefits the segmentation results. For RBFLE, the performance is inferior even the similarities are measured by geodesic metric and kernel method. Because the

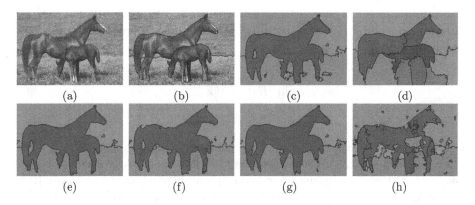

(a)   (b)   (c)   (d)

(e)   (f)   (g)   (h)

Fig. 1. Influence of different covariance descriptors to RBFLE and LRR: (a) original image; (b) ground truth; (c) result of CovI + RBFLE; (d) result of CovI + LRR; (e) result of CovII + RBFLE; (f) result of CovII + LRR; (g) result of CovIII + RBFLE; (h) result of CovIII + LRR.

inner noises (due to multi-collinearity) of the covariance descriptors may distort the true data values. Moreover from Table 2, we notice that the performance of RBFLE goes up with the growing of the entries in the covariance descriptor while the result of LRR varies. One possible reason is that we use extrinsic metric in the LRR algorithm, which may influence the performance.

In addition, Figure 1 displays one result of the algorithms with different covariance descriptors. It can be found that both algorithms are benefits from the extra information given by the add-in dimensions of the descriptors although those add-ins also bring noises.

5   Conclusion

The multi-collinearity usually happens when constructing covariance descriptors. It brings redundancy and noise into the covariance descriptors, which can distort the true data.

We present two approaches for reducing the effect of multi-collinearity. One is to measure the distance between covariance descriptors by a RBF kernel with a particular geodesic distance; another is to apply low rank representation algorithm on the Riemannian manifold. Our empirical experiments show that LRR method is good for covariance matrix based segmentation since it captures the subspace structure of the data set which is less effected by the noises.

However, the LRR algorithm in this paper is based on an extrinsic metric of the manifold. In the future, we will explore the LRR algorithm with the intrinsic properties of the manifold, i.e. by a geodesic distance.

Appendix: Solution of Eq. (4)

The solution of Eq. (4) is partly refer to the work of Wang et al. [24], but the distance induced by *Frobenius* norm is not geodesic. The problem is rephrased as follows.

Find a matrix Z that satisfied,

$$\min_{E,Z} \|E\|_F^2 + \lambda \|Z\|_*,$$

$$s.t. \quad \mathcal{X} = \mathcal{X}_{\times_3} Z + E$$

where, $\mathcal{X}$ is a 3-order tensor stacking by covariance matrices $(X_i)_{d\times d}$, $i = 1, 2, ..., n$; $\|\cdot\|_F$ is the *Frobenius* norm; $\|\cdot\|_*$ is the nuclear norm; λ is the balance parameter; $\times_3$ means mode-3 multiplication of a tensor and matrix [15].

For the error term E, we have $\|E\|_F^2 = \|\mathcal{X} - \mathcal{X}_{\times_3} Z\|_F^2$, and we can rewrite $\|E\|_F^2$ as,

$$\|E\|_F^2 = \sum_i^N \|E_i\|_F^2,$$

where, $E_i = X_i - \sum_j^N z_{ij} X_j$, i.e. the *i-th* slice of E.

Note that for matrix A, it holds $\|A\|_F^2 = tr(A^T A)$, and X_i is symmetric, so, the above equation can be expanded as,

$$\|E_i\|_F^2 = tr[(X_i - \sum_j^N z_{ij}X_j)^T(X_i - \sum_j^N z_{ij}X_j)]$$

$$= tr(X_i^T X_i) - tr(X_i^T \sum_j^N z_{ij}X_j) - tr(\sum_j^N z_{ij}X_j^T X_i)$$

$$+ tr(\sum_{j_1}^N z_{ij_1}X_{j_1}^T \sum_{j_2}^N z_{ij_2}X_{j_2})$$

$$= tr(X_i X_i) - 2tr(\sum_j^N z_{ij}X_i X_j) + tr(\sum_{j_1,j_2}^N z_{ij_1}z_{ij_2}X_{j_1}X_{j_2}).$$

Let Δ be a symmetric matrix of size $N \times N$, whose entries are $\Delta_{ij} = \Delta_{ji} = tr(X_i X_j)$. Because X_i is a symmetric matrix, Δ_{ij} can be written as $\Delta_{ij} = vec(X_i)^T vec(X_j)$, where $vec(\cdot)$ is an operator that vectorized a matrix. As a Gram matrix, Δ is positive semidefinite. So, we have,

$$\|E_i\|_F^2 = \Delta_{ii} - 2\sum_{j=1}^N z_{ij}\Delta_{ij} + \sum_{j_1}^N \sum_{j_2}^N z_{ij_1}z_{ij_2}\Delta_{j_1 j_2}$$

$$= \Delta ii - 2\sum_{j=1}^N z_{ij}\Delta_{ij} + \mathbf{z}_i \Delta \mathbf{z}_i^T.$$

For $\Delta = PP^T$,

$$\|E\|_F^2 = \sum_{i=1}^N \Delta_{ii} - 2tr[Z\Delta] + tr[Z\Delta Z^T]$$

$$= C + \|ZP - P\|_F^2,$$

Then, the optimization is equivalent to:

$$\min_Z \|ZP - P\|_F^2 + \lambda\|Z\|_*.$$

Let Δ be a symmetric matrix, whose entries are $\Delta_{ij} = \Delta_{ji} = tr(X_i X_j)$, and $P = \Delta^{\frac{1}{2}}$. First, we transform the above equation into an equivalent formulation

$$\min_Z \frac{1}{\lambda}\|ZP - P\|_F^2 + \|J\|_*,$$

$$s.t. \quad J = Z.$$

Then by ALM, we have,

$$\min_{Z,J} \frac{1}{\lambda}\|ZP - P\|_F^2 + \|J\|_* + <Y, Z - J> + \frac{\mu}{2}\|Z - J\|_F^2,$$

where, Y is the Lagrange coefficient, λ and μ are scale parameters.

The above problem can be solved by the following two subproblems [17],

$$J_{k+1} = \min_J(\|J\|_* + <Y, Z_k - J> +\frac{\mu}{2}\|Z_k - J\|_F^2)$$

and,

$$Z_{k+1} = \min_Z(\frac{1}{\lambda}\|ZP - P\|_F^2 + <Y, Z - J_k> +\frac{\mu}{2}\|Z - J\|_F^2).$$

Fortunately according to [3], the solutions for the above subproblems have the following close forms,

$$J = \Theta(Z + \frac{Y}{\mu}),$$

$$Z = (\lambda\mu J - \lambda Y + 2\Delta)(2\Delta + \lambda\mu I)^{-1},$$

where, $\Theta(\cdot)$ is the singular value thresholding operator [3].

Thus, by iteratively updating J and Z until the converge conditions are satisfied, a solution for Eq. (4) can be found.

References

1. Arbelaez, P., Maire, M., Fowlkes, C., Malik, J.: Contour detection and hierarchical image segmentation. TPAMI **33**(5), 898–916 (2011)
2. Arsigny, V., Fillard, P., Pennec, X., Ayache, N.: Fast and Simple Computations on Tensors with Log-euclidean Metrics, Phd thesis, INRIA (2005)
3. Cai, J.-F., Candès, E.J., Shen, Z.: A singular value thresholding algorithm for matrix completion. SIAM J. Optim. **20**(4), 1956–1982 (2010)
4. Candès, E.J., Li, X., Ma, Y., Wright, J.: Robust principal component analysis? J. ACM (JACM) **58**(3), 11 (2011)
5. Chen, J., Yang, J.: Robust subspace segmentation via low-rank representation. IEEE Trans. Cybern. **44**(8), 1432–1445 (2014)
6. Comaniciu, D., Meer, P.: Mean shift: a robust approach toward feature space analysis. IEEE Trans. Pattern Anal. Mach. Intell. **24**(5), 603–619 (2002)
7. Felzenszwalb, P.F., Huttenlocher, D.P.: Efficient graph-based image segmentation. Int. J. Comput. Vis. **59**(2), 167–181 (2004)
8. Freixenet, J., Muñoz, X., Raba, D., Martí, J., Cufí, X.: Yet another survey on image segmentation: region and boundary information integration. In: Heyden, A., Sparr, G., Nielsen, M., Johansen, P. (eds.) ECCV 2002, Part III. LNCS, vol. 2352, pp. 408–422. Springer, Heidelberg (2002)
9. Fu, Y., Gao, J., Hong, X., Tien, D.: Low rank representation on Riemannian manifold of symmetric positive definite matrices. In: Proceedings of SDM. SIAM (2015)
10. Ganesh, A., Lin, Z., Wright, J., Wu, L., Chen, M., Ma, Y.: Fast algorithms for recovering a corrupted low-rank matrix. In: 2009 3rd IEEE International Workshop on Computational Advances in Multi-Sensor Adaptive Processing (CAMSAP), pp. 213–216. IEEE (2009)
11. Gu, X., Deng, J.D., Purvis, M.K.: Improving superpixel-based image segmentation by incorporating color covariance matrix manifolds. In: 2014 IEEE International Conference on Image Processing (ICIP), pp. 4403–4406. IEEE (2014)

12. Habiboğlu, Y.H., Günay, O., Çetin, A.E.: Covariance matrix-based fire and flame detection method in video. Mach. Vis. Appl. **23**(6), 1103–1113 (2012)
13. Harandi, M.T., Sanderson, C., Wiliem, A., Lovell, B.C.: Kernel analysis over Riemannian manifolds for visual recognition of actions, pedestrians and textures. In: 2012 IEEE Workshop on Applications of Computer Vision (WACV), pp. 433–439. IEEE (2012)
14. Jayasumana, S., Hartley, R., Salzmann, M., Li, H., Harandi, M.: Kernel methods on Riemannian manifolds with Gaussian RBF kernels. IEEE Trans. Pattern Anal. Mach. Intell. **37**(12), 2464–2477 (2015). IEEE
15. Kolda, T.G., Bader, B.W.: Tensor decompositions and applications. SIAM Rev. **51**(3), 455–500 (2009)
16. Li, Z., Wu, X.-M., Chang, S.-F.: Segmentation using superpixels: a bipartite graph partitioning approach. In: 2012 IEEE Conference on Computer Vision and Pattern Recognition (CVPR), pp. 789–796. IEEE (2012)
17. Lin, Z., Chen, M., Ma, Y.: The augmented Lagrange multiplier method for exact recovery of corrupted low-rank matrices (2010). arXiv preprint arXiv:1009.5055
18. Liu, G., Lin, Z., Yan, S., Sun, J., Yu, Y., Ma, Y.: Robust recovery of subspace structures by low-rank representation. IEEE Trans. Pattern Anal. Mach. Intell. **35**(1), 171–184 (2013)
19. Liu, G., Yan, S.: Latent low-rank representation for subspace segmentation and feature extraction. In: 2011 IEEE International Conference on Computer Vision (ICCV), pp. 1615–1622. IEEE (2011)
20. Martin, D., Fowlkes, C., Tal, D., Malik, J.: A database of human segmented natural images and its application to evaluating segmentation algorithms and measuring ecological statistics. In: ICCV 2001, vol. 2, pp. 416–423 (2001)
21. Meilă, M.: Comparing clusterings: an axiomatic view. In: ICML 2005, pp. 577–584. ACM (2005)
22. Unnikrishnan, R., Pantofaru, C., Hebert, M.: Toward objective evaluation of image segmentation algorithms. TPAMI **29**(6), 929–944 (2007)
23. Wang, B., Hu, Y., Gao, J., Sun, Y., Yin, B.: Kernelized low rank representation on grassmann manifolds (2015). arXiv preprint arXiv:1504.01806
24. Wang, B., Hu, Y., Gao, J., Sun, Y., Yin, B.: Low rank representation on grassmann manifolds: an extrinsic perspective (2015). arXiv preprint arXiv:1504.01807
25. Wang, X., Li, H., Masnou, S., Chen, L.: Sparse coding and mid-level superpixel-feature for ℓ_0-graph based unsupervised image segmentation. In: Wilson, R., Hancock, E., Bors, A., Smith, W. (eds.) CAIP 2013, Part II. LNCS, vol. 8048, pp. 160–168. Springer, Heidelberg (2013)
26. Wright, J., Ganesh, A., Rao, S., Peng, Y., Ma, Y.: Robust principal component analysis: exact recovery of corrupted low-rank matrices via convex optimization. In: Advances in Neural Information Processing Systems, pp. 2080–2088 (2009)
27. Xie, Y., Ho, J., Vemuri, B.: On a nonlinear generalization of sparse coding and dictionary learning. In: Proceedings of the International Conference on Machine Learning, p. 1480. NIH Public Access (2013)

Predictive Analytics for Critical Care (PACC)

Normalized Cross-Match: Pattern Discovery Algorithm from Biofeedback Signals

Xueyuan Gong[1(✉)], Simon Fong[1], Yain-Whar Si[1], Robert P. Biuk-Aghai[1],
Raymond K. Wong[2], and Athanasios V. Vasilakos[3]

[1] Department of Computer and Information Science,
University of Macau, Macau, China
{yb47453,ccfong,fstasp,robertb}@umac.mo
[2] School of Computer Science and Engineering,
University of New South Wales, Sydney, Australia
wong@cse.unsw.edu.au
[3] Department of Computer Science, Electrical and Space Engineering,
Lulea University of Technology, Lulea, Sweden
athanasios.vasilakos@ltu.se

Abstract. Biofeedback signals are important elements in critical care applications, such as monitoring ECG data of a patient, discovering patterns from large amount of ECG data sets, detecting outliers from ECG data, etc. Because the signal data update continuously and the sampling rates may be different, time-series data stream is harder to be dealt with compared to traditional historical time-series data. For the pattern discovery problem on time-series streams, Toyoda proposed the CrossMatch (CM) approach to discover the patterns between two time-series data streams (sequences), which requires only $O(n)$ time per data update, where n is the length of one sequence. CM, however, does not support normalization, which is required for some kinds of sequences (e.g. EEG data, ECG data). Therefore, we propose a normalized-CrossMatch approach (NCM) that extends CM to enforce normalization while maintaining the same performance capabilities.

Keywords: Pattern discovery · CrossMatch · NCM · Time-series streams

1 Introduction

Biofeedback signals in the form of time-series data are significant to critical care applications. For example, monitoring electrocardiogram (ECG) data of patient (ECG data is a kind of time-series data stream) helps to save human resources to monitor the ECG of the patient, discovering common patterns from large amount of ECG data sets may find specific pattern which represents the body condition of the patient, detecting outliers from ECG data helps to discover the

---

The original version of this chapter was revised: The spelling of the fourth author's name was corrected. The erratum to this chapter is available at DOI: 10.1007/978-3-319-42996-0_24

H. Cao et al. (Eds.): PAKDD 2016 Workshops, LNAI 9794, pp. 169–180, 2016.
DOI: 10.1007/978-3-319-42996-0_14

problem of human health, etc. In general, most healthcare applications would have to deal with time-series, for analysis, matching, comparison and so forth. Other applications include but not limit to financial data, web click-stream data, motion capture data, and sensor network data. A number of different approaches for dealing with data streams have been proposed in the literature, e.g. subsequence matching [6,16], pattern discovery [17–19], and outlier detection [3,4].

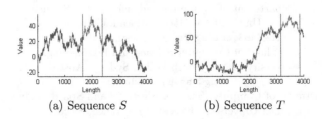

(a) Sequence S (b) Sequence T

Fig. 1. Discovered patterns in time-series data streams (Color figure online)

The objective of pattern discovery in data streams is to find common patterns among n data streams. Hence, the basis of the problem is to find common patterns between two data streams. Figure 1 shows an example of pattern discovery between two data streams. The red lines in Fig. 1 represent the patterns discovered in two respective sequences. Toyoda et al. [19] proposed an approach called CrossMatch (CM) to solve this problem. CM is based on the dynamic time warping (DTW) distance measure. CM is very efficient with respect to time and space complexity, which only requires $O(w)$ per data update and $O(wn)$ in total, where w is a parameter to constrain the warping window and n is the length of the data streams (assuming that the two data streams are of the same length).

Nevertheless, the original version of CM does not consider normalization. Normalization is required [8,14] to report meaningful patterns for many data sets. In other words, CM does not support normalization and it does not support many data sets, e.g. biosignals. Moreover, CM cannot discover the patterns shown in Fig. 1.

Because CM is very effective and efficient and uses a simple algorithm, in this paper we propose an algorithm called normalized-CrossMatch (NCM), which extends CM to support normalization while preserving its advantages.

The remainder of this paper is organized as follows: In Sect. 2, we discuss the related works on DTW and the relevant pattern discovery approaches. The naive solution (NS) and NCM are introduced in Sect. 3. The experimental results and analysis are then provided in Sect. 4. Finally, Sect. 5 concludes the paper.

2   Related Work

In this section, we review the literature on DTW and then review the existing pattern discovery approaches.

There are two popular similarity measure approaches for comparing the similarities between two time series, namely, Euclidean distance (ED) and DTW. According to previous works [1,20], DTW is superior to ED in terms of effectiveness. Yet, the time complexity of DTW is $O(n^2)$ whereas that of ED is $O(n)$. Therefore, DTW has significant research potential and numerous studies have focused on accelerating it. Warping window constraints are proposed to constrain the path of DTW to reduce the calculation of the DTW distances [7,15]. Keogh and Ratanamahatana [9] proposed a lower bounding approach to efficiently calculate a bound to avoid the expensive DTW distance calculation. Keogh et al. [10] proposed an early abandoning approach to eliminate unnecessary calculation of the DTW distance.

Although DTW is effective, ED has the advantage of efficiency. Accordingly, a number of pattern discovery approaches based on ED have been proposed in the literature. Chiu et al. [5] first proposed the motif (pattern) discovery approach. The smart brute-force (SBF) approach [12] was then proposed to calculate smartly the distance between neighboring subsequences to reduce the computational time. Mueen et al. [13] proposed the Mueen-Keogh (MK) approach, which uses a reference index to prune unnecessary calculations. Recently, Li et al. [11] proposed the Quick-Motif (QM) approach to combine the locality of neighboring subsequences with the pruning of unnecessary calculations. However, the objective of motif discovery is slightly different from that of pattern discovery. Specifically, the goal of motif discovery is to find the most similar subsequence pair between two time series, whereas the aim of pattern discovery is to find all of the similar subsequence pairs between two time series. In addition, motif discovery requires the length of the motif to be fixed while pattern discovery allows the length of the pattern to be within an available range. Therefore, as the focus of motif discovery is different from that of pattern discovery, we do not compare our approach with the motif discovery approaches.

The other branch of pattern discovery is the DTW-based approaches. Toyoda et al. [18] first tried to discover the patterns between two time series by only calculating a matrix. Toyoda and Sakurai [17] then proposed a cross-similarity method for the pattern discovery. Later, the CM approach [19] was proposed to effectively and efficiently discover the patterns in time-series data streams. Yet, none of these approaches consider normalization. In contrast, all of the ED-based motif discovery approaches consider normalization. Therefore, in this paper, we propose the NCM approach to make the pattern discovery problem more applicable.

3   Proposed Method

In this section, we first introduce the notations and problem definition. Next, the naive solution (NS) is introduced as a straightforward way to solve the pattern discovery problem. Then, the NCM approach is proposed as an improved solution to the pattern discovery problem.

3.1 Notation and Problem Definition

We first define the key terms used in this paper and then define the problem definition. First, the data streams (sequences) are defined: Sequence $S = \{s_1, s_2, \ldots, s_n\}$ and $T = \{t_1, t_2, \ldots, t_m\}$ are two ordered sets, where s_i and t_i represent the i-th value of S and T, respectively. The lengths of S and T are denoted as $|S| = n$ and $|T| = m$, respectively. With sequences S and T, the aim of the pattern discovery problem is to discover similar subsequences between S and T. A subsequence is defined: Subsequences $S_{i,j}$ and $T_{i',j'}$ are two subsequences of S and T, respectively, where $S_{i,j}$ starts from s_i and ends at s_j ($1 \leq i \leq j \leq n$), while $T_{i',j'}$ starts from $t_{i'}$ and ends at $t_{j'}$ ($1 \leq i' \leq j' \leq m$). Now, we are in position to define the problem based on the definitions of a sequence and subsequence.

Problem Definition. Given two sequences S and T, find all similar subsequence pairs $S_{i,j}$ and $T_{i',j'}$ between S and T, where the distance of $S_{i,j}$ and $T_{i',j'}$ is smaller than or equal to a threshold ε times $(|S_{i,j}| + |T_{i',j'}|)/2$, denoted as $Dist(S_{i,j}, T_{i',j'}) \leq \varepsilon(|S_{i,j}| + |T_{i',j'}|)/2$. In addition, $|S_{i,j}|$ and $|T_{i',j'}|$ are defined to be bigger or equal to a minimum length l_{min}, denoted $|S_{i,j}| \geq l_{min}$ and $|T_{i',j'}| \geq l_{min}$.

The reason for defining a minimum length l_{min} is to limit the number of trivial patterns to be discovered. As the lengths of $S_{i,j}$ and $T_{i',j'}$ are defined to be variable, many patterns with very short lengths will be discovered, e.g. $|S_{i,j}| = 3$ and $|T_{i',j'}| = 4$ while $|S| = 20000$ and $|T| = 18000$. Therefore, we define l_{min} to make it applicable to the algorithm.

3.2 Naive Solution (NS)

Given two sequences S and T, the NS will exhaustively compare all pairs $S_{i,j}$ and $T_{i',j'}$ between S and T, regardless of the limitation of l_{min}. For each length of interest, denoted as w, of the subsequence pairs, the required time complexity is $O(nmw^2)$. In detail, the computational time to calculate the distance of $S_{i,j}$ and $T_{i',j'}$ is $O(w^2)$ (DTW distance) as the length of each $S_{i,j}$ and $T_{i',j'}$ is w. Moreover, all $S_{i,j}$ ($n - w$, which is approximately equal to n) are compared with $T_{i',j'}$ ($m - w$, which is approximately equal to m), and thus the time complexity is $O(nm)$. In conclusion, the time complexity is $O(nmw^2)$. Moreover, to prune trivial subsequence pairs that are too short, there is no need to search for all possible lengths of interest w. Suppose there are θ lengths of interest w, then the time complexity becomes $O(\theta nmw^2)$.

3.3 Normalized-CrossMatch

Calculate Normalized Value. Before introducing the NCM algorithm, the approach to calculate the normalized values s'_j and $t'_{j'}$ should be introduced. Equation (1) illustrates the method to calculate s'_j and $t'_{j'}$.

$$s'_j = \frac{s_j - \mu^s_{i,j}}{\sigma^s_{i,j}} \qquad t'_{j'} = \frac{t_{j'} - \mu^t_{i',j'}}{\sigma^t_{i',j'}} \tag{1}$$

where $\mu^s_{i,j}$ and $\mu^t_{i',j'}$ are the means of $S_{i,j}$ and $T_{i',j'}$, while $\sigma^s_{i,j}$ and $\sigma^t_{i',j'}$ are the standard deviations of $S_{i,j}$ and $T_{i',j'}$, respectively. μ and σ can be calculated as follows:

$$\mu_{i,j} = \frac{1}{j-i+1} \sum_{r=i}^{j} x_r \qquad \sigma_{i,j} = \sqrt{\frac{1}{j-i+1} \sum_{r=i}^{j} x_r^2 - \mu_{i,j}^2} \tag{2}$$

Note that the form of the equation that calculates $\sigma_{i,j}$ is changed to reduce the computational time. Here, we calculate $\mu_{i,j}$ and $\sigma_{i,j}$ by the sums of x_r and x_r^2, respectively, which takes O(n) time to compute. The two sum values A and $A2$ are shown below:

$$A_{i,j} = \sum_{r=i}^{j} x_r \qquad A'_{i,j} = \sum_{r=i}^{j} x_r^2 \tag{3}$$

Based on Eq. (3), it is possible to calculate $\mu_{i+1,j+1}$ and $\sigma_{i+1,j+1}$ in O(1) rather than O(n). We can have $\mu_{i,j} = A_{i,j}/(j-i+1)$ and $\sigma_{i,j} = \sqrt{A'_{i,j}/(j-i+1) - \mu_{i,j}^2}$ from Eq. (3). Thus, $\mu_{i+1,j+1}$ and $\sigma_{i+1,j+1}$ can be calculated as follows:

$$\mu_{i+1,j+1} = \frac{1}{j-i+1}(A_{i,j} - x_i + x_{j+1})$$
$$\sigma_{i+1,j+1} = \sqrt{\frac{1}{j-i+1}(A'_{i,j} - x_i^2 + x_{j+1}^2) - \mu_{i+1,j+1}^2} \tag{4}$$

According to Eq. (4), the computational time is only O(1). In detail, the two sum values $A_{i,j}$ and $A'_{i,j}$ are calculated according to Eq. (2), which takes O(n) time. Then, whenever new data are updated, $A_{i,j}$ and $A'_{i,j}$ can be calculated according to Eq. (4), which takes O(1) time.

Algorithm of NCM. According to the CM algorithm proposed in [19], we propose an extended algorithm called NCM, which supports normalization while ensuring the advantages of CM, i.e. low space and time complexity.

Given sequences S and T, we first define a similarity metric score [17,19] to combine threshold ε with distance. The equation is given below:

$$Scr(S_{i,j}, T_{i',j'}) = \varepsilon(|S_{i,j}| + |T_{i',j'}|)/2 - Dist(S_{i,j}, T_{i',j'}) \tag{5}$$

Then, the criterion to discover patterns is changed from $Dist(S_{i,j}, T_{i',j'}) \leq \varepsilon(|S_{i,j}| + |T_{i',j'}|)/2$ to $\varepsilon(|S_{i,j}| + |T_{i',j'}|)/2 - Dist(S_{i,j}, T_{i',j'}) \geq 0$. Next, we define a matrix called the normalized score matrix which is extended from the score matrix [17] to calculate $SCR(S_{i,j}, T_{i',j'})$. Thus, by calculating the matrix we are able to discover the patterns between S and T rather than exhaustively comparing all of the subsequence pairs between S and T. Each entry of the matrix is denoted as $SM(j, j')$ (j and j' are the indices of the end points of $S_{i,j}$ and $T_{i',j'}$). Then, $Scr(S_{i,j}, T_{i',j'})$ can be calculated as follows:

$$Scr(S_{i,j}, T_{i',j'}) = SM(j, j') \tag{6}$$

$$SM(j, j') = -||s'_j - t'_{j'}|| + \max \begin{cases} 0 \\ \varepsilon/2 + M(j, j' - 1) \\ \varepsilon/2 + M(j - 1, j') \\ \varepsilon + M(j - 1, j' - 1) \end{cases} \tag{7}$$

where $M(0,0) = M(j,0) = M(0,j') = 0$ ($j = 1, 2, \ldots, n$ and $j' = 1, 2, \ldots, m$) and s'_j and $t'_{j'}$ are normalized values of s_j and t_j, respectively. However, the normalized score matrix cannot record the indices of the start points of $S_{i,j}$ and $T_{i',j'}$. Thus, another matrix is needed to keep the start points of $S_{i,j}$ and $T_{i',j'}$, which is called the position matrix [17,19]. Each entry of the position matrix is $PM(j, j')$ and the equation of the position matrix is given below:

$$PM(j, j') = \begin{cases} PM(j - 1, j') & \text{If } M(j - 1, j') \neq 0 \text{ and} \\ & (\varepsilon/2 + M(j - 1, j')) \text{ is max in Eq. (7)} \\ PM(j, j' - 1) & \text{If } M(j, j' - 1) \neq 0 \text{ and} \\ & (\varepsilon/2 + M(j, j' - 1)) \text{ is max in Eq. (7)} \\ PM(j - 1, j' - 1) & \text{If } M(j - 1, j' - 1) \neq 0 \text{ and} \\ & (\varepsilon + M(j - 1, j' - 1)) \text{ is max in Eq. (7)} \\ (j, j') & \text{otherwise} \end{cases} \tag{8}$$

In conclusion, three kinds of information are recorded by the score matrix SM and the position matrix PM, namely, the score (the similarity metric), the start position, and the end position. Note that the end position is implied by j and j' in Eq. (7) when two similar subsequences are found. Thus, it is possible to discover patterns between S and T.

Parameters Set in NCM. After introducing the method to efficiently calculate the normalized value (Sect. 3.3) and presenting the method for calculating the two matrices (Sect. 3.3), a contradictory issue still needs to be solved. Specifically, the length of the subsequence should be known in advance before calculating the normalized value of the subsequence as implied in Sect. 3.3, namely, i and j should be determined before calculating $\mu_{i,j}$ and $\sigma_{i,j}$. However, it is impossible to know the starting positions i and i' before the similar subsequence pairs are found according to Eq. (7). Therefore, a parameter l_e is set to determine the expected length of subsequence $\mu_{i,j}$, and $\sigma_{i,j}$ can be successfully calculated based on l_e. A second parameter l_w is also set to determine the minimum length of subsequence l_{min}, where $l_{min} = l_e - l_w$. Moreover, the threshold ε (Sect. 3.1), which is proportional to the length of the subsequence, is set. Thus, the similar subsequence pairs should satisfy Eq. (9) as shown below:

$$Scr(S_{i,j}, T_{i',j'}) \geq \varepsilon(l_e - l_w) \tag{9}$$

Therefore, it is possible to compute $\mu_{i,j}$ and $\sigma_{i,j}$ without the start positions i and i'. Thus, Eq. (3) can be written as follows:

$$A_{j-l_e+1,j} = \sum_{r=j-l_e+1}^{j} x_r \qquad A'_{j-l_e+1,j} = \sum_{r=j-l_e+1}^{j} x_r^2 \qquad (10)$$

In this way, the start positions i and i' are ignored and thus Eq. (4) is changed as follows:

$$\mu_{j-l_e+2,j+1} = \frac{1}{l_e}(A_{j-l_e+1,j} - x_{j-l_e+1} + x_{j+1})$$

$$\sigma_{j-l_e+2,j+1} = \sqrt{\frac{1}{l_e}(A'_{j-l_e+1,j} - x^2_{j-l_e+1} + x^2_{j+1}) - \mu^2_{j-l_e+2,j+1}} \qquad (11)$$

Based on Eqs. (10) and (11), Eq. (1) is changed to the style shown below:

$$s'_j = \frac{s_j - \mu^s_{j-l_e+1,j}}{\sigma^s_{j-l_e+1,j}} \qquad t'_{j'} = \frac{t_{j'} - \mu^t_{j'-l_e+1,j'}}{\sigma^t_{j'-l_e+1,j'}} \qquad (12)$$

Hence, s'_j and $t'_{j'}$ in Eq. (7) can be calculated successfully according to Eq. (12).

Pattern Discovery Procedure in NCM. We are now ready to introduce the procedure for pattern discovery in NCM, which is similar to the CM algorithm in [19] but slightly different in that NCM supports normalization. First, two variables are initialized, $C' = \{C'_{scr}, C'_{sp}, C'_{ep}\}$ and CS, where C' denotes a candidate of a subsequence pair (C'_{scr} represents the score of the subsequence pair, C'_{sp} represents the start positions of the subsequence pair, and C'_{ep} represents the end positions of the subsequence pair) and CS denotes a set of candidates of the subsequence pair.

Next, as long as new normalized data s'_j or $t'_{j'}$ are calculated, C' will be updated by the Eqs. (7) and (8). Then, as long as $C'_{scr} \geq \varepsilon(l_e - l_w)$, C' will be added to CS if C'_{sp} does not exist in CS or C' will substitute the current one if $C'_{scr} \geq C_{scr}$. Finally, if a candidate C in CS satisfies $(\forall_r, SP(j,r) \neq C_{sp}) \wedge (\forall_r, SP(r,j') \neq C_{sp})$, C is regarded as a similar subsequence pair (discovered pattern).

4   Experimental Results

In this section, we carry out experiments on synthetic data to demonstrate that the execution time of NCM can be nearly seven orders of magnitude faster than NS. Moreover, the execution time of NCM is of the same order of magnitude as CM, while NCM supports normalization and CM does not. Our experiments are conducted on a computer equipped with an Intel Xeon E5-1650 CPU at 3.5 GHz, 64 GB memory, and the Windows 7 operating system. The programming language is C++ and the development environment is Microsoft Visual Studio 2013.

4.1   Test on Synthetic Data Sets

We create synthetic data to test the execution times of NCM, NS, and CM on sequences of different lengths. The synthetic data generation algorithm is adopted from [2,11,13], which is given in Eq. (13).

$$s_{i+1} = s_i + N(0,1) \tag{13}$$

where $N(0,1)$ is a function to generate random values subject to a normal distribution. The mean and the standard deviation of the normal distribution are set to 0 and 1, respectively.

Based on Eq. (13), we generate four pairs of sequences with different lengths, i.e. 2000, 4000, 8000, and 16000 data points. We then insert a pattern (the length of which is 760 and is shown in Fig. 2) deliberately into two sequences of each pair. Finally, the NCM, NS, and CM algorithms are tested on these four pairs of sequences to check the execution time and whether they can find the testing pattern correctly.

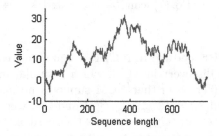

Fig. 2. Pattern inserted into synthetic data

Before proceeding to the results of the experiment, we need to emphasize that NS is too slow to obtain a result. Therefore, NS is only tested on the synthetic data with a length of 2000. For synthetic data with a length of 4000, we estimate that it is at least two times slower than synthetic data with a length of 2000. Specifically, it requires at least 1.1×10^7 s, which equals nearly 127.3 days. Hence, we omit the experiments of NS for synthetic data with lengths of 4000, 8000, and 16000 for convenience. The parameters used in NCM, NS, and CM are summarized in Table 1.

Now, we are in position to introduce the results of the experiments, which are shown in Table 2. For better illustration, the execution times of NCM, NS, and CM are also given in Fig. 3.

As shown in Table 2, NCM and NS can successfully retrieve the inserted pattern, while CM cannot retrieve any of the pattern. Yet, NCM has a nearly $3\% \sim 16\%$ bias, which is compromised for speed as the length of the pattern retrieved by NCM is variant. However, $3\% \sim 15\%$ inaccuracy is acceptable as the execution time is at least seven orders of magnitude faster than NS.

Table 1. Parameters used in NCM, NS, and CM

Parameter	NCM	NS	CM
eps	0.01	0.0001	0.01
eL	800	800	/
dL	300	300	/
wL	4000	/	/
mL	/	/	500

Note that NS will retrieve many trivial patterns that neighbor each other, as the neighboring subsequences are, of course, similar. Therefore, we choose one pattern with the least DTW distance from the overlapped patterns. As expected, CM cannot retrieve any of the inserted pattern because of the normalization-support problem.

Table 2. Results of NCM, NS, and CM on synthetic data sets

Method	Length	Discovered pattern	Score/distance	Wall clock time (sec)
NCM	2000	$S_{939,1572}$ $T_{1238,1863}$	6.13	0.279
	4000	$S_{1661,2376}$ $T_{3155,3868}$	6.65	1.247
	8000	$S_{4577,5394}$ $T_{6575,7381}$	7.36	3.899
	16000	$S_{11639,12374}$ $T_{12640,13385}$	6.44	10.868
NS	2000	$S_{805,1564}$ $T_{1105,1864}$	0.0001	5.46×10^6
CM	2000	/	/	0.198
	4000	/	/	0.943
	8000	/	/	3.182
	16000	/	/	9.746

Figure 3 gives a more straightforward depiction of the execution times of NCM, NS, and CM, where the dashed line represents NS, the straight line represents NCM, and the dotted line represents CM. There is only one point on the line of NS and the line is dashed, which means we only test the NS on synthetic data with a length of 2000 and the trend is estimated by analysis of the NS algorithm. According to Table 2, the execution times of NCM and NS are 0.279 and 5.46×10^6, respectively. Therefore, NCM is $5.46 \times 10^6/0.279 = 1.96 \times 10^7$ times faster than NS, which is seven orders of magnitude faster. In addition, NCM and CM overlap as they are of the same order of magnitude. Thus, we zoom-in on their lines in Fig. 3(b) to better illustrate their relationship. As shown in Fig. 3(b), NCM is slightly slower than CM, but they are still of the same order of magnitude, which indicates that NCM preserves the time efficiency of CM while extending CM to support normalization.

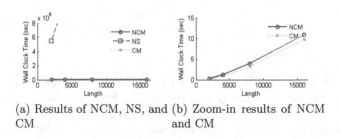

(a) Results of NCM, NS, and CM

(b) Zoom-in results of NCM and CM

Fig. 3. Execution time of NCM, NS, and CM

Synthetic data with a length of 8000 are chosen as an example to illustrate the results, which are given in Fig. 4. The red line in Fig. 4 represents the discovered pattern, which has nearly 7.5 % inaccuracy. Obviously, the discovered pattern is similar to the original pattern (Fig. 2). Thus, the effectiveness of NCM is acceptable, although with some inaccuracy. Note that all of the synthetic data sets require normalization and thus CM cannot discover any patterns in any of the synthetic data sets.

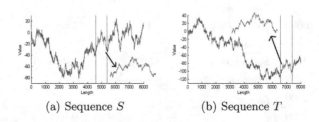

(a) Sequence S (b) Sequence T

Fig. 4. Discovered patterns in synthetic data with length 8000 (Color figure online)

5   Conclusion

In this paper, we propose the NCM approach, which supports normalization, after reviewing the shortcomings of CM with respect to normalization. NCM not only supports normalization but also preserves the time and space complexity of CM, which are O(nm) in total, where n and m are the lengths of two sequences. The focus of NCM is on time-series data streams rather than on traditional stored data.

In the near future, we plan to do more experiments on NCM to test the applicability of NCM to real bio-data sets, e.g. EEG data, ECG data, EDA data. Additionally, we also plan to apply several accelerating techniques used in the data mining and database community that have not yet been applied to NCM.

Acknowledgments. The authors are thankful for the financial supports by the Macao Science and Technology Development Fund under the research project (No. 126/2014/A3), titled A Scalable Data Stream Mining Methodology: Stream-based Holistic Analytics and Reasoning in Parallel, by the University of Macau and the Macau SAR government.

References

1. Aach, J., Church, G.M.: Aligning gene expression time series with time warping algorithms. Bioinformatics **17**, 495–508 (2001)
2. Agrawal, R., Faloutsos, C., Swami, A.: Efficient similarity search in sequence databases. In: Lomet, D.B. (ed.) FODO 1993. LNCS, vol. 730, pp. 69–84. Springer, Heidelberg (1993)
3. Angiulli, F., Fassetti, F.: Detecting distance-based outliers in streams of data. In: Proceedings of the 16th Conference on Information and Knowledge Management (CIKM), pp. 811–820 (2007)
4. Bu, Y., Chen, L., Fu, A.W.-C., Liu, D.: Efficient anomaly monitoring over moving object trajectory streams. In: Proceedings of the 15th International Conference on Knowledge Discovery and Data Mining (SIGKDD), pp. 159–168 (2009)
5. Chiu, B., Keogh, E., Lonardi, S.: Probabilistic discovery of time series motifs. In: Proceedings of the 9th International Conference on Knowledge Discovery and Data Mining (SIGKDD), pp. 493–498 (2003)
6. Gong, X., Si, Y.-W., Fong, S., Mohammed, S.: NSPRING: normalization-supported SPRING for subsequence matching on time series streams. In: IEEE 15th International Symposium on Computational Intelligence and Informatics (CINTI), pp. 373–378 (2014)
7. Itakura, F.: Minimum prediction residual principle applied to speech recognition. IEEE Trans. Acoust. Speech Signal Process. **23**, 67–72 (1975)
8. Keogh, E., Kasetty, S.: On the need for time series data mining benchmarks: a survey and empirical demonstration. Data Min. Knowl. Discov. **7**, 349–371 (2003)
9. Keogh, E., Ratanamahatana, C.A.: Exact indexing of dynamic time warping. Knowl. Inf. Syst. **7**, 358–386 (2005)
10. Keogh, E., Wei, L., Xi, X., Vlachos, M., Lee, S.-H., Protopapas, P.: Supporting exact indexing of arbitrarily rotated shapes and periodic time series under euclidean and warping distance measures. Int. J. Very Large Data Bases **18**, 611–630 (2009)
11. Li, Y., Leong Hou, U., Yiu, M.L., Gong, Z.: Quick-motif: an efficient and scalable framework for exact motif discovery. In: Proceedings of the International Conference on Data Engineering (ICDE) (2014)
12. Mueen, A.: Enumeration of time series motifs of all lengths. In: IEEE 13th International Conference on Data Mining (ICDM), pp. 547–556 (2013)
13. Mueen, A., Keogh, E.J., Zhu, Q., Cash, S., Westover, M.B.: Exact discovery of time series motifs. In: SDM, pp. 473–484 (2009)

14. Rakthanmanon, T., Campana, B., Mueen, A., Batista, G., Westover, B., Zhu, Q., Zakaria, J., Keogh, E.: Searching and mining trillions of time series subsequences under dynamic time warping. In: Proceedings of the 18th International Conference on Knowledge Discovery and Data Mining (SIGKDD), pp. 262–270 (2012)
15. Sakoe, H., Chiba, S.: Dynamic programming algorithm optimization for spoken word recognition. IEEE Trans. Acoust. Speech Signal Process. **26**, 43–49 (1978)
16. Sakurai, Y., Faloutsos, C., Yamamuro, M.: Stream monitoring under the time warping distance. In: IEEE 23rd International Conference on Data Engineering (ICDE), pp. 1046–1055 (2007)
17. Toyoda, M., Sakurai, Y.: Discovery of cross-similarity in data streams. In: IEEE 26th International Conference on Data Engineering (ICDE), pp. 101–104 (2010)
18. Toyoda, M., Sakurai, Y., Ichikawa, T.: Identifying similar subsequences in data streams. In: Bhowmick, S.S., Küng, J., Wagner, R. (eds.) DEXA 2008. LNCS, vol. 5181, pp. 210–224. Springer, Heidelberg (2008)
19. Toyoda, M., Sakurai, Y., Ishikawa, Y.: Pattern discovery in data streams under the time warping distance. VLDB J. **22**, 295–318 (2013)
20. Yi, B.-K., Jagadish, H., Faloutsos, C.: Efficient retrieval of similar time sequences under time warping. In: Proceedings of the 14th International Conference on Data Engineering (ICDE), pp. 201–208 (1998)

Event Prediction in Healthcare Analytics:
Beyond Prediction Accuracy

Lina Fu[(✉)], Faming Li, Jing Zhou, Xuejin Wen, Jinhui Yao,
and Michael Shepherd

PARC, A Xerox Company, Palo Alto, USA
{lina.fu,faming.li,jing.zhou,xuejin.wen,jinhui.yao,
michael.shepherd}@parc.com

Abstract. During the recent few years, the United States healthcare
industry is under unprecedented pressure to improve outcome and reduce
cost. Many healthcare organizations are leveraging healthcare analytics,
especially predictive analytics in moving towards these goals and bringing
better value to the patients. While many existing event prediction models
provide helpful predictions in terms of accuracy, their use are typically
limited to prioritizing individual patients for care management at fixed
time points. In this paper we explore Enhanced Modeling approaches
around two important aspects: (1) model interpretability; (2) flexible prediction window. Better interpretability of the model will guide us towards
more effective intervention design. Flexible prediction window can provide a higher resolution picture of patients' risks of adverse events over
time, and thereby enable timely interventions. We illustrate interpretation and insights from our Bayesian Hierarchical Model for readmission
prediction, and demonstrate flexible prediction window with Random
Survival Forests model for prediction of future emergency department
visits.

Keywords: Healthcare analytics · Predictive modeling · Bayesian
Hierarchical Model · Random Survival Forests

1   Introduction

The current healthcare system in United States is unsustainable due to the ever
rising cost. Particularly the cost in United States is nearly twice as high as in
most other developed countries [1].The rapid cost growth is driven by aging
population, the pervasiveness of chronic diseases, the shortage of primary care
physician and nursing, inefficiency and lack of quality. Healthcare providers and
payers are also under increasing pressure from consumers to improve quality
and deliver better outcomes. In response, healthcare industry is experiencing
fundamental transformation as it moves from a volume-based business to a value-
based business. The ongoing payment reform strategies that incentivize value

---

L. Fu and F. Li—Equal contribution.

© Springer International Publishing Switzerland 2016
H. Cao et al. (Eds.): PAKDD 2016 Workshops, LNAI 9794, pp. 181–189, 2016.
DOI: 10.1007/978-3-319-42996-0_15

such as accountable care and bundling (a payment approach in which providers are asked to deliver a set of services for a predefined price) are intended to motivate organizations to improve the efficiency of their care.

One strategy that healthcare organizations start to deploy is leveraging their healthcare data to gain insights for optimizing their operation. With rapid adoption of electronic health records (EHRs) in healthcare systems, it is possible for data scientists to access unprecedented amount of clinical data. For example, a large integrated healthcare system such as Kaiser Permanente, with approximately nine million members, may manage up to forty-four petabytes of data through its EHR system alone [2]. Currently, the healthcare organizations are looking more toward predictive analytics, which enable them to "see" future events using historical data. Ultimately, organizations will want to be able to take advantage of prescriptive analytics to provide decision makers with sophisticated recommendations for optimal future outcomes.

2   Current Methods for Event Prediction

In healthcare there are various needs for predictive analytics. The majority of them involve predicting future adverse events based on observed historical information. Examples of adverse events include hospital admission [3], hospital readmission [4,5], emergency department (ED) visit [4], disease onset [6], critical events that occur in intensive care units (ICUs) [7], cardiac arrest [8], and mortality [9].

The typical event prediction in healthcare analytics is formulated as a classification question: predict whether a future event will occur during a fixed future time window, given historic data from an observation period. A example is to predict whether a patient will visit the emergency department in the next six month or not, given observed data from the past year. A variety of classification methods have been used for this type of questions. Billings et al. used a collection of multivariate logistic regressions to predict hospital admission and readmission in England [3]. Kartoun et al. used logistic regression with the adaptive LASSO to predict the likelihood of 30 day readmission following an index congested heart failure admission [5]. Somanchi et al. used Support vector machine and logistic regression with LASSO penalty to predict if a patient will go into cardiac arrest in hospital.

The classification models have provided useful prediction in most cases in terms of accuracy. However, the interpretability and actionable insights from predictive models can be as important, if not more, in practical applications. The widely used Logistic regression provides limited interpretability. Care providers can see which risk factors are contributing to an individual patients' high risk score, and tailor interventions around these risk factors. However, logistic regression falls short when it comes to explaining a large number of multilevel categorical variables. To address this limitation, we will discuss Bayesian Hierarchical Model (BHM) for predicting hospital readmission in Sect. 3. BHM is a statistical model in hierarchical form that estimates the parameters of the posterior distribution using the Bayesian method. Another limitation in existing event prediction models for healthcare is the fixed prediction window. Typically a separate model is required for each prediction window. In Sect. 4, we will illustrate the use of Random Survival Forests (RSF) to generate a continuous prediction of probability for future emergency department visits. RSF is an ensemble tree method for the analysis of right censored survival data. In our studies we used claim data from one US state Medicaid program, which include around 50 hospitals.

3   Hospital Readmission Prediction with Bayesian Hierarchical Model

Current readmission risk prediction are helpful for care providers to prioritize their efforts in managing higher-risk patients. However, they are not necessarily adequate in providing insights to some of the deeper drivers and guiding system-level interventions or policies. For example, healthcare agencies are often interested in comparing entities, such as hospitals, geographical regions, in a statistically risk-adjusted fashion, so that they could scrutinize the worse performing entities while identifying best practices among the better performing ones. Unfortunately, logistic regression does not allow one to estimate the individual effects of different groups reliably, especially when the number of groups are large. Bayesian Hierarchical Model (BHM) [10], on the other hand, estimates fixed-effects across groups as well as random effects by different groups. This approach performs partial pooling among the groups, and thereby reduces the uncertainties in parameter estimates for groups with small sample size. As a result, it enables us to model categorical variables involving a large number of groups. Also, in logistic regression, the coefficients for categorical variables are estimated with respect to a reference group in the category, it is generally difficult to look for outlier groups in that category with statistical significance. And when multiple categorical variables are modeled, interpreting the effects for each group become extremely awkward, if not impossible. Whereas in BHM, since the coefficients are estimated relative to the average group effect, it's much easier to interpret and compare the contribution of different groups and identify outliers.

The outcome variable of our model is the rate of all-cause, unplanned readmission or death within 30 days of discharging from an acute index hospital admission, while using features shown in Table 1 as predictors. The majority of features are selected using logistic regression with LASSO penalty. Specifically Major Diagnosis Category has 17 levels, insurer has 5 levels, ethnicity has 8 levels, and hospital has 42 levels. With logistic regression, essentially a separate intercept is estimated for each unique combination of these subgroups. Our training data has a decent size of close to 20,000 samples. But as one might imagine, for some of these subgroups, the numbers of samples are very limited, leading to large variance in the corresponding coefficient estimates. The partial pooling BHM performs improves these estimates significantly.

Before we proceed to interpret the BHM and compare the group effects, we should mention that BHM does not sacrifice the prediction performance in terms

Table 1. Features used in Bayesian Hierarchical Model for readmission prediction

Index stay	Length of stay
	Major diagnosis category
Demographic & administrative	Age
	Ethnicity
	Insurer
	Hospital
Encounter history	Number of emergency room visits in the past 6 months
	Number of acute admissions in the past year
	Number of readmissions in the past year
	Total length of acute hospital stay in the past year
Comorbidity	Chronic obstructive pulmonary disease
	Liver disease
	Hemiplegia or paraplegia
	Malignancy and tumor

of C statistic. The C statistic reported for all-cause readmission are in the range of 0.64 to 0.78 for studies using claim data ([11,12]). We have achieved a C statistic of 0.78 with logistic regression, and 0.75 when we excluded planned readmission (ICD-9 diagnosis code V58.11, Encounter for antineoplastic chemotherapy) as defined in this study. The BHM also produces C statistic of 0.75.

As an example of comparing effects of different groups on readmission risks, first let's take a look at the ethnicities groups. Figure 1(a) shows the coefficient means and standard deviations of ethnicity groups 1 through 8. Ethnicity group 3 and 6 are shown to be significantly higher risk than average, with more than 84 % of the subpopulation having higher than average readmission risk (mean is at least one standard deviation above zero). In fact, from the MCMC simulation traces in estimating BHM, we could find a fairly accurate estimate of the percentage of population in each group that have higher than average readmission risk. Therefore, one could adjust the detection threshold for identifying outlier groups depending on the application needs. For comparison, Fig. 1(b) shows the readmission rates by ethnicity group directly from the data. We can see BHM

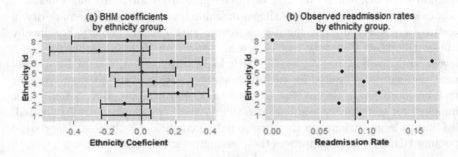

Fig. 1. Ethnicity coefficients in BHM, compared with readmission rates by ethnicity group.

is consistent with the data in identifying the two outlier groups, but adjusts the comparison by accounting for other readmission risk factors, and also provides more detailed information on the magnitude and variance of the contributions of these groups.

As a second example, we examine the comparison of different hospitals in terms of readmission risk. Figure 2(a) shows the coefficient means and standard deviations of Hospitals 1 through 42. As highlighted in the figure, Hospitals 13 and 23 are shown to be significantly lower risk than average, while Hospital 28 has significantly higher risk than average. For comparison, Fig. 2(b) shows the readmission rates by hospital directly from the data. Again we see BHM is consistent with the data in identifying the three outlier groups, while adjusting the comparison by accounting for other readmission risk factors as well as sample sizes in each hospital. For instance, Hospital 31 has a readmission rate of zero. However, its sample size of 29 is not large enough for us to conclude that it is associated with a significant lower than average readmission risk. Therefore, in Fig. 2(a) it does not stand out as an outlier.

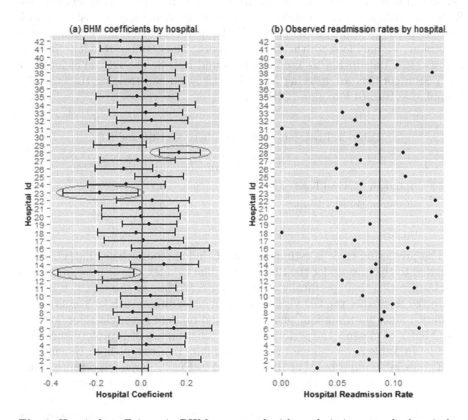

Fig. 2. Hospital coefficients in BHM, compared with readmission rates by hospital.

4   ED Visit Prediction with Random Survival Forests

The ED predictive modeling estimates the risk (probability) of a patient visiting hospital emergency department within a future timeframe. Sometime it is preferred to pinpoint the risk at any time point. For instance, a care provider would like to know when a patient will have high risk so as to plan for intervention coordinately. To acquire a continuous risk trajectory of individual patient, we adopted survival analysis instead of using classification method which requires a fixed time window.

When it comes to survival analysis, the default choice is Cox regression analysis due to its convenience. The Cox model can easily interpret the relationship of the hazard function to predictors. But it needs to impose parametric or semi-parametric constraints on the underlying distributions. Extensions of the random forest [13] to survival analysis provide an alternative way to build a time to event prediction model that automatically deal with high-level interactions and higher-order terms in variables and allows for better accuracy. Since we also applied random forest to predict future ED in a fixed prediction window, the Random Survival Forests provides an appropriate comparison against the classification method. Although ED visit could happen multiple times within a given timeframe, we only look for the first occurrence. The detail of Random Survival Forests (RSF) algorithm we used can be found in [14]. The central elements of the RSF algorithm are growing a survival tree and constructing the ensemble Cumulative Hazard Function (CHF).

Table 2. Error rate comparison between RSF and RF

	3 months error rate	6 months error rate
Random Survival Forests	0.23	0.21
Random Forest Classifer	0.21	0.20

The prediction error is estimated with C-index (concordance index), which is related to the area under the ROC curve. The C-index can be interpreted as a misclassification that specifically accounts for censoring. In practice, it is usually interested to predict the ED visit in different timeframes, such as 3 months and 6 months. Since both random survival tree and random forest classifier both use the C-index to measure the performance, we can compare their performance side-by-side. In Table 2, we can see they have similar error rate at both timeframes.

The variable importance of RSF is listed in Fig. 3. Large importance values indicate variables with high predictive ability, whereas zero or negative values identify non-predictive variables to be filtered. Under the C-index, one can interpret variable importance in terms of misclassification. The variable importance of feature x measures the increase (or drop) in misclassification error on the test data if x were not available. This is directly comparable to the variable importance of RF classifier. There are overlap among the top important variables,

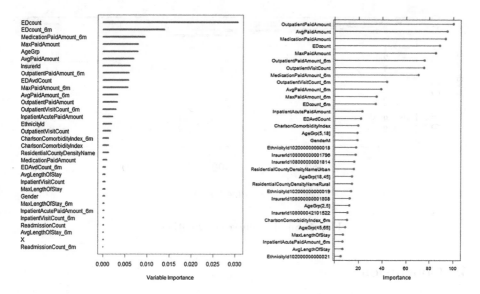

Fig. 3. Top important variables in RSF survival analysis (left) and RF classifier (right).

such as EDcount, which is the total historical ED visits in the past 3 years; MedicationPaidAmount_6m is the total medication cost in the past 6 months, MaxPaidAmount is the maximum cost of an individual claim in the past 3 years. We notice that EDcount is much more important than EDcount_6m in both RSF and RF. It indicates that the long term ED utilization history is more important for future ED prediction. We also notice that there is no a single leading predictor in RF classifier and cost in different categories as well as ED history are similar top predictors. On the other hand, the variable importance of 3 years ED history far exceeds any other predictors in RSF survival analysis (almost twice as the second predictor). Comparing RF classifier and RSF survival analysis, we can see that the ED history is most predictive to tell when a future ED could happen while overall costs in various categories are more predictive to tell if a future ED could happen within a given timeframe.

The main advantage of survival analysis over classifier is its ability to project the continuous risk curve. Figure 4 shows the survival curves of 9 patients. We can see patient 2 developed elevated risk after about 3 months. We compared the prediction to the test data and observed that patient 2 indeed had a ED visit about 4 months later. With a good estimation of when a patient's risk may elevate, care provider can make individualized plan and prioritize resource among different patients. In contrast, with a ED prediction classifier, a care provider has to decide a prediction window. If the prediction window is too small, a patient like patient 2 may be neglected. If the prediction window is too large, care provider may not have enough resource for intervention.

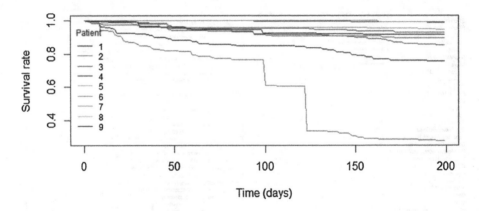

Fig. 4. Survival curves of 9 patients.

5 Conclusion

In this paper, we have developed two event prediction models to address two practical issues in existing classification based prediction model: interpretability and fixed prediction window. In many healthcare applications, the classification models have achieved excellent prediction accuracy. But in some cases, the aforementioned issues can limit the adoption of prediction models in practical use. We have demonstrated in hospital readmission prediction that BHM can improve the interpretability over logistic regression when there are a large number of multilevel categorical variables. We also have demonstrated in ED visit prediction that RSF survival analysis can achieve accuracy comparable to RF classifier while generate a continuous probability curve for a future event.

References

1. Davis, K.: 2012 Annual Report: President's Message—Health Care Reform: A Journey. Commonwealth Fund, New York (2012)
2. Cusack, C.M., Hripcsak, G., Bloomrosen, M., Rosenbloom, S.T., Weaver, C.A., Wright, A., et al.: The future state of clinical data capture and documentation: a report from AMIA's 2011 policy meeting. J. Am. Med. Inform. Assoc. **20**(1), 134–140 (2013)
3. Billings, J., Georghiou, T., Blunt, I., et al.: Choosing a model to predict hospital admission: an observational study of new variants of predictive models for case finding. BMJ Open **3**, e003352 (2013). doi:10.1136/bmjopen-2013-003352
4. Zhou, J., Shepherd, M., Li, F., Fu, L., et al.: Delivering actionable insights on population risk to improve health outcomes and reduce healthcare costs. In: International Conference on Health Informatics and Medical Systems (2015)
5. Kartoun, U., Kumar, V., Brettman, A., Yu, S., Liao, K., et al.: A risk model for 30-day heart failure readmission using electronic medical records. In: 2015 Joint Summits on Translational Science, San Francisco, CA, March 2015

6. Krishnan, R., Razavian, N., Choi, Y., Nigam, S., Blecker, S., Schmidt, A., Sontag, D.: Early detection of diabetes from health claims. In: Machine Learning in Healthcare Workshop, NIPS (2013)
7. Bhattacharya, S., Rajan, V., Huddar, V.: A novel classification method for predicting acute hypotensive episodes in critical care. In: 5th ACM Conference on Bioinformatics, Computational Biology and Health Informatics (ACM BCB 2014), Newport Beach, USA (2014)
8. Somanchi, S., Adhikari, S., Lin, A., Eneva, E., Ghani, R.: Early prediction of cardiac arrest (code blue) using electronic medical records. In: 21st ACM SIGKDD International Conference on Knowledge Discovery and Data Mining (2015)
9. Kartoun, U., Corey, K., Zheng, H., Shaw, S.: A prediction model to assess mortality risk in cirrhosis. In: 2016 Joint Summits on Translational Science, San Francisco, CA, March 2016
10. Gelman, A., Hill, J.: Data Analysis Using Regression and Multi-level/Hierarchical Models, 1st edn. Cambridge University Press, Cambridge (2006)
11. Kansagara, D., Englander, H., Salanitro, A., Kagen, D., et al.: Risk prediction models for hospital readmission: a systematic review. JAMA **306**(15), 1688–1698 (2011)
12. Walraven, C.V., Wong, J., Forster, A.J.: LACE+ index: extension of a validated index to predict early death or urgent readmission after hospital dischargeusing administrative data. Open Med. **6**(3), e80–90 (2012)
13. Breiman, L.: Random forests. Mach. Learn. **45**, 5–32 (2001)
14. Ishwaran, H., Kogalur, U., Blackstone, E., Lauer, M.: Random survival forestss. Ann. Appl. Stat. **2**(3), 841–860 (2008)

Clinical Decision Support for Stroke Using Multi–view Learning Based Models for NIHSS Scores

Vaibhav Rajan[1]([✉]), Sakyajit Bhattacharya[1], Ranjan Shetty[2], Amith Sitaram[3], and G. Vivek[2]

[1] Xerox Research Centre India, Bengaluru, India
vaibhav.rajan@xerox.com
[2] Kasturba Medical College, Manipal University, Manipal, India
[3] University Hospital, Zurich, Switzerland

Abstract. Cerebral stroke is a leading cause of physical disability and death in the world. The severity of a stroke is assessed by a neurological examination using a scale known as the NIH stroke scale (NIHSS). As a measure of stroke severity, the NIHSS score is widely adopted and has been found to also be useful in outcome prediction, rehabilitation planning and treatment planning. In many applications, such as in patient triage in under–resourced primary health care centres and in automated clinical decision support tools, it would be valuable to obtain the severity of stroke with minimal human intervention using simple parameters like age, past conditions and blood investigations. In this paper we propose a new model for predicting NIHSS scores which, to our knowledge, is the first statistical model for stroke severity. Our multi–view learning approach can handle data from heterogeneous sources with mixed data distributions (binary, categorical and numerical) and is robust against missing values – strengths that many other modeling techniques lack. In our experiments we achieve better predictive accuracy than other commonly used methods.

1 Introduction

Stroke is the second leading cause of death and a major cause of neurological disability in the world [15]. Annually, 15 million people worldwide suffer a stroke. Of these, 5 million die and another 5 million are left permanently disabled [15]. Stroke is not limited to western or high–income countries only: about 85 % of all stroke deaths are registered in low– and middle–income countries.

After a stroke occurs, one of the first steps undertaken by a neurologist is to ascertain the severity of the stroke and its effects on the patient. The National Institute of Health (NIH) Stroke Scale (NIHSS) is a standardized scale used to assess

This work was supported by an Open Innovation Grant from Xerox Research Centre India.

H. Cao et al. (Eds.): PAKDD 2016 Workshops, LNAI 9794, pp. 190–199, 2016.
DOI: 10.1007/978-3-319-42996-0_16

and quantify the level of neurological impairment of a stroke patient. The NIHSS score is widely used and is a consistent measure of stroke severity. It has been extensively studied and found to be an effective predictor of patient outcome and hospital disposition. It is also used in treatment and dosage planning for stroke patients.

In the absence of a trained neurologist, in under–resourced health care centres as well as in other clinical decision support systems there is a need for obtaining the stroke severity using simple easily obtained predictors and with minimal human intervention. In this paper we develop such a model for stroke severity by modeling NIHSS scores. The model uses easily usable predictors such as blood investigation results, past conditions of the patient, medications being taken and demographic factors such as age, gender, socio–economic status etc. To the best of our knowledge, a study of how these factors affect stroke severity has not been conducted earlier and no statistical model for stroke severity exists today. While being of scientific merit in itself, since it reveals risk factors that distinguish a mild stroke from a severe stroke, the model has several practical applications in treatment planning, hospital resource management and automated clinical decision support systems in general.

Many statistical modeling techniques suffer from two serious limitations: they cannot (i) model heterogeneous data types with different data distributions (binary, categorical and numeric), and (ii) handle missing values, both of which are common in medical data. We describe a multi–view learning approach based on collective matrix factorization [10] that efficiently addresses both these challenges, and further opens up the opportunity to integrate, in the future, any other type of data that may be useful in stroke severity prediction. This approach also has significantly better predictive ability compared to other predictive models.

2   Background

A stroke occurs when blood flow to a part of the brain stops. If blood flow is stopped for longer than a few seconds, the brain cannot get blood and oxygen. Brain cells can die, causing permanent damage. Stroke impairs many critical neurological functions, causing a large number and broad range of physical and social disabilities. The final outcome of a stroke can vary considerably–from complete recovery to permanent disability and death.

2.1   Stroke Severity and the NIHSS Score

The NIHSS score is computed by a 11–item manual neurological examination to evaluate the effect of stroke on the levels of consciousness, language, neglect, visual–field loss, extraocular movement, motor strength, limb ataxia, dysarthria, and sensory loss. Each item is associated with a specific set of activities and/or questions and is scored based on the responses of the patient. The individual scores from each item are summed to calculate a patient's final NIHSS score that can lie between 0 and 42. The NIHSS score is widely accepted as a measure of stroke severity mainly due its consistency demonstrated in inter–examiner and in test–retest scenarios [12]. NIH [14] suggests an interpretation of the score as shown in Table 1.

Table 1. NIHSS score for stroke severity

NIHSS score	Stroke severity
0	No stroke symptoms
1–4	Minor stroke
5–15	Moderate stroke
16–20	Moderate to severe stroke
21–42	Severe stroke

The NIHSS score is used in several contexts:

Outcome Prediction: The NIHSS score has been found to strongly predict the patient's outcome and likelihood of recovery after stroke [1,3,6,13]. The score is calculated usually at the onset of stroke symptoms and is repeated at regular intervals. This sequence of scores can be utilized to monitor the effectiveness of treatment methods and quantify a patient's improvement [8]. It has also been used to predict complications [16,17].

Rehabilitation Planning: Due to its predictive value, the NIHSS score can help in planning a patient's rehabilitation or long–term care needs such as in planning hospital disposition [18] and cost of stroke care [4].

Treatment Planning: A major role of the NIHSS score is in treatment planning. Minimum and maximum NIHSS score have been set for a number of treatment options to assist physicians in choosing a treatment plan [5]. The effectiveness of Tissue plasminogen activator (tPA), a proven treatment for acute ischemic strokes, is strongly dependent on the delay between stroke onset and the drug administration [7]. Since NIHSS is a reliable quantifier of stroke severity, it is frequently used as an indicator of tPA treatment, particularly in Emergency Care.

3   A New Model for NIHSS Scores

In this paper, we propose a new statistical model for predicting the NIHSS scores from clinical investigations. The model has a number of practical uses:

1. The model can be used for patient triage in rural/understaffed primary care centres to automatically (i.e. without the need for trained personnel) identify and efficiently direct severe cases of stroke to tertiary care centres with minimal human intervention.

2. Given the criticality of deciding the stroke severity for administering tPA for acute ischemic strokes in emergency care, an automatic method can significantly speed up the decision–making and hence improve care delivery and patient outcome.
3. The model can be used for predicting patient outcomes and recovery likelihood automatically at the onset of stroke symptoms or at admission time.
4. The model can also be used in automatic treatment planning tools and for automatic budget and rehabilitation planning in hospitals.

4   Subjects and Data

We retrospectively study 230 stroke patients admitted to the Kasturba Medical College, Manipal. The data corresponds to patient conditions at admission time, unless mentioned otherwise. The following details were collected from the case records of the patients.

- NIHSS score at the time of admission (NIHSS)
- Non–clinical variables: Age in years, Sex, Education, Occupation
- Past Conditions: Hypertension, Diabetes Mellitus, Heart Disease
- Addictions: Alcohol, Smoking
- Blood Investigations: Haemoglobin (Hb), Random Blood Sugar (RBS), Creatinine (Cr), Sodium (Na), Albumin (Alb), Platelet (Plt), Total Counts (TC)
- Medications: Statins, Anti Epileptics, Beta Blockers, Anti Diabetics, Heparin, Clopidogrel, Other Oral Anticoagulants

Most of these variables are categorical: past conditions, medications and addictions are encoded as binary (0/1) variables indicating the presence/absence of the corresponding condition/intake of medication/addiction; education and occupation are encoded into 6 categories. In addition, for some patients reports from radiological investigations (Echo, CT and MRI) are available which are encoded as binary variables indicating Abnormal/Normal reports. The variables used for building a model for NIHSS scores can be grouped as shown in Fig. 1. There are 27 features in total with binary, categorical and numerical features:

Standard univariate analysis shows that past hypertension and heart disease as well as intake of aspirin and clopidogrel are associated with the severity of stroke. Abnormal total blood counts is found to have significant effect on the severity of the stroke.

5   Multi–view Learning for NIHSS Scores

Measurements from heterogeneous sources for the same subject, also called views, are commonly presented as co–occurring samples. For example, blood investigations, past medical conditions, radiological investigations etc. present multiple views for the same subject in our study. Multi–view learning assumes

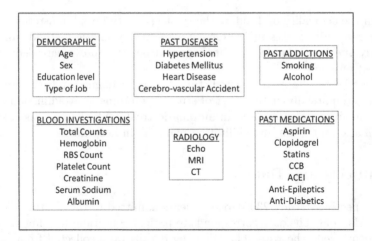

Fig. 1. Groups of features in our data

that the measurement process for each view differs and hence the noise model and the signal–to–noise ratio in each view also differs.

A naïve way to learn from such multiple views is to concatenate them and use the concatenation as a single data set. But a view may have variations or information that is not related to the NIHSS score which needs to be identified and excluded. Several studies in the past have illustrated the benefits of principled techniques of exploring multi–view data by a combined analysis of the views [9]. In this work, we use a multi–view learning approach that combines multiple data sets by finding shared information between them. Such approaches assume that the information shared between views is more interesting than information specific to each of the sources. For instance, [19] proposed a data fusion approach based on canonical correlation analysis (CCA), which is a classical method to find linear relationship between two sets of variables. Multi–view approaches by modeling shared information has been an active research area in recent times, for example, classical CCA has been extended to a probabilistic formulation [2], to a Bayesian formulation [11] and a multi–view generalization of Bayesian CCA is given in [20].

While CCA–based formulations work for co–occurring data sets with a given noise distribution, the data sets in our case belong to different distribution types, namely, binary, categorical and numerical. Recently, Klami et al. [10] proposed a generic multi–view learning approach for arbitrary collection of matrices. The new collective matrix factorization solution (CMF) models both the information shared by views and information that is specific to each view, and can also handle multiple data distributions. We thus use CMF to find a low–rank representation of patients shared across all data sets, and consequently use it to predict stroke severity. We will briefly describe the CMF method as proposed by [10].

CMF finds low–rank representations for arbitrary collection of matrices with shared entities. The idea is to capture shared information between data matrices in the low–rank representations. Klami et al. [10] uses variational Bayesian

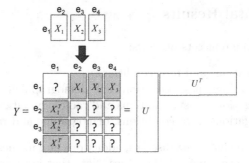

Fig. 2. Illustration of the CMF technique for multi–view learning

approximation to learn the model which not only captures the shared information but also captures information specific to a given matrix or a subset of matrices. Suppose we have M matrices $X_m = [x_{ij}^{(m)}]$ representing E sets of entities, each with cardinality d_e. Let r_m and c_m denote the entity sets corresponding to the rows and columns of matrices. In this work, row entities (i.e. patients) are shared across all data matrices and column entities represent feature types such as past medication, blood investigation etc. The goal of CMF is to approximate each matrix with a rank–K product plus additional row and column bias terms. As shown in [10], the element corresponding to the row i and column j of the mth matrix can be written as (Fig. 2):

$$x_{ij}^{(m)} = \sum_{k=1}^{K} u_{ik}^{(r_m)} u_{jk}^{(c_m)} + b_i^{(m,r)} + b_j^{(m,c)} + \varepsilon_{ij}^{(m)} , \tag{1}$$

where $\mathbf{U}_e = [u_{ik}^{(e)}] \in \mathbb{R}^{d_e \times K}$ is the low–rank matrix related to the entity set e, $b_i^{(m,r)}$ and $b_j^{(m,c)}$ are the bias terms for the mth matrix, and $\varepsilon_{ij}^{(m)}$ is element–wise independent noise. The low–rank approximation of entity sets corresponding to the patients can be used as a combined representation of patients shared across all data sets.

5.1 Classification of NIHSS Scores

We build classification models that can predict the NIHSS score range for a given data vector consisting of values of the predictor variables. The two classes are based on NIHSS Score ranges: [1–6] and [7–42] indicating mild and severe stroke respectively. Standard binary classifiers – K–Nearest Neighbors, Logistic Regression and Random Forests – are trained to classify each input vector into one of these two classes. We measure the classification accuracy using leave–one–out cross validation: for each observation, we train the classifier on the remaining data and use the classifier to predict the NIHSS score range of the observation left out. The classification accuracy reported is the proportion of the predictions that are correct. As a baseline, we use the column–wise concatenation of all the data with the same standard classifiers, denoted by *Org*.

6   Experimental Results

We consider four different sets of views:

V1: Blood Investigations and past conditions
V2: Blood Investigations, past conditions and demographic data
V3: Blood Investigations, past conditions and radiology data
V4: Blood Investigations, past conditions, demographic and radiology data

Past conditions include past diseases, addictions and medications (see Fig. 1) and these features have binary (0/1) values. Note that in views V2, V3 and V4, there are missing values, in radiology and demographic data, that have been imputed during the transformation and these features cannot be used in Org dataset without imputation.

Using logistic regression or KNN for classification, when the concatenated data (Org) is used directly for classification, we obtain ~59 % classification accuracy whereas the same classifier on the transformed representation of V1 gives ~65 % accuracy, an increase of almost 10 %. With random forest, the increase in accuracy is nearly 15 %. These results are shown in Fig. 3 for 3 different classifiers – K–Nearest Neighbors, Logistic Regression and Random Forest – on the original data (concatenated datasets) and on the transformed data from each of the four views. In each case, transforming the data improves the classification accuracy by 10 % or more.

We observe that the accuracy remains the same even in the absence of radiology data suggesting that the model effectively predicts the severity with simple predictors like blood investigations and past conditions. The overall accuracy is around 70 % on this dataset, which is still useful in applications like patient triage in rural/under–resourced centres where it can be used to automatically identify severe patients and re–direct them to tertiary care centres. Note that our data has just 203 observations and with more data, which we will collect in the future, we expect the accuracy to increase further; and regression models that can exactly predict the NIHSS score can also be designed to be used in other applications.

Robustness Against Missing Values. To test for robustness against missing values, we artificially add missing values to our datasets. We take the original dataset without any missing values (V1) and remove values from the data in steps such that upto 25 % of the values are missing. In each case, after deleting the values, we transform the data during which missing values are imputed. As before, we train three classifiers on the original data (without missing values) and on the transformed data (after deleting a percentage of values). Classification accuracy obtained by the classifiers are shown in Fig. 4. We observe that the missing values do not deteriorate the performance of the classification after the transformation that imputes the missing values.

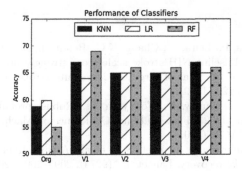

Fig. 3. Leave–one–out CV classification accuracy on the original concatenated data (Org) and on four transformed views: V1, V2, V3, V4. Classifiers used are: K–Nearest Neighbors (KNN), Logistic Regression (LR), Random Forest (RF).

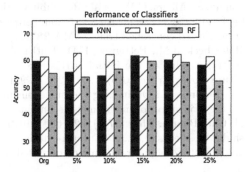

Fig. 4. Leave–one–out CV classification accuracy on the original data (Org) and on the transformed data after artificially deleting a fixed percentage of values ranging from 5 % to 25 %. Classifiers used are: K–Nearest Neighbors (KNN), Logistic Regression (LR), Random Forest (RF).

7   Conclusion

Most healthcare datasets are heterogeneous, contains missing values and consists of different kinds of datatypes. Our multi–view learning approach handles all these challenges in a principled manner that enhances predictive learning. We believe that the modeling technique can be usefully applied in many other contexts, particularly in healthcare. We present a new model for NIHSS scores based on multi–view learning. The model for NIHSS scores can be used to predict the severity of a stroke and numerous applications of such a model in clinical decision support systems are discussed. To our knowledge this is the first work that discusses a statistical model for NIHSS scores and its applications.

Acknowledgment. We thank Abhishek Tripathi who helped us with our experiments while he was at Xerox Research Centre India.

References

1. Adams, H., Davis, P., Leira, E., Chang, K.C., Bendixen, B., Clarke, W., Woolson, R., Hansen, M.: Baseline NIH stroke scale score strongly predicts outcome after stroke: a report of the trial of Org 10172 in acute stroke treatment (TOAST). Neurology **53**(1), 126 (1999)
2. Archambeau, C., Delannay, N., Verleysen, M.: Robust probabilistic projections. In: Proceedings of the 23rd International Conference on Machine Learning, ICML 2006, pp. 33–40. ACM (2006)
3. Baird, A.E., Dambrosia, J., Janket, S.J., et al.: A three-item scale for the early prediction of stroke recovery. Lancet **357**(9274), 2095–2099 (2001)
4. Caro, J.J., Huybrechts, K.F., Kelley, H.E., for the Stroke Economic Analysis Group: Predicting treatment costs after acute ischemic stroke on the basis of patient characteristics at presentation and early dysfunction. Stroke **32**(1), 100–106 (2001)
5. Clark, W.M., Wissman, S., Albers, G.W., et al.: Recombinant tissue-type plasminogen activator (alteplase) for ischemic stroke 3 to 5 hours after symptom onset: the atlantis study: a randomized controlled trial. JAMA **282**(21), 2019–2026 (1999)
6. DeGraba, T.J., Hallenbeck, J.M., Pettigrew, K.D., Dutka, A.J., Kelly, B.J.: Progression in acute stroke: value of the initial NIH stroke scale score on patient stratification in future trials. Stroke **30**(6), 1208–1212 (1999)
7. Eissa, A., Krass, I., Bajorek, B.: Optimizing the management of acute ischaemic stroke: a review of the utilization of intravenous recombinant tissue plasminogen activator (tPA). J. Clin. Pharm. Ther. **37**(6), 620–629 (2012)
8. Furlan, A., Higashida, R., Wechsler, L., et al.: Intra-arterial prourokinase for acute ischemic stroke: the proact ii study: a randomized controlled trial. JAMA **282**(21), 2003–2011 (1999)
9. Hardoon, D., Szedmak, S., Shawe-Taylor, J.: Canonical correlation analysis: an overview with application to learning methods. Neural Comput. **16**(12), 2639–2664 (2004)
10. Klami, A., Bouchard, G., Tripathi, A.: Group-sparse embeddings in collective matrix factorization. In: International Conference on Learning Representations (2014)
11. Klami, A., Virtanen, S., Kaski, S.: Bayesian canonical correlation analysis. J. Mach. Learn. Res. **14**(1), 965–1003 (2013)
12. Goldstein, L.B., Bertels, C., Davis, J.N.: Interrater reliability of the NIH stroke scale. Arch. Neurol. **46**, 660–662 (1989)
13. Lyden, P., Lu, M., Jackson, C., Marler, J., Kothari, R., Brott, T., Zivin, J.: Underlying structure of the national institutes of health stroke scale: results of a factor analysis. Stroke **30**(11), 2347–2354 (1999)
14. NIH: Stroke scale. http://www.ninds.nih.gov/doctors/NIH_Stroke_Scale.pdf
15. World Health Organization: The world health report 2000 health systems: improving performance. http://www.who.int/cardiovascular_diseases/en/cvd_atlas_15_burden_stroke.pdf
16. Rocco, A., Pasquini, M., Cecconi, E., Sirimarco, G., Ricciardi, M.C., Vicenzini, E., Altieri, M., Di Piero, V., Lenzi, G.L.: Monitoring after the acute stage of stroke: a prospective study. Stroke **38**(4), 1225–1228 (2007)
17. Saposnik, G., Guzik, A.K., Reeves, M., Ovbiagele, B., Johnston, S.C.: Stroke prognostication using age and NIH stroke scale: SPAN-100. Neurology **80**(1), 21–28 (2013)

18. Schlegel, D., Kolb, S.J., Luciano, J.M., Tovar, J.M., Cucchiara, B.L., Liebeskind, D.S., Kasner, S.E.: Utility of the NIH stroke scale as a predictor of hospital disposition. Stroke **34**(1), 134–137 (2003)
19. Tripathi, A., Klami, A., Kaski, S.: Simple integrative preprocessing preserves what is shared in data sources. BMC Bioinform. **9**(1), 111 (2008)
20. Virtanen, S., Jia, Y., Klami, A., Darrell, T.: Factorized multi-modal topic model. In: Proceedings of the Twenty-Eighth Conference Annual Conference on Uncertainty in Artificial Intelligence (UAI 2012), pp. 843–851. AUAI Press (2012)

Data Mining in Business and Finance (WDMBF)

A Music Recommendation System Based on Acoustic Features and User Personalities

Rui Cheng[1]([✉]) and Boyang Tang[2]

[1] University of Arizona, Tucson, AZ, USA
ruicheng@email.arizona.edu
[2] Technology University of Delft, Delft, The Netherlands
B.Tang@student.tudelft.nl

Abstract. Music recommendation attracts great attention for music providers to improve their services as the volume of new music increases quickly. It is a great challenge for users to find their interested songs from such a large size of collections. In the previous studies, common strategies can be categorized into content-based music recommendation and collaborative music filtering. Content-based recommendation systems predict users' preferences in terms of the music content. Collaborative filtering systems predict users' ratings based on the preferences of the friends of the targeting user. In this study, we proposed a hybrid approach to provide personalized music recommendations. This is achieved by extracting audio features of songs and integrating these features and user personalities for context-aware recommendation using the state-of-the-art support vector machines (SVM). Our experiments show the effectiveness of this proposed approach for personalized music recommendation.

Keywords: Music recommendation system · Audio feature · User personality · Support vector machine

1 Introduction

Nowadays, people have difficulty in getting music they want from online music stores and streaming services (e.g. Spotify, ITunes) as the volume of new music goes up rapidly. Music recommendation systems play a vital role for this purpose. It provides listeners with new music that matches their tastes, and enables online music providers to provide the music to the right customer.

Although many researches made great efforts on music recommendation system, most of them only rely on user behaviors: the combination of user-based song rating scores and relevance of songs/items to each other. This is called collaborative filtering approach.

Collaborative filtering (CF) is used by researchers to discover the relations between users and items. It can be model-based or memory-based. Model-based recommender system [2] uses machine learning techniques to represent user preferences by a set of rating scores. Memory-based recommender system [6, 19, 24] finds an active user's nearest neighbors using a massive number of explicit user votes. Then it aggregates the neighbors' ratings to predict the active user's ratings of relevant items.

© Springer International Publishing Switzerland 2016
H. Cao et al. (Eds.): PAKDD 2016 Workshops, LNAI 9794, pp. 203–213, 2016.
DOI: 10.1007/978-3-319-42996-0_17

Another approach is to recommend music based on available metadata: information such as the album, artist, and year of release is usually known. However, this approach is not always useful to recommend songs by artists that the user is known to enjoy, because it disregards the fact that the repertoire of an artist is rarely homogenous: listeners may enjoy particular songs more than others [23].

Generally, CF-based recommendation system outperforms content-based recommendation system in predicting rating scores [21]. However, collaborative filtering is applicable only when usage data is available. Besides, CF-based recommendation system suffers from the cold start problem. For example, it cannot recommend new songs that have not been rated, and it cannot provide recommendation to new users who have not rated any songs. Additionally, songs that are only of interest to a niche audience are more difficult to recommend because usage data is scarce. Especially in music recommendation, they comprise the majority of the song, because the user's rated patterns follow a power law [11]. However, content-based recommendation system is not affected by these issues.

Thus, many researchers have developed hybrid recommendation systems, combining both collaborative filtering and content-based algorithms to make more accurate prediction. The experiment results of Wang's and Yoshii's experiments [24, 25] showed that hybrid methods outperform individual approaches. However, limitations existed that many of them only take into consideration attributes of items (e.g. singer, genre, etc.), which have a gap with high level music concepts, rather than acoustic features.

Besides, in music recommendation domain, context information is useful in predict user preferences [1]. For example, when users are searching music, the location, the time, and their mood would affect their preferences. And the changes of context information make it impossible for recommendation system to make correct predictions every time.

To solve these problems, some researches [21] showed that similarity of audio signals can be a bridge between a song and its' high-level tags such as genre, mood, and instrumentation. In addition, Rentfrow and Gosiling's experiments [18] showed that preferences for music styles are related to a wide array of personality dimensions (e.g., Openness), self-views (e.g., political orientation), and cognitive abilities (e.g., verbal IQ), which can be treat as a partially unchangeable observable context factors.

In this paper, we designed a hybrid music recommendation system that considered the user personalities and audio features of song. In order to solve the sparsity of preference ratings problem and cold start problem, we proposed the use of the support vector machine (SVM) [5]. Because unlike other learning methods, SVM's performance is not related to the number of features in the system, but to the margin with which it separates the data. Experimentally, SVM has achieved superior performance on a number of high-dimensional datasets [9]. We compare the proposed system to the collaborative filtering approach. Our experiments show that the proposed music recommendation system outperforms the collaborative filtering approach in predicting user rates.

The rest of this paper is organized as follows: Sect. 2 describes our hybrid recommendation system that considered both content and context information, followed by a brief introduction to the SVM. Section 3 describes the evaluation results of our model. The last section gives concluding remarks.

2 Hybrid Music Recommendation System

In our hybrid music recommendation system, we considered both the content information of songs (audio features) and partially unchangeable observable context factors (user personalities). In previous content-based music recommendation system, music information is extracted from the available music descriptions such as singers and albums. Users' preferences are predicted by analyzing the relationship between the music ratings given by individuals and the corresponding music attributes. A rudimentary way is simple music tags matching. However, using music tags suffers from the well-known problems of synonymy and polysemy in information retrieval [10]. Another popular technique used to represent music content information is catch music audio information. Many of the previous researches extract data from MIDI (Musical Instrument Digital Interface) corpora, where the files are symbolized by musical scores. However, considering the popularity of MP3 (MPEG Layer 3) digital music archives, we built our system based on audio features extracted from MP3 music files.

2.1 Content Information

Musical genre classification by using audio signals has been studied by many researchers [13, 22], giving us hints in selecting audio features to represent music objects in our recommendation system. We grouped these feature into three group to represent timbre texture, rhythmic and pitch content. The performance and relative importance of the proposed features were examined by our system using real-world MPEG audio corpus.

Timbral texture features are based on the standard features proposed for music-speech discrimination [22]. The following specific features are used to represent timbral texture in our system:

- *Mel Frequency Cepstral Coefficients (MFCC):* They are perceptually motivated features and provide a compact representation of the spectral envelope such that most of the signal energy is concentrated in the first coefficients.
- *Spectral Centroid:* It is the balancing point of the subband energy distribution and determines the frequency area around which most of the signal energy concentrates. To formulize:

$$C(t) = \frac{\sum_{i=0}^{I-1} (i+1) s_i(t)}{\sum_{i=0}^{I-1} s_i(t)}$$

- *Spectral rolloff point:* It is used to distinguish voice speech from unvoiced music, which has a higher rolloff point because their power is better distributed over the subband range. To formulize:

$$\sum_{i=0}^{R} s_i(t) = 0.85 \sum_{i=0}^{I-1} s_i(t)$$

- *Spectral Flux:* It determines changes of spectral energy distribution of two successive windows. To formulize:

$$\Delta(t,t+1) = \sqrt{\sum_{i=0}^{I-1} \left| \frac{s_i(t)}{\max\left(s_j(t)\right):0 \leq j \leq I-1} - \frac{s_i(t+1)}{\max\left(s_j(t+1)\right):0 \leq j \leq I-1} \right|}$$

Rhythmic Content Features used to represent rhythm structure are based on detecting the most salient periodicities of the signal. Gorge's method [22] is applied to construct the beat histogram, from which six features are calculated to represent rhythmic content:

- *A0, A1:* relative amplitude of the first and second histogram peak.
- *RA:* ratio of the amplitude of the second peak divided by the amplitude of the first peak.
- *P1, P2:* period of the first, second peak in bpm.
- *SUM:* overall sum of the histogram (indication of beat strength).

Pitch content features describe the melody and harmony information about music signals. They are extracted using various pitch detection techniques [22]. Basically the dominant peaks of the autocorrelation function are calculated via the summation of envelopes of each frequency band obtained by decomposing the signal. Then they are accumulated into pitch histograms from which the pitch content features are extracted. The pitch content features typically include the amplitudes and periods of maximum peaks in the histogram, pitch intervals between the two most prominent peaks, and the overall sums of the histograms. Because the different magnitudes of features, we normalized all audio features into 0–1.

2.2 Context Information

Context-aware recommendation systems assumed that some additional information is available that influences the rating behavior such as when a rating behavior happened or where users listened the music. In our music recommendation system, we used user personalities as the context information which is unchanged during comparatively short time (e.g. openness, emotional stability, wealthy, intelligent).

We define context as variable $c \in C$ and content as variable $d \in D$, if multiple context $C_3, \ldots C_m$ and content $D_1, \ldots D_m$ are allowed. The task is to estimate the following rating function:

$$y: U \times I \times C_3 \ldots \times C_m \times D_1 \ldots \times D_m \to \mathbb{R}$$

Note that we start the index of the context variables with 3 because from technical point of view, users and items can be seen as the first and second 'context'.

Figure 1 shows an example of how we create prediction matrix. There are users U with personalities C_3 listening music items I that have content features $\mathcal{D}$.

$$U = \{Tom, Lily, Ben\}$$
$$I = \{Someone\ like\ you,\ Be\ with\ you,\ This\ is\ us\}$$
$$C_3 = \{intelligence,\ wealthy,\ openness\}$$
$$\mathcal{D} = \{mean\ of\ pitch,\ variance\ of\ pitch,\ mean\ of\ tempo\}$$

The first tuple in Fig. 1 states that Tom, who has 3 scores in intelligence, 4 scores in wealthy and 5 scores in openness, give "Someone like you" 3 scores, whose mean pitch is 648, mean tempo is 0.62, and variance of pitch is 79794.

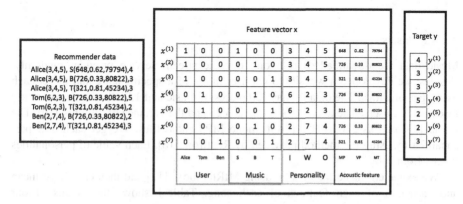

Fig. 1. Creating real value feature × using actual users' data

Figure 1 shows how we framed our data into the matrix. In the first row, the first three columns represent who rated the music. The following three columns represent which is the music. The next three columns show the personalities of the given person, and the last three column shows the acoustic features of the specific music.

2.3   Support Vector Machine

The support vector machine is a supervised classification system that finds the maximum margin hyperplane separating two classes of data. If the data are not linearly separable in the feature space, as is often the case, they can be projected into a higher dimensional space by means of a Mercer kernel. In fact, only the inner products of the data points in this higher dimensional space are necessary. Thus the projection can be implicit if such an inner product can be computed directly [15].

In this study, we adopt the support vector regression (SVR) model, which applies a regression technique to the SVM to predict numerical values of users' preference of a specific song, because SVM has performed very well in a number of high-dimensional data sets even without feature selection [9]. For example, it outperforms radial basis networks on recognizing the US postal service database of handwritten digits (using 16×16 bitmap as input) [20]. Promising results are also reported in face detection (where the input dimensionality is 283 [17] and text categorization (where the input dimensionality is over 10,000) [10].

3 Experimental Evaluation

Experiments were carried out to observe the recommendation performance of our approach. We compared it with collaborative filtering methods and factorization machine, by using accuracy of user rating prediction. First we compared the results of SVM with different Kernel functions. Then we put different combination of content and context information into model and compared the results. Last we compared our hybrid music recommendation system model with other recommendation models.

3.1 Datasets

Music data are downloaded from online-music stream service provider randomly. Besides, we developed a website to get user rating of a specific song and to get each users' personalities. The data set has 120 pieces of music and 1,050 rating (1 to 5 stars) made by 102 users. The average of rating is 3.23 and the variance of rating is 1.30. The music is stored as 22050 Hz, 16-bit, mono MP3 audio files. We get each user personalities by using the method provided by Rentfrow [18]. Each value of personalities ranges from 1–7.

We extracted music features by using MIRtoolbox[1] [12] and then calculated mean and variances of each features of each song. Table 1 shows the details of our parameters.

3.2 Evaluation Metrics

Decision support accuracy and Mean Absolute Error (MAE) [4] are two classic evaluation indicators of the accuracy of recommendation system. In this study, we chose both metrics as our evaluation standards. Specifically, decision support accuracy assumes the prediction process as a binary operation: users like or dislike a song. Predicted and actual scores above 2.5 out of 5 are considered "like". And MAE is calculated by averaging the absolute errors in rating prediction pairs as follows:

$$MAE = \frac{\sum_{j=1}^{N} |P_{i,j} - R_{i,j}|}{N}$$

where $P_{i,j}$ is system's rating (prediction) of item j for user i, and $R_{i,j}$ is the rating of user i for item j in the test data. N is the number of rating-prediction pairs between the test data and the prediction result. A lower MAE means a greater accuracy. If we use the average of ratings to predict user ratings, the MAE would be 1.22. If we use "like" to

---

[1] https://www.jyu.fi/hum/laitokset/musiikki/en/research/coe/materials/mirtoolbox.

tag all user ratings in this dataset, the accuracy would be 0.68. In our experiments, we randomly left out 20 % rating record. Notice that this used somewhat less data than required, but allowed us to use a single model to evaluate the performance of recommendation system convincingly. We applied the cross-validate procedure by repeating 10 times with different random seeds. The reported numbers are the mean of the results.

Table 1. Parameters

Category	Parameter
User personalities	Extraversion
	Agreeableness
	Conscientiousness
	Emotional stability
	Openness
	Social dominance
	Depression
	Self-esteem
	Intelligence
Acoustic feature (mean and variance)	Centroid
	Flux
	MFCC
	Pitch
	Rolloff
	Rhythm

3.3 Prediction Result

Because SVM performs well in a number of high-dimensional data sets even without feature selection, we put all of the features into SVM with different kernel function to train our model. We found that Radius Basis Function (RBF) is the best kernel function in this case. There are two important parameters in it. One is gamma which defines how far the influence of a single training example reaches, and another is C, which trades off misclassification of training examples against simplicity of the decision surface. In this experiment, we search the best parameters (gamma and C) by their cross-validation accuracy, and we explore them in a normal large grid, which is 10^3 to 10^{-3}. The results are shown in Table 2 (Fig. 2).

Table 2. Result of SVM with different kernel function

Kernel type	MAE	Direction accuracy (rounded)
Linear	0.8947	75.5 %
Polynomial	0.8559	75.2 %
Radius basis	0.8284	76.2 %
Sigmoid	0.8448	75.2 %

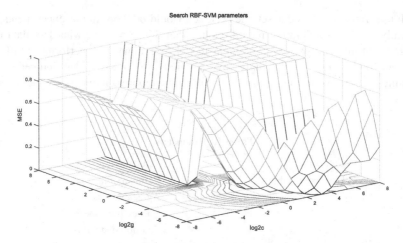

Fig. 2. Search RBF-SVM parameters

Next, we defined our features into three groups. Hybrid feature group contained both the music audio features and the user personalities; content-based feature group, which represented the content-based music recommendation system, only contained the music content information; context-based feature group only contained the user personality matrix. The results are shown as follows:

Table 3. MAE of direction accuracy of different combination of features

Feature group	MAE	Direction accuracy (rounded)
Hybrid feature	0.8149	89.7 %
Content-based feature	0.8497	75.2 %
User personality feature	0.8866	77.9 %

Table 3 shows that our hybrid music recommendation model has lower MAE and higher direction accuracy than other two models. And we found that user personality features play more important role in predict whether a user like or dislike a song, while music audio features contributes more on sores accuracy. This result indicated that these two set of features benefit our model from different aspects.

Finally, we compared our approach with collaborative filtering method, which is based on finding users with similar likes as the target user. We first used all of the training datasets to train the two models. Then we calculated the prediction MAE of our model with respect to the size of training sets. As shown in following figure and table, our approach performed much better than collaborative filtering approach in MAE and direction accuracy. With only 100 training data point, our approach can achieve 0.94 MAE in predicting 394 unknown users' ratings (Fig. 3 and Table 4).

Table 4. Compare collaborative filtering with our method

Method	MAE	Direction accuracy
Collaborative filtering	1.12	70.2 %
Our approach	0.8149	89.7 %

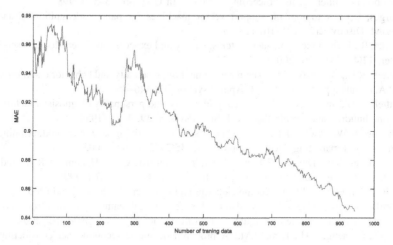

Fig. 3. MAE in SVM with respect to number of training data

4 Conclusion and Discussions

In this paper we described a hybrid music recommendation system for online music stream providers. The system is based on SVM model, which is faster than traditional recommendation algorithms and can solve matrix sparse and cold start problems. By using the audio features and user personalities information, this model can take content and context information, rather than only user ratings, into consideration.

Our experiments showed that RBF-SVM is suit for music recommendation compare to other kind of SVM. Combining the content and context information can reduce the MAE and improve the decision accuracy or prediction. In addition, our approach can predict users' preference well with only a small data set.

Future research would collect more data to test whether the model still performs well with large data sets to overcome the disadvantage of using limited scale of datasets. Furthermore, additional context features such as time and location will also be conserved to improve the model.

References

1. Adomavicius, G., Tuzhilin, A.: Context-aware recommender systems. In: Ricci, F., Rokach, L., Shapira, B., Kantor, P.B. (eds.) Recommender Systems Handbook, pp. 217–253. Springer, US (2011)

2. Adomavicius, G., Tuzhilin, A.: Toward the next generation of recommender systems: a survey of the state-of-the-art and possible extensions. IEEE Trans. Knowl. Data Eng. **17**(6), 734–749 (2005)

3. Arnett, J.: The soundtrack of recklessness: musical preferences and reckless behavior among adolescents. J. Adolesc. Res. **7**, 313–331 (1992)

4. Breese, J.S., Heckerman, D., Kardie, C.: Empirical analysis of predictive algorithms for collaborative filtering. In: Proceedings of the 14th UAI, pp. 43–52 (1998)

5. Burges, C.J.: A tutorial on support vector machines for pattern recognition. Data Min. Knowl. Discov. **2**(2), 121–167 (1998)

6. Burke, R.: Hybrid recommender systems: survey and experiments. User Model. User-Adap. Inter. **12**(4), 331–370 (2002)

7. Cattell, R.B., Anderson, J.C.: The measurement of personality and behavior disorders by the I.P.A.T. music preference test. J. Appl. Psychol. **37**, 446–454 (1953)

8. Cattell, R.B., Saunders, D.R.: Musical preferences and personality diagnosis: a factorization of one hundred and twenty themes. J. Soc. Psychol. **39**, 3–24 (1954)

9. Cheung, K.W., Kwok, J.T., Law, M.H., Tsui, K.C.: Mining customer product ratings for personalized marketing. Decis. Support Syst. **35**(2), 231–243 (2003)

10. Deerwester, S.C., Dumais, S.T., Landauer, T.K., Furnas, G.W., Harshman, R.A.: Indexing by latent semantic analysis. J. Am. Soc. Inf. Sci. **41**(6), 391–407 (1990)

11. Celma Herrada, Ò.: Music recommendation and discovery in the long tail (2009)

12. Lartillot, O., Toiviainen, P.: A Matlab toolbox for musical feature extraction from audio. In: International Conference on Digital Audio Effects, pp. 237–244, September 2007

13. Li, Q., Myaeng, S.H., Kim, B.M.: A probabilistic music recommender considering user opinions and audio features. Inf. Process. Manag. **43**(2), 473–487 (2007)

14. Little, P., Zuckerman, M.: Sensation seeking and music preferences. Pers. Individ. Differ. **7**, 575–577 (1986)

15. Mandel, M.I., Ellis, D.P.: Song-level features and support vector machines for music classification. In: ISMIR 2005: 6th International Conference on Music Information Retrieval: Proceedings: Variation 2: Queen Mary, University of London & Goldsmiths College, University of London, 11–15 September 2005, pp. 594–599. Queen Mary, University of London (2005)

16. McCown, W., Keiser, R., Mulhearn, S., Williamson, D.: The role of personality and gender in preferences for exaggerated bass in music. Pers. Individ. Differ. **23**, 543–547 (1997)

17. Osuna, E., Freund, R., Girosi, F.: Training support vector machines: an application to face detection. In: Proceedings of 1997 IEEE Computer Society Conference on Computer Vision and Pattern Recognition, pp. 130–136. IEEE, June 1997

18. Rentfrow, P.J., Gosling, S.D.: The do re mi's of everyday life: the structure and personality correlates of music preferences. J. Pers. Soc. Psychol. **84**(6), 1236 (2003)

19. Sarwar, B., Karypis, G., Konstan, J., Riedl, J.: Item-based collaborative filtering recommendation algorithms. In: Proceedings of the 10th International Conference on World Wide Web, pp. 285–295. ACM, April 2001

20. Schölkopf, B., Sung, K.K., Burges, C.J., Girosi, F., Niyogi, P., Poggio, T., Vapnik, V.: Comparing support vector machines with Gaussian kernels to radial basis function classifiers. IEEE Trans. Sig. Process. **45**(11), 2758–2765 (1997)

21. Slaney, M., Weinberger, K., White, W.: Learning a metric for music similarity. In: International Symposium on Music Information Retrieval (ISMIR), September 2008

22. Tzanetakis, G., Cook, P.: Music genre classification of audio signals. IEEE Trans. Speech Audio Process. **10**(5), 293–302 (2002)

23. Van den Oord, A., Dieleman, S., Schrauwen, B.: Deep content-based music recommendation. In: Advances in Neural Information Processing Systems, pp. 2643–2651 (2003)
24. Wang, J., De Vries, A.P., Reinders, M. J.: Unifying user-based and item-based collaborative filtering approaches by similarity fusion. In: Proceedings of the 29th Annual International ACM SIGIR Conference on Research and Development in Information Retrieval, pp. 501–508. ACM, August 2006
25. Yoshii, K., Goto, M., Komatani, K., Ogata, T., Okuno, H.G.: Hybrid collaborative and content-based music recommendation using probabilistic model with latent user preferences. In: ISMIR, vol. 6, 7th (2006)

A Social Spam Detection Framework via Semi-supervised Learning

Xianchao Zhang, Haijun Bai, and Wenxin Liang[(✉)]

Dalian University of Technology, Dalian, China
xczhang@dlut.edu.cn, 408927717@mail.dlut.edu.cn, wxliang@dlut.edu.cn

Abstract. With the increasing popularity of social networking websites such as Twitter, Facebook, Sina Weibo and MySpace, spammers
on them are getting more and more rampant. Social spammers always
create a mass of compromised or fake accounts to deceive users and lead
them to access malicious websites which contain illegal, pornography or
dangerous information. As we all know, most of the studies on social
spam detection are based on supervised machine learning which requires
plenty of annotated datasets. Unfortunately, labeling a large number
of datasets manually is a complex, error-prone and tedious task which
may costs a lot of human efforts and time. In this paper, we propose a
novel semi-supervised classification framework for social spam detection,
which combines co-training with k-medoids. First we utilize k-medoids
clustering algorithm to acquire some informative and presentative samples for labelling as our initial seeds set. Then we take advantage of the
content features and behavior features of users for our co-training classification framework. In order to illustrate the effectiveness of k-medoids,
we compare the performance with random selecting strategy. Finally, we
evaluate the effectiveness of our proposed detection framework compared
with several classical supervised algorithms.

Keywords: Semi-supervised learning · Social spam · Co-training ·
k-medoids

1 Introduction

Social networking websites such as Twitter, Facebook, Sina Weibo and MySpace
have gained more and more popularity and attentions around the world in recent
years. Twitter, as a microblogging site, is the fastest growing one than any
other social networking site and allows users to post their latest updates and
share messages using no more than 140 characters, known as tweets. Users could
communicate and stay in touch with their friends through the exchange of tweets.

Accompanied by the popularity of social networks, spam as an indelible by-
product threatens users and social network websites with different forms and

This work was supported by National Science Foundation of China (No. 61272374,
61300190) and 863 Project (No. 2015AA015463).

H. Cao et al. (Eds.): PAKDD 2016 Workshops, LNAI 9794, pp. 214–226, 2016.
DOI: 10.1007/978-3-319-42996-0_18

definitions. For example, spammers often use Twitter as a tool to post malicious links, send unsolicited messages to legitimate users, and hijack trending topics. Social spammers always create a mass of compromised or fake accounts to deceive users and lead them to access malicious websites which contain much illegal, pornography or dangerous information. Sometimes, the spammers disguise themselves as normal users and imitate the behavior of legitimate users. This kind of spammers are hardly to be discovered and also very harmful to legitimate users and social networks. As a countermeasure, Twitter has its own detection methods and rules against spam and abuse. Users who violate the rules will be suspended permanently. Furthermore, legitimate users can report spam to Twitter. For example, if users discover spam messages, they can click the "report as spam" link on their homepages of Twitter and then the reports will be submitted to Twitter for further investigating. Also users can post a tweet in the format of "@spam@username", where the @username is to account for the spammer's username. Even so, there are still a lot of spam users on Twitter.

In order to improve the quality of user experience and reduce the websites' load of dealing with unwanted and sometimes dangerous content, a multiple researches have been done so far. For example, the studies in [14,18], create honey-profile accounts to be followed by spammers, and then analyze the behavior of the spammers. Some of the studies describe the relationship between users in graphs, and use a graph algorithm to extract features for detection [19,22]. It is known that most of the studies on social spam detection are based on supervised machine learning [1,7,14,22], which requires plenty of annotated datasets. Benevenuto et al. [3] discussed video spammers by extracting some features in YouTube. Unfortunately, labeling a large number of datasets manually is a complex, error-prone and tedious task which may costs a lot of human efforts and time. Moreover, co-training is a good paradigm of semi-supervised learning, which has drawn considerable attentions and interests recently [26].

In this paper, a novel semi-supervised classification framework was proposed for social spam detection, which combines co-training with k-medoids.

The main contributions of this paper are as follows:

- We proposed a novel semi-supervised classification framework which combines the co-training approach with k-medoids clustering algorithm for social spam detection.
- We presented to utilize content features and behavior features of users for co-training.
- We evaluated the effectiveness of our framework on a large scale dataset derived from Twitter.

The remainder of this paper is organized as follows. The related work is stated in Sect. 2. We present our classification framework in Sect. 3. Section 4 shows the performance of our framework and we draw a conclusion in the last Section.

2 Related Work

On the heels of spammer detection in traditional platforms like Email and Web [5], some efforts have been devoted to detect spammers in various social networking sites, such as Twitter [1,10,19], Sina Weibo [7,17], Facebook [8,21]. Heymann et al. made a survey of approaches and future challenges about defeating spam in social networks [11]. A plenty of researchers extract all kinds of user features such as profile feature, content feature, network feature and so on, and then adopt different classification algorithms or frameworks to detect spammers. Lin et al. [17] utilized the URL rate and the interaction rate as the main features for detecting the long-surviving Twitter spam accounts effectively. Ahmed et al. identified a set of 14 generic statistical features for spam detection in online social networks. Wang et al. [20] focused on the detection of spam tweets, solely making the most of the tweet-inherent features.

Some other studies focus on spam campaigns detection based on unsupervised approaches. Gao et al. [8] presented a solution to firstly build similarity graph based on the URLs and description texts, then quantified and characterized spam campaigns launched using accounts on online social networks. Lee et al. [13] proposed a content-driven framework to extract campaigns from large-scale social media but didn't categorize the campaigns according to their cooperation purpose. Zhang et al. [24] promoted the campaigns detection by a novel similarity information entropy. Zhang et al. [23] proposed RP-LDA to extract user features and find user groups within which users share similar retweeting behavior in order to detect spamming groups in microblogging services.

Nevertheless, there are only a few researchers absorbed in social spam detection based on semi-supervised approaches. Recently, Li et al. [16] proposed a semi-supervised framework for social spammer detection(SSSD), which utilizes a ranking scheme based on the social graph to detect social spammers. The semi-supervised approaches are paid more and more attentions by all kinds of researchers, of course we are no exceptions.

Among the existing semi-supervised learning methods, co-training proposed by Blum and Mitchell [4] in 1998, is attracting more and more attentions. The standard co-training assumes that the data can be described by two views satisfy the sufficiency and independence assumptions. Goldman and Zhou [9] proposed an algorithm which used two different supervised learning algorithms to train the two classifiers. Zhou and Li [25] proposed the tri-training approach, which uses three classifiers generated from bootstrap samples of the original training set. Du et al. [6] got the conclusions that co-training 's effectiveness are mixed. Kiritchenko and Matwin [12] adopted the co-training methods to address the email classification problem. They trained the classifiers using SVM and Naive Bayes, and the results showed that SVM was a better choice. As far as I know, co-training has not been applied to social spam detection. Furthermore, to tackle the lackness of labeled tweets and take advantages of multiple unlabeled datasets, we proposed the semi-supervised classification framework for social spam detection, which combines co-training with k-medoids.

3   The Proposed Framework

In this section, we first introduce the problem of spam detection and the overview of semi-supervised framework, and then introduce features for classification. Finally, we present the details of our semi-supervised detection framework.

3.1   Framework Overview

We usually formulate users as a set of features. Let $A = \{\mathbf{x_i}\}^n$ be the user account feature set, where $\mathbf{x_i}$ is the feature vector of user i and n is the total number of users. Also we define $L = \{(\mathbf{x_i}, y_i)\}^l$ denotes the labeled data set, where l is the number of labeled data, and $y_i \in \{+1, -1\}$ is the label of user i ($+1$ denotes the spam user, and -1 denotes the legitimate user). Meanwhile, we define $U = \{\mathbf{x_j}\}^{(n-l)}$ denotes the unlabeled instances. Generally, the problem of social spam detection is to train a classifier f using labeled data L, and predict whether a user in unlabeled data U is a spammer or not. The proposed semi-supervised classification framework is shown in Fig. 1.

As shown in the framework, our semi-supervised classification framework for social spam detection uses only a few labeled samples which were selected by k-medoids and then utilizes a large number of unlabeled samples via co-training framework. Specifically, we first propose a cluster analysis approach which we use to make the detection framework more robust and could select the diverse and representative samples to label. Then we split the features into two views, $view1$ uses the content feature set $x1$, and $view2$ uses the behavior feature set $x2$. We trained two classifiers $C1$ and $C2$ based on the two views. At last, we augment the confident users as new labeled data to the opposite classifier to boost the classification performance. Also we add these confident users to our final classifier C for retraining the classifier. Our framework iteratively runs the whole steps until the classifier could not be refined any further.

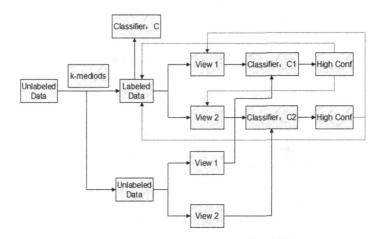

Fig. 1. Social spam detection framework

3.2 Identifying Features of Spammer

Co-training is a good paradigm of semi-supervised, which requires the data to be described by two views of features. For example, we could detect social spammers from two views, the content features and the behavior features of users. Either of views is sufficient for the detection of social spammers if we had enough labeled data. However, labeling a large number of datasets manually is a complex, error-prone and tedious task which may costs a lot of human efforts and time. So we propose a efficient semi-supervised spam detection framework combines co-training with k-medoids. The features we used are defined as followings:

- **Content features**. We extract the content features from posted tweets, url links, @mentions and *hashtags*.
- **Behavior features**. We extract the behavior features from following behavior and other social network behavior, also including some other metrics of graph, such as *clusteringcoefficient, eccentricity, closeness* and *betweenness*.

Table 1. User features

Category	Features in our study	Used/proposed in study
content	Account age	[14, 22]
	Number of tweets	[22]
	Number of recent tweets	[16]
	Tweets rate	[14, 22]
	Tweets similarity	[1, 2, 14, 22]
	Average neighbors' tweets	[22]
	Re-tweet count/rate	[2, 14, 19]
	Url count/rate/unique	[1, 2, 14, 19]
	Ratio of one url	[14, 22]
	@*mention* count/rate/unique	[1, 2, 14]
	Hashtag count/rate	[2, 19]
behavior	Number of followers	[2, 14, 19]
	Number of followings	[2, 14, 19, 22]
	F-F ratio	[1, 2, 14, 22]
	Following rate	[22]
	Average neighbors' followers	[22]
	FMNF	[22]
	Bi-links	[14]
	Bi-links ratio	[22]
	Clustering Coefficient	[22]
	Eccentricity	[16]
	Closeness	[16]
	Betweenness	[22]

The specific features for two views are listed in Table 1. Ultimately we collect 23 features in total, 11 for content features and 12 for behavior features.

3.3   Semi-supervised Social Spammer Detection

The details of the detection framework are presented in Algorithm 1.

Algorithm 1. Semi-Supervised Spammer Detection

Input:
    U: a set of unlabeled users;
    L: a set of labeled users;
Output:
    C : the classification Model;
    $p \leftarrow 10, k \leftarrow 50$;
    $\tau \leftarrow 0.5, n \leftarrow 20$;
    while True **do**
        Use L to train a classifier C based on both the content view and behavior view;
        Use L to train a classifier $C1$ based on the content view $x1$;
        Use L to train a classifier $C2$ based on the behavior view $x2$;
        Select the high confidence($\geq \tau$) users from $C1$, such as top p spam users and top k legitimate users, and then add them to $C2$ and L;
        Select the high confidence($\geq \tau$) users from $C2$, such as top p spam users and top k legitimate users, and then add them to $C1$ and L;
        if number of iterators $> n$ or no enough users whose classify result confidence is larger than the threshold τ to be selected **then**
            break
        end if
    end while
    return C;

At first, we initialize the variables: The parameter K is the number of clustering, also it is the initial number of labeled users. We use 2500 initial seeds, so K is set to be 2500. The confidence threshold τ is set to be 0.5, which means we would select the users whose confidence is larger than or equal to 0.5. The threshold τ is an empirical parameter, which is usually set like this in other studies. With the improvement of classification performance, the classifier can recognize samples with high confidence threshold, which could be utilize to adjust the threshold. At each iteration, we select top p spam users and top k legitimate users from the unlabeled data, while p is set to be 10 and k is set to be 50 in order to balance the ratio of spammers, and then we augment them to the other classifier to boost the classification performance. The parameter n is the maximum iteration number, which is set to be 20 originally for facilitating our experiments, if the iterator number is larger than n or there is no enough users whose classify result confidence is larger than threshold to be selected, the circle will be terminated.

Then, we learn the initial classification model C using learning algorithm SVM and labeled data L. Also we train a classifier $C1$ that only considers the content view $x1$, meanwhile we train a classifier $C2$ that only considers the behavior view $x2$. The two classifications predict the unlabeled data and select top p spam users and top k legitimate users from the unlabeled data separately, and then add them to the other classification to improve the performances of the classifications. Our framework also augment the selected high confidence users to labeled data L in order to enlarge our training set and boost the classification performance of classification model C.

Finally, when there is no more users to be selected whose classify result confidence is larger than the threshold or the iteration number is large than the maximum iteration number, the circle will be terminated and will obtain the final training set and the final classification C. We also can rerun the iterations when classifier C finished in order to adjust the initial points and improve classification performance.

The differences between our proposed algorithm and other algorithms are as following: we combine clustering algorithm with co-training for social spammer detection; we extract content features and behavior features for co-training algorithm.

4   Experiments

In this section, we first introduce the dataset which we use to demonstrate our framework, then we evaluate the effectiveness of our proposed detection framework, at last we compare the detection result of our semi-supervised frame with supervised models.

4.1   Dataset

Twitter, as a microblogging site, is the fastest growing one than any other social networking site, allows users to utilize *tweets*, *mentions*, *hashtag* and *retweet* for sharing information with their friends.

- **Tweets**: This feature allows users to post their latest updates and share messages using no more than 140 characters.
- **@mentions**: This feature facilitates users to directly address someone by using @username methodology. If A mentions B in a tweet, B can see the tweet, even though B is not A's follower. So spammers often use mention to propagate their spam messages, while they have rare followers.
- **Hash-tags**: This feature allows users to keep track of tweets related to certain keywords. Therefor, users can get updates of their interest by looking for tweets via hashtags.
- **Retweet**: This feature facilitates users to share someone's tweet with all of their followers.

We use the UDI-Twitter dataset [15] for our semi-supervised classification framework combines co-training with k-medoids clustering algorithm, a subset of Twitter containing 50 million tweets for 140 thousand users and 284 million following relationships collected at May 2011. Then we extract all features listed in Table 1 of 140 thousand users based on their profiles and tweets content.

How do we spot the spammers? A user was marked as spammer if only the evidence of spamming behavior was found. Spammers often post malicious URLs or phishing URLs which direct users to illegal or fake websites. Therefor, if a user post at least one malicious or phishing URL, we will label the user as a spmmmer. Also, if a user always post plenty of advertisements for products promotion, we label the user as a spammer. There are some users who post a lot of pornographic information or URL links directed to pornographic websites, we label them as spammers as well. Some other spammers go further by copying personal tweets and photos from other users making them more similar to real users, we can identify them by searching for the information like tweets and photos, and then compare the watermarks in photos and timestamps. We invite 50 volunteers to identify the spammers by majority vote. Eventually, we extracted 2615 spammers from 140,000 users and sampled 11194 legitimate users as our dataset. The data processing of our experiment is similar with other studies, we label samples for evaluating or as initial training set.

4.2 Evaluation of Performance

We use 10-fold cross validation to improve the reliability of classifier evaluation in our experiments. In 10-fold cross validation, the original samples are randomly divided into 10 equally-sized sub-samples, 9 sub-samples are used as a training set and the remaining one is used as test set. The evaluations are executed 10 times to ensure that each sub-sample is used as a testing set once in each evaluation. The final evaluation is generated by averaging the results of 10 evaluations. Given a classification algorithm, we consider its confusion matrix as in Table 2.

Where a represents the number of spam users that were correctly classified, b represents the spam users that were falsely classified as legitimate users, c represents the number of legitimate users that were falsely classified as spam users, and d represents the number of legitimate users that were correctly classified. We used the standard metrics such as precision, recall, accuracy, and the F1-measure for performance metrics. Specifically, the precision is $P = a/(a+c)$, the recall is $R = a/(a+b)$, and the F-measure is defined as $F1 = 2PR/(P+R)$. We focus on the F1-measure as it is the trade-off of precision and recall.

Table 2. Confusion matrix

		Prediction	
		Spammer	Legitimate
Actual	Spammer	a	b
	Legitimate	c	d

4.3   Experimental Setup

In order to prove that our semi-supervised classification framework is effective, we made some powerful comparisons.

Firstly, we conducted our experiments on different initial labeled dataset with different seeds selection strategies. Secondly, we compared the performance of our framework with classical supervised algorithm such as *NaiveBayes*, *J48*, *RandomForest*, *Logistic* and so on, which were implemented by weka. In supervised algorithms, we use 10-fold cross validation on 2500 labeled data which are the initial seeds we selected in our framework. We used the standard metrics such as precision, recall, accuracy, and the F1-measure for performance metrics which are mainly measured for spammers.

4.4   Experiments on Different Initial Labeled Data

We utilize k-medoids clustering algorithm to acquire some informative and presentative initial labeled data. K-means is also a classical clustering algorithm which takes the average of all the data points as the center point, that is to say, the center point may not be a substantial point but a virtual position. However, we need to select a specific sample as initial data to label. So, we use k-medoids to attain the substantial center point which is informative and presentative for labeling. To illustrate the effectiveness of this kind of selecting approach, we compare the performance with randomly selected strategy in Fig. 2, where the size of initial seeds ranges from 100 to 2500 and the interval number of seeds is 200. In order to make our semi-supervised classification framework more effective and robust, the initial labeled dataset should cover a diverse set of samples. If we randomly select some samples to label for our initial training set, the selected samples may not be diverse and representative especially with a small number of samples. So we propose to utilize k-medoids clustering algorithm to select the representative informative users to label.

The comparison results of k-medoids and random selecting strategy are shown in Fig. 2(a) shows the detection accuracies of k-medoids and random selecting strategy with different initial seeds. From the figure, we can see that

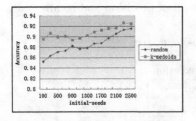 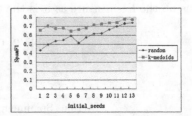

(a) Accuracy of different initial seeds   (b) F1 of different initial seeds

Fig. 2. Comparison of different initial seeds

both of the two selecting strategies present a rising trend in general with the increase of number of initial seeds set. The accuracy of the k-medoids approach is always higher than that of the random selecting approach with the same initial seeds set. Figure 2(b) shows the F1-measures of two seeds selecting strategies. Also the F1 value of k-medoids is higher than that of the random selecting approach. Noting that two measure metrics tend to be stable when the size of initial seeds reaches 2500, we suppose that with our seeds selecting scheme it can provide sufficient information for training when it reaches a threshold. So, we use 2500 initial seeds for our experiment.

4.5 Experimental Results

In this subsection, we comprehensively demonstrated the performance of our framework. We know present our experiment results.

At the beginning, Fig. 3 shows the iteration process of our framework. With the number of iterations increasing, F1-measure and Accuracy are rising except for the slightly falling at first, which is because that our semi-supervised co-training framework gets more and more stable. When the 20th iteration ends, the accuracy is 92.72 % and the F1-measure is 0.7824. If we expand the maximum number of iteration to a larger value and make the iteration process ends with that there is no more hight confident samples to be selected, the accuracy is 94.72 % and the F1-measure is 0.758.

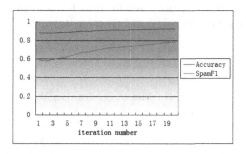

Fig. 3. The result of each iteration (Color figure online)

To illustrate the effectiveness of our semi-supervised co-training framework, we compare it with some standard classification algorithms shown as Table 3, as we can see, the Precision, F1-Measure and Accuracy of our framework are higher than those of any other classification algorithm. The NaiveBayes performs best in terms of the Recall, while our classification framework outperforms the other classifications except for NaiveBayes.

5 Conclusion

In this paper, we have presented the design and implementation of our semi-supervised classification framework for social spammer detection, which

Table 3. Performance results

	Precision	Recall	F1-Measure	Accuracy
NaiveBayes	0.383	**0.825**	0.523	79.36 %
JRip	0.551	0.516	0.533	87.60 %
J48	0.563	0.557	0.56	88.00 %
LogitBoost	0.615	0.35	0.446	88.08 %
Bagging	0.635	0.466	0.538	89.00 %
RandomForest	0.621	0.516	0.564	89.04 %
Logistic	0.645	0.455	0.533	89.08 %
Decorate	0.628	0.516	0.566	89.16 %
FT	0.618	0.589	0.603	89.36 %
Our classification	**0.813**	0.71	**0.758**	**94.72%**

combines co-training with k-medoids clustering algorithm. We take advantage of k-medoids to select some informative and presentative samples as our initial seeds set. Experimental results demonstrated its effectiveness compared with typical supervised learning strategies. We also used content feature set and behavior feature set as the two views of co-training, either of them is sufficient for the detection of social spammers if we had enough labeled dataset. In the future, we will extract more features for our classification framework and integrate more technologies such as active learning and transfer learning.

References

1. Amleshwaram, A.A., Reddy, N., Yadav, S., Gu, G., Yang, C.: Cats: characterizing automation of Twitter spammers. In: 2013 Fifth International Conference on Communication Systems and Networks (COMSNETS), pp. 1–10. IEEE (2013)
2. Benevenuto, F., Magno, G., Rodrigues, T., Almeida, V.: Detecting spammers on Twitter. In: Collaboration, Electronic Messaging, Anti-Abuse and Spam Conference (CEAS) (2010)
3. Benevenuto, F., Rodrigues, T., Almeida, V., Almeida, J., Gonçalves, M.: Detecting spammers and content promoters in online video social networks. In: Proceedings of the 32nd International ACM SIGIR Conference on Research and Development in Information Retrieval (SIGIR), pp. 620–627. ACM (2009)
4. Blum, A., Mitchell, T.: Combining labeled and unlabeled data with co-training. In: Proceedings of the Eleventh Annual Conference on Computational Learning Theory, pp. 92–100. ACM (1998)
5. Chen, F., Tan, P., Jain, A.: A co-classification framework for detecting web spam and spammers in social media web sites. In: Proceedings of the 18th ACM Conference on Information and Knowledge Management (CIKM), pp. 1807–1810. ACM (2009)
6. Du, J., Ling, C.X., Zhou, Z.H.: When does cotraining work in real data? IEEE Trans. Knowl. Data Eng. **23**(5), 788–799 (2011)

7. Fu, H., Xie, X., Rui, Y.: Leveraging careful microblog users for spammer detection. In: Proceedings of the 24th International Conference on World Wide Web Companion, pp. 419–429. International World Wide Web Conferences Steering Committee (2015)
8. Gao, H., Hu, J., Wilson, C., Li, Z., Chen, Y., Zhao, B.: Detecting and characterizing social spam campaigns. In: Proceedings of the 10th Annual Conference on Internet Measurement (IMC), pp. 35–47. ACM (2010)
9. Goldman, S., Zhou, Y.: Enhancing supervised learning with unlabeled data. In: ICML, pp. 327–334. Citeseer (2000)
10. Grier, C., Thomas, K., Paxson, V., Zhang, M.: @ spam: the underground on 140 characters or less. In: Proceedings of the 17th ACM Conference on Computer and Communications Security (CCS), pp. 27–37. ACM (2010)
11. Heymann, P., Koutrika, G., Garcia-Molina, H.: Fighting spam on social web sites: a survey of approaches and future challenges. IEEE Internet Comput. 11(6), 36–45 (2007)
12. Kiritchenko, S., Matwin, S.: Email classification with co-training. In: Proceedings of the 2011 Conference of the Center for Advanced Studies on Collaborative Research, pp. 301–312. IBM Corp. (2011)
13. Lee, K., Caverlee, J., Cheng, Z., Sui, D.: Content-driven detection of campaigns in social media. In: Proceedings of the 20th ACM International Conference on Information and Knowledge Management (CIKM), pp. 551–556. ACM (2011)
14. Lee, K., Caverlee, J., Webb, S.: Uncovering social spammers: social honeypots+machine learning. In: Proceeding of the 33rd International ACM (SIGIR) Conference on Research and Development in Information Retrieval, pp. 435–442. ACM (2010)
15. Li, R., Wang, S., Deng, H., Wang, R., Chang, K.C.C.: Towards social user profiling: unified and discriminative influence model for inferring home locations. In: KDD, pp. 1023–1031 (2012)
16. Li, Z., Zhang, X., Shen, H., Liang, W., He, Z.: A semi-supervised framework for social spammer detection. In: Cao, T., Lim, E.-P., Zhou, Z.-H., Ho, T.-B., Cheung, D., Motoda, H. (eds.) PAKDD 2015. LNCS, vol. 9078, pp. 177–188. Springer, Heidelberg (2015)
17. Lin, C., He, J., Zhou, Y., Yang, X., Chen, K., Song, L.: Analysis and identification of spamming behaviors in sina weibo microblog. In: Proceedings of the 7th Workshop on Social Network Mining and Analysis, p. 5. ACM (2013)
18. Stringhini, G., Kruegel, C., Vigna, G.: Detecting spammers on social networks. In: Proceedings of the 26th Annual Computer Security Applications Conference, pp. 1–9. ACM (2010)
19. Wang, A.: Don't follow me: spam detection in Twitter. In: Proceedings of the 2010 International Conference on Security and Cryptography (SECRYPT), pp. 1–10. IEEE (2010)
20. Wang, B., Zubiaga, A., Liakata, M., Procter, R.: Making the most of tweet-inherent features for social spam detection on Twitter. arXiv preprint arXiv:1503.07405 (2015)
21. Wang, D., Irani, D., Pu, C.: A social-spam detection framework. In: Proceedings of the 8th Annual Collaboration, Electronic Messaging, Anti-Abuse and Spam Conference (CEAS), pp. 46–54. ACM (2011)
22. Yang, C., Harkreader, R., Gu, G.: Empirical evaluation and new design for fighting evolving twitter spammers. IEEE Trans. Inf. Forensics Secur. 8(8), 1280–1293 (2013)

23. Zhang, Q., Zhang, C., Cai, P., Qian, W., Zhou, A.: Detecting spamming groups in social media based on latent graph. In: Sharaf, M.A., Cheema, M.A., Qi, J. (eds.) ADC 2015. LNCS, vol. 9093, pp. 294–305. Springer, Heidelberg (2015)
24. Zhang, X., Zhu, S., Liang, W.: Detecting spam and promoting campaigns in the Twitter social network. In: Proceedings of the 2012 IEEE 12th International Conference on Data Mining, pp. 1194–1199. IEEE Computer Society (2012)
25. Zhou, Z.H., Li, M.: Tri-training: exploiting unlabeled data using three classifiers. IEEE Trans. Knowl. Data Eng. 17(11), 1529–1541 (2005)
26. Zhou, Z.H., Li, M.: Semi-supervised learning by disagreement. Knowl. Inf. Syst. 24(3), 415–439 (2010)

A Hierarchical Beta Process Approach for Financial Time Series Trend Prediction

Mojgan Ghanavati[1,2(✉)], Raymond K. Wong[1], Fang Chen[1,2],
Yang Wang[2], and Joe Lee[3]

[1] School of Computer Science and Engineering,
University of New South Wales, Sydney, Australia
{mojgang,wong}@cse.unsw.edu.au
[2] National ICT Australia (NICTA), Sydney, Australia
{fang.chen,yang.wang}@nicta.com.au
[3] Novel Approach Limited, Hong Kong, China
joe.lee@novelapp.net

Abstract. An automatic stock market categorization system would be invaluable to investors and financial experts, providing them with the opportunity to predict a stock price changes with respect to the other stocks. In recent years, clustering all companies in the stock markets based on their similarities in shape of the stock market has increasingly become popular. However, existing approaches may not be practical because the stock price data are high-dimensional data and the changes in the stock price usually occur with shift, which makes the categorization more complex. In this paper, a hierarchical beta process (HBP) based approach is proposed for stock market trend prediction. Preliminary results show that the approach is promising and outperforms other popular approaches.

Keywords: Stock trend prediction · Hierarchical beta process · GARCH-based clustering

1 Introduction

Time series analysis is finding the correlations in data. The most significant challenges faced by time series analysts include defining the shape of time series, forecasting their future trends and classifying them to different categories. Solving these tasks can significantly help the economy and society. These tasks are actively applied in the stock market section. Malkiel and Fama believe that historical stock prices can be efficiently used to predict their future trend [5]. However, stock market analysis is a complicated task due to the large, high-dimensional, non-normally-distributed and non-stationary time series. Non-stationary means that the statistical properties such as mean, variance and/or autocovariance, change over time. New theories and methods are needed to handle these settings. In particular, forecasting a stock market price movement trend has been a great challenge for a long time. Lots of works have been done on mining the financial time series [12,13,15,16].

© Springer International Publishing Switzerland 2016
H. Cao et al. (Eds.): PAKDD 2016 Workshops, LNAI 9794, pp. 227–237, 2016.
DOI: 10.1007/978-3-319-42996-0_19

Huang et al. [6] used a wrapper approach to choose the best feature subset of 23 technical indices and then combined different classification algorithms to predict the future trend of Korea and Taiwan stock markets. Yu et al. [19] proposed a support vector machine (SVM) based model called least squares support vector machine (LSSVM) to predict stock market trends. They have used genetic algorithm, first to select the input features for LSSVM and then to optimize LSSVM parameters. To evaluate efficiency of the proposed model, $S\&P500$ index, Dow Jones industrial average (DJIA) index, and New York stock exchange (NYSE) index, have been used as testing targets. Patel et al. [14] compared the application of four models including artificial neural network (ANN), SVM, random forest and naive-bayes for stock market trend prediction. Two different approaches have been taken to provide the inputs of these models. In the first approach, ten technical parameters are computed based on stock price data while the second approach focuses on representing these technical parameters as trend deterministic data. To evaluate the efficiency of these models, 10 years historical data of two stocks namely Reliance Industries and Infosys Ltd., and two stock price indices CNX Nifty and S&P Bombay Stock Exchange (BSE) Sensex have been used. Li et al. [7] proposed a supervised regression approach to discover the patterns between stock movements and different information sources.

However stock condition assessment needs further prediction accuracy since any wrong investment may cost thousands to million dollars. In addition, most of the developed models for stock market prediction are parametric or semi-parametric (e.g. [1]). Parametric models usually have a fixed model structure based on a priori assumptions on the data behaviour. Also, they are mostly unable to adjust the model to the complexity of problem. Considering these limitations, we adopt a Bayesian nonparametric model to predict the stock future trend. Nonparametric models provide a more flexible strategy that requires fewer assumptions about model structure. In particular, we consider the beta process (BP) which provides a Bayesian nonparametric prior for statistical models that involves binary prediction results. In our case, the prediction results include up and down trends which are presented with 1 and -1 respectively. Therefore, the model is used to predict the next trend of stocks more accurately by capturing specific patterns of different stock groups. To the best of our knowledge, the flexibility of using Bayesian non-parametric methods for stock market trend prediction has not been investigated. In the literature there are relatively few works that specifically address the classification of financial time series with a non-parametric approach [10]. In the current work we try to fill this gap providing an HBP-based method suitable to predict the stock market condition and also providing useful insight for further investigation.

2   Method

2.1   Feature Selection and Pre-clustering

To find a group of moving objects that are travelling together, first, all the objects are pre-clustered in each timestamp. We collected various financial indicators that affect the stock market trend prediction considering the previous studies. However some indicators may have more contribution on the stock future trends [18]. Therefore, we applied a correlation-based SVM following the work of Lin et al. [11], to find an optimum subset of financial indicators for the pre-clustering step. The importance of these indicators shown in Table 1, is because they can give us clues about the actual trend of the stock market. For example, first two indicators are moving averages. A simple moving average is an indicator that calculates the average price of a stock over a specified number of periods. If a stock is exceptionally volatile, then a moving average will help to smooth the data. A moving average filters out random noise and offers a smoother perspective of the price action. All the indicators are calculated for all the trading days considering weekly averages and their values are normalised between -1 and 1. Some of the indicators called leading indicators are designed to lead price movements. Some of the more popular leading indicators include commodity channel index (CCI), momentum, relative strength index (RSI), stochastic oscillators (K%, D%) and

Table 1. Selected technical indicators and their formulas.

Name of indicators	Formulas
Simple n-day moving average	$\dfrac{C_t + C_{t-1} + \ldots + C_{t-n}}{n}$
Weighted n-day moving average	$\dfrac{(n \times C_t) + ((n-1) \times C_{t-1}) + \ldots + C_n}{n + (n-1) + \ldots + 1}$
Momentum	$C_t - C_{t-n}$
Stochastic K%	$\dfrac{C_t - LL_{t-n}}{HH_{t-n} - LL_{t-n}} \times 100$
Stochastic D%	$\dfrac{\sum\limits_{i=0}^{n-1} K_{t-i}\%}{n}$
RSI (Relative Strength Index)	$100 - \dfrac{100}{1 + (\sum\limits_{i=0}^{n-1} \frac{Up_{t-i}}{n})/(\sum\limits_{i=0}^{n-1} \frac{Dw_{t-i}}{n})}$
MACD (Moving Average Convergence Divergence)	$MACD(n)_{t-1} + 2/n + 1 \times (DIFF_t - MACD(n)_{t-1})$
Larry William's R%	$\dfrac{H_n - C_t}{H_n - L_n} \times 100$
A/D (Accumulation/Distribution) oscillator	$\dfrac{H_n - C_{t-1}}{H_n - L_n}$
CCI (Commodity Channel Index)	$\dfrac{M_t - SM_t}{0.015 D_t}$
Volume average	$\dfrac{V_t + V_{t-1} + \ldots + V_{t-n}}{n}$
Adj close momentum	$AC_t - AC_{t-n}$

Larry Williams R%. CCI measures the difference between a stock's price change and its average price change. In this manner, CCI can be used to identify over-bought and oversold levels. High positive readings indicate that prices are well above their average, which is a show of strength. Low negative readings indicate that prices are well below their average, which is a show of weakness. Momentum measures the rate-of-change of a stock's price. As the price of a stock rises, price momentum increases. RSI compares the average price change of the advancing periods with the average change of the declining periods. An oscillator is an indicator that fluctuates above and below a center line or between set levels as its value changes over time. Stochastic oscillator is a momentum indicator that measures the price of a security relative to the high/low range over a set period of time. The indicator oscillates between 0 and 100, with readings below 20 considered oversold and readings above 80 considered overbought. A 14-period stochastic oscillator reading of 30 would indicate that the current price was 30 % above the lowest low of the last 14 days and 70 % below the highest high. Williams R% reflects the level of the close relative to the highest high for the look-back period. Accumulation distribution (A/D) oscillator is a momentum indicator that relates price changes with volume. The closer the close price is to the high price, the more volume is added to the cumulative total.

2.2   GARCH-Based Distance

We aim to adjust HBP to predict each individual stock movement by capturing the movement patterns of different stock groups. Therefore the first step will be clustering the stocks. In financial time series clustering, a suitable distance measurement is crucial [4]. Assume that there is a distance $D_{(i,j)}$ between $stock_i$ and $stock_j$ that measures the difference between $stock_i$ and $stock_j$. To compute the distance of different stocks, we treat each stock as a time series.

Some of the popular time series distance quantifying methods are shape based, edit based and feature based distances. The shape based and edit based distances can be used when the time series have stable variances since the time series pairs with the closer distance will more likely have a relatively closer distance in the future trend. However, in case of financial time series, there are some empirical regularity to be considered to derive a suitable distance measure. First, financial time series are generally non-stationary, the squared values of time series are autocorrelated and there is a non-linear relationships between subsequent observations of the squared values. The issue of heteroskedastic gave birth to autoregressive conditional heteroskedasticity (ARCH) model which is a significant step in financial time series modelling. The ARCH model can be defined as:

$$\sigma = \alpha_0 + \alpha_1 \epsilon_{t-1}^2 + \ldots + \alpha_q \epsilon_{t-q}^2 = \alpha_0 + \sum_{i=1}^{q} \alpha_i \epsilon_{t-i}^2 \qquad (1)$$

where ϵ_t is a zero mean heteroskedastic univariate process that is defined as:

$$\epsilon_t = u_t \sqrt{h_t} = u_t \sigma_t \qquad (2)$$

where u_t is a univariate noise process with zero mean and variance σ_u^2 and h_t is a univariate stochastic process independent from u_t, $\alpha_0 > 0$ and $0 \leq \alpha_i < 1$, $i > 0$. On top of that, Bollerslev [2] introduced generalized autoregressive conditional heteroskedasticity (GARCH) model that uses values of the past squared observations and past variances to model the variance at time t. GARCH(p, q) is defined as:

$$h_t = \alpha_0 + \alpha_1 \epsilon_{t-1}^2 + \ldots + \alpha_p \epsilon_{t-p}^2 + \beta_1 h_{t-1} + \ldots + \beta_q h_{t-q} = \alpha_0 + \sum_{i=1}^{p} \alpha_i \epsilon_{t-i}^2 + \sum_{j=1}^{q} \beta_j h_{t-i} \qquad (3)$$

where $\alpha_0 > 0$, $0 \leq \alpha_i < 1, 0 \leq \beta_j < 1, (i = 1, \ldots p; j = 1, \ldots q), (\sum_{i=1}^{p} \alpha_i + \sum_{j=1}^{q} \beta_j) < 1$. We adopt a GARCH-based method following the work of D'Urso et al. [4] to measure the distance between financial time series. This distance metric is based on the estimated GARCH parameters and their estimated covariance. Considering GARCH(p, q) for a pair of time series x and y, the distance measure is defined as follows:

$$d_{GARCH} = (L_x - L_y)'(V_x + V_y)^{-1}(L_x - L_y) \qquad (4)$$

where $V_x = \begin{pmatrix} \sigma_{\hat{\alpha}_x}^2 & Cov(\hat{\alpha}_x, \hat{\beta}_x) \\ Cov(\hat{\beta}_x, \hat{\alpha}_x) & \sigma_{\hat{\beta}_x}^2 \end{pmatrix}$ and $V_y = \begin{pmatrix} \sigma_{\hat{\alpha}_y}^2 & Cov(\hat{\alpha}_y, \hat{\beta}_y) \\ Cov(\hat{\beta}_y, \hat{\alpha}_y) & \sigma_{\hat{\beta}_y}^2 \end{pmatrix}$ are estimated covariance of $GARCH(p, q)$ for each pair of time series and $L_x = (\hat{\alpha}_x, \hat{\beta}_x)$ and $L_y = (\hat{\alpha}_y, \hat{\beta}_y)$ are estimated parameters. D'Urso et al. [4] showed that by defining $V = V_x + V_y = \begin{pmatrix} \sigma_{\hat{\alpha}}^2 & Cov(\hat{\alpha}, \hat{\beta}) \\ Cov(\hat{\beta}, \hat{\alpha}) & \sigma_{\hat{\beta}}^2 \end{pmatrix}$ where $\sigma_{\hat{\alpha}}^2 = \sigma_{\hat{\alpha}_x}^2 + \sigma_{\hat{\alpha}_y}^2 /$, $\sigma_{\hat{\beta}}^2 = \sigma_{\hat{\beta}_x}^2 + \sigma_{\hat{\beta}_y}^2$ and $Cov(\hat{\alpha}, \hat{\beta}) = Cov(\hat{\beta}, \hat{\alpha}) = (Cov(\hat{\alpha}_x, \hat{\beta}_x), Cov(\hat{\beta}_x, \hat{\alpha}_x))$, and by if $Cov(\hat{\alpha}, \hat{\beta})/\sigma_{\hat{\alpha}}, \sigma_{\hat{\beta}} = 0$, the distance reduces to the squared Euclidean distance between the standardized estimated coefficients of the GARCH model. Therefore the distance (4) can be rewritten as:

$$d_{GARCH} = \frac{(\hat{\alpha}_x - \hat{\alpha}_y)^2}{\sigma_{\hat{\alpha}}^2} + \frac{(\hat{\beta}_x - \hat{\beta}_y)^2}{\sigma_{\hat{\beta}}^2} \qquad (5)$$

2.3   GARCH-Based Clustering for Financial Time Series

SWARM clustering method [8] is modified and used to cluster the stocks over time using GARCH based coefficient distance on daily return. SWARM was proposed to cluster moving objects with arbitrary shape of clusters in loosely consecutive timestamps. The SWARM clustering method inputs are objects' trajectories and two parameters. The parameters indicate the minimum number of objects in each cluster (min_o), and minimum number of timestamps (min_t). Each cluster (called swarm) is defined as $swarm = O_{j...k}$, where:

$|(O_{j...k})| > min_o$: There should be at least min_o objects.
$|(T_{h...l})| > min_t$: Objects in O are in the same cluster for at least min_t.
$C_{t_i}(o_{i_1}) \cap C_{t_i}(o_{i_2}) \cap ... \cap C_{t_i}(o_{i_p}) \neq \emptyset$

where $o_1, o_n \subset O_{db}$, $\{t_1, t_2, t_m\} \subset T_{db}$; O_{db} is a set of all moving objects, T_{db} is a set of all timestamps in the database and $C_{t_i}(o_j)$ is the set of clusters that object o_j is in at timestamp t_i.

To accelerate the process of clustering, three pruning rules are applied:

RULE 1. Prune if $|T_{max}(O)| < min_t$ ($T_{max}(O)$ is a maximal timeset of objectset O).

RULE 2. Exclude O if there is an O' such that O' is generated by adding an object o into the set O and O' is a swarm.

RULE 3. Exclude (O, T) if there is an object set O' such that O' is generated by adding an object o into O, and $|T_{max}(O')| = |T_{max}(O)|$. $|T_{max}(O)|$ is the maximal timeset of objectset O where:
 1. $C_{t_i}(o_{i_1}) \cap C_{t_i}(o_{i_2}) \cap ... \cap C_{t_i}(o_{i_m}) \neq \emptyset$, $\forall t_j \in T$,
 2. $\nexists t_x \in T_{db} \setminus T$, s.t. $C_{t_i}(o_{i_1}) \cap C_{t_i}(o_{i_2}) \cap ... \cap C_{t_i}(o_{i_m}) \neq \emptyset$

The problem of SWARM is that, it only specifies the overall density, but it has no restriction on density of segments. For example, if parameters set to $Min_t = 60, Min_0 = 2$ for data from week 0 to week 100, the two stocks in Fig. 1 would be wrongly accepted as a SWARM.

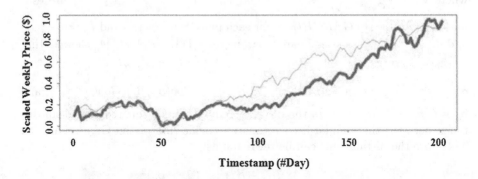

Fig. 1. Weekly prices of two stocks in two years

To address this problem, two more parameters $|Seg|$ and S_{min_o} are introduced which denote the number of segments and minimum number of common timestamps within each segment, respectively. Figure 2 presents the modified SWARM clustering algorithm.

Algorithm 1 Swarm($O, T_{max}, o_{last}, min_o, min_t, |O_{DB}|, |T_{DB}|, C_{DB}, |Seg|, Smin_o$)

Input:

list: O: current object;

T_{max}: maximal timeset of O;

o_{last}: lastest object added into O;

min_o and min_t: minimum threshold parameters;

$|O_{DB}|$: number of objects in database;

$|T_{DB}|$: number of timestamps in database;

C_{DB}: clustering snapshots at each time stamp

$|Seg|$: number of segments

Output: (O, T_{max}) if it is a closed swarm.

if **APruning**($T_{max}, |Seg|, min_t$) is FALSE then

   return;

if **BPruning**($o_{last}, O, T_{max}, C_{CB}$) then

   forward = true;

   for o = next(o_{last}) to last(O_{DB}) do

     $O' = O$.add(o);

     T'_{max} = **GetCommonTimeStamp**($o, o_{last}, T_{max}, C_{CB}$);

     if $|T_{max}| = |T'_{max}|$ then

       forward = false;

     end if

     Swarm($O', T', o, min_o, min_t, |O_{DB}|, |T_{DB}|, C_{CB}$);

   Loop

   if foward and $|O| \geq min_o$ then

     output pair(O, T) as a closed swarm;

   end if

end if

APruning($T_{max}, |Seg|, min_t, T_{DB}$)

Flag = true

For i = 1 to $|Seg|$

   if $\left|T_{seg_i}[T_{max}]\right| < \dfrac{min_t}{|seg|}$ then

     return false;

   end if;

loop;

BPruning($o_{last}, O, T_{max}, C_{DB}$)

for o in $O_{DB} - O$ and $o < o_{last}$

   if $C_t(o) \subseteq C_t(O), t \in T_{max}$ then

   return false;

   end if

return true;

GetCommonTimeStamp($o, o_{last}, T_{max}, C_{CB}$)

for t in T_{max}

   if $C_t(o) \cap C_t(O) \neq \emptyset$ then

   $T'_{max} = T'_{max} + t$;

   end if

return T'_{max};

Fig. 2. Modified SWARM clustering algorithm

2.4   Hierarchical Beta Process for Stock Market Movement Prediction

Hierarchical beta process (HBP) is applied on the clustered stocks to predict the future stock trends. A beta process, $B \sim BP(c, B_0)$, is a positive random measure on a space Ω, where c, the concentration function, is a positive function over Ω, and B_0, the base measure, is a fixed measure on Ω. If B_0 is discrete, $B_0 = \sum_k q_k \delta_{w_k}$, then B has atoms at same locations $B = \sum_k p_k \delta_{w_k}$, where $p_k \sim Beta(c(w_k)q_k, c(w_k)(1 - q_k))$, and each $q_k \in [0, 1]$. An observation data X could be modelled by a Bernoulli process with the measure B, $X \sim BeP(B)$, where $X = \sum_k z_k \delta_{w_k}$, and each z_k is a Bernoulli variable, $z_k \sim Ber(pk)$. Furthermore, when there exists a set of categories, and each data belongs to one of them, hierarchical beta process could be used to model the data. Within each category, the atoms and the associated atom usage are modelled by a beta process. Meanwhile a beta process prior is shared by all the categories. More details could be found in Thibaux and Jordan [17]. For a stock market, denote $\pi_{k,i}$ as the probability of price going up for the ith stock in the kth group. Considering hierarchical construction for stock market assessment,

$$q_k \sim Beta(c_0 q_0, c_0(1 - q_0)), \quad where \quad k = 1, 2, \ldots, K,$$
$$\pi_{k,i} \sim Beta(c_k q_k, c_k(1 - q_k)), \quad where \quad i = 1, \ldots, n_k, \qquad (6)$$
$$z_{k,i,j} \sim Ber(\pi_{k,i}), \quad where \quad j = 1, \ldots, m_{k,i}.$$

q_k and c_k are the mean and concentration parameters for the kth group. q_0 and c_0 are hyper parameters for the hierarchical beta process. $z_{k,i} = z_{k,i,j}|j = 1, \ldots, m_{k,i}$ is the history of ith stock in the kth group. $z_{k,i,j} = 1$ means the stock price has been increased in the jth timestamp, otherwise $z_{k,i,j} = 0$. For hierarchical beta process, a set of q_k are used to describe increasing rates of stock prices in different groups. Following the work of [9], we consider both mean and concentration parameters, which is important for more effective assessment.

Algorithm 2.

Input: Stock up trend history $\{z_{i,j,k}\}$, $k = 1, \ldots, K$; $i = 1, \ldots, n_k$; $j = 1, \ldots, m_{k,i}$; hyper parameters c_0 and q_0

Output: The probability of price increasing $\pi_{k,i}$ for each stock.

for t=1,2,...,T,

$$q_k = \frac{c_0 q_0 + \sum_i s_{i,k}}{c_0 + \sum_i s_{i,k} + \sum_i \sum_{l=0}^{m_k - 1 - s_{i,k}} \frac{c_k}{1 + c_k}}, \quad where \ s_{i,k} = \sum_j z_{i,j,k};$$

$$\pi_{i,k}^{(t)} = \frac{c_k^{(t)} q_k^{(t)} + \sum_j z_{i,j,k}}{c_k^{(t)} + m_{i,k}};$$

end for

calculate $\bar{\pi}_{i,k} = \frac{1}{T} \sum_{t=1}^{T} \pi_{i,k}^{(t)}$

return $\bar{\pi}_{i,k}$.

Fig. 3. Hierarchical beta process for stock market trend prediction

Therefore, for each group, given both c_k and q_k, we have:

$$\pi_{k,i}|q_k, c_k, z_{k,i} \sim Beta(c_k q_k + \sum_j z_{k,i,j}, c_k(1 - q_k) + m_{k,i} - \sum_j z_{k,i,j}) \quad (7)$$

The approximate inference algorithm is shown in Fig. 3.

3   Experiments and Results

In this section, the proposed HBP method is evaluated and compared with popular trend prediction methods. Five years data of 1328 stocks in Hong Kong is used to evaluate the proposed trend prediction method. The historical data is daily and covers the period between June 2010 and June 2015. To predict the trend of stocks for a given month, all the available records before that month are used as training data that is a popular way of using HBP for prediction. The stock market trend prediction problem is defined as a binary classification problem where 1 and −1 represent the up and down trends respectively. Table 2 shows the performance diagnostics including sensitivity, specificity, f-measure and AUC by different methods. Similar indicators have been considered in all models for fair comparison.

Table 2. Performance of different methods for Stock market trend prediction

	Recall	Specificity	FScore	GMean	AUC
HBP+SWARM	0.54	0.32	0.52	0.55	0.55
HBP	0.53	0.32	0.51	0.52	0.52
SVM(Linear)	0.51	0.33	0.49	0.43	0.44
SVM(Polynomial)	0.50	0.37	0.48	0.41	0.42
LMNN	0.33	0.51	0.28	0.30	0.22

To investigate the significance of the results shown in Table 2, Friedman and Nemenyi tests [3] have been chosen to further analyse the results. Friedman test is used to compare different classification results according to their similarity. Friedman test, as a non-parametric test, is more suitable than parametric tests when more than two classifiers are involved [3]. Friedman test compares the average ranks of algorithms under a *null*-hypothesis. The *null*-hypothesis assumes that all the algorithms perform the same and hence their output ranks should be the same. Table 3(a) presents the results of Friedman test and hence we reject the hypothesis, i.e., the algorithms do not perform the same. Friedman test has been performed considering the results of 10 times performing all three methods on stock market data. The χ_F^2 values namely Chi-Square more than 0 with $p < 0.05$ for all the performance diagnostics suggest that there are significant differences between performance measurements values of these three methods (HBP, SVM(Linear) and LMNN). In other words, these results illustrate that even if we perform these methods several times on different data samples, the performance will not be similar and their performances can be ranked.

When the *null*-hypothesis is rejected, we can proceed with a post-hoc test. Nemenyi tests are used here to show the difference between each pair of the algorithms and rank the methods based on their performance. In other words, Nemenyi test is a post-hoc test for pairwise comparisons (Table 3(b)) that are used after Friedman test. Nemenyi test is to test the same hypothesis as Friedman's but just between two methods at a time. As shown in the comparison between HBP and SVM(Linear) in Table 3(b), critical value (q) more than 0 with $p < 0.05$ rejects the *null*-hypothesis. This means that HBP performs better than SVM with linear kernel on all measurements. Similarly, as shown in the comparison between HBP and LMNN in Table 3(b), q more than 0 with $p < 0.05$ implies that KDFuzzyML outperforms Weibull. The higher the critical value is, the bigger difference between their performances is. For instance, for AUC, the critical value from Nemenyi on HBP and LMNN is 6.53, which is larger than the critical value from Nemenyi on HBP and SVM(Linear) (i.e., 5.99). This implies that for AUC, HBP performs the best, followed by SVM(Linear) and then LMNN. This is consistent with the results shown in Table 2.

Table 3. Comparison between the proposed method and other methods using (*a*) Friedman test and then (*b*) Nemenyi test

(a) Friedman test		(b) Nemenyi test		
Metrics	Critical values	Metrics	HBP vs. SVM(Linear)	HBP vs. LMNN
Sensitivity	$\chi^2_F = 12.15$, p < 0.05	Sensitivity	q $= 3.53$, p < 0.05	q $= 4.48$, p < 0.05
Specificity	$\chi^2_F = 13.14$, p < 0.05	Specificity	q $= 4.43$, p < 0.05	q $= 5.24$, p < 0.05
FScore	$\chi^2_F = 23.22$, p < 0.05	FScore	q $= 7.94$, p < 0.05	q $= 7.78$, p < 0.05
AUC	$\chi^2_F = 16.37$, p < 0.05	AUC	q $= 5.99$, p < 0.05	q$=6.53$, p < 0.05

4   Conclusion

This paper proposes the use of a Bayesian nonparametric learning approach to predict stocks future trend from existing infrastructure data. Compared to traditional statistical modelling approaches, nonparametric modelling is not limited by a fixed model structure and is able to adjust the model complexity adaptively according to the complexity of historical data. SWARM clustering algorithm is adjusted and used to group the stocks. Then a hierarchical beta process based approach is proposed to predict stock market trend in each group. Our experiment results show that nonparametric modelling outperforms previous parametric modelling for stock market trend prediction. Our ongoing work includes more extensive experiments (including data from other stock exchanges and comparisons with more specific, related methods) and further optimization of the proposed approach.

References

1. Ausín, M.C., Galeano, P., Ghosh, P.: A semiparametric Bayesian approach to the analysis of financial time series with applications to value at risk estimation. Eur. J. Oper. Res. **232**(2), 350–358 (2014)
2. Bollerslev, T.: Generalized autoregressive conditional heteroskedasticity. J. Econ. **31**(3), 307–327 (1986)
3. Demšar, J.: Statistical comparisons of classifiers over multiple data sets. J. Mach. Learn. Res. **7**, 1–30 (2006)
4. D'Urso, P., Cappelli, C., Lallo, D., Massari, R.: Clustering of financial time series. Phys. A Stat. Mech. Appl. **392**(9), 2114–2129 (2013)
5. Fama, E.F.: Efficient capital markets: a review of theory and empirical work*. J. Finan. **25**(2), 383–417 (1970)
6. Huang, C.J., Yang, D.X., Chuang, Y.T.: Application of wrapper approach and composite classifier to the stock trend prediction. Expert Syst. Appl. **34**(4), 2870–2878 (2008)
7. Li, Q., Jiang, L., Li, P., Chen, H.: Tensor-based learning for predicting stock movements. In: Twenty-Ninth AAAI Conference on Artificial Intelligence (2015)
8. Li, Z., Ding, B., Han, J., Kays, R.: Swarm: mining relaxed temporal moving object clusters. Proc. VLDB Endowment **3**(1–2), 723–734 (2010)
9. Li, Z., Zhang, B., Wang, Y., Chen, F., Taib, R., Whiffin, V., Wang, Y.: Water pipe condition assessment: a hierarchical beta process approach for sparse incident data. Mach. Learn. **95**(1), 11–26 (2014)
10. Lin, A., Shang, P., Feng, G., Zhong, B.: Application of empirical mode decomposition combined with k-nearest neighbors approach in financial time series forecasting. Fluctuation Noise Lett. **11**(02), 1250018 (2012)
11. Lin, Y., Guo, H., Hu, J.: An SVM-based approach for stock market trend prediction. In: The 2013 International Joint Conference on Neural Networks (IJCNN), pp. 1–7. IEEE (2013)
12. Montgomery, D.C., Jennings, C.L., Kulahci, M.: ntroduction to Time Series Analysis and Forecasting. Wiley, Hoboken (2015)
13. Moskowitz, T.J., Ooi, Y.H., Pedersen, L.H.: Time series momentum. J. Financ. Econ. **104**(2), 228–250 (2012)
14. Patel, J., Shah, S., Thakkar, P., Kotecha, K.: Predicting stock and stock price index movement using trend deterministic data preparation and machine learning techniques. Expert Syst. Appl. **42**(1), 259–268 (2015)
15. Qian, X.Y., Liu, Y.M., Jiang, Z.Q., Podobnik, B., Zhou, W.X., Stanley, H.E.: Detrended partial cross-correlation analysis of two nonstationary time series influenced by common external forces. Technical report, arXiv.org (2015)
16. Shumway, R.H., Stoffer, D.S.: Time Series Analysis and Its Applications. Springer, New York (2013)
17. Thibaux, R., Jordan, M.I.: Hierarchical beta processes and the indian buffet process. In: International Conference on Artificial Intelligence and Statistics, pp. 564–571 (2007)
18. Xing, H.J., Ha, M.H., Hu, B.G., Tian, D.Z.: Linear feature-weighted support vector machine. Fuzzy Inf. Eng. **1**(3), 289–305 (2009)
19. Yu, L., Chen, H., Wang, S., Lai, K.K.: Evolving least squares support vector machines for stock market trend mining. IEEE Trans. Evol. Comput. **13**(1), 87–102 (2009)

Efficient Iris Image Segmentation for ATM Based Approach Through Fuzzy Entropy and Graph Cut

Shibai Yin[1(✉)], Yibin Wang[2], and Tao Wang[1]

[1] School of Economic Information Engineering, Southwestern University
of Finance and Economics, Chengdu, China
{Shibaiyin, cnuwt}@swufe.edu.cn
[2] School of Automation, Northwestern Polytechnical University, Xi'an, China
Yibeen.wong@gmail.com

Abstract. In order to realize accurate personal identification in the ATMS, an efficient iris image segmentation approach based on the fuzzy 4-partition entropy and graph cut is presented which can not only yield noisy segmentation results but short the running time. In this paper, an iterative calculation scheme is presented for reducing redundant computations in fuzzy 4-entropy evaluation. Then the presented algorithm uses the probabilities of 4 fuzzy events to define the costs of 4 label assignments (iris, pupil, background and eyelash) for each region in the graph cut. The final segmentation result is computed using graph cut, which produces smooth segmentation result and yields noise. The experimental results demonstrate the presented iterative calculation scheme can greatly reduce the running time. Quantitative evaluations over 20 classic iris images also show that our algorithm outperforms existing iris image segmentation approaches.

Keywords: Iris segmentation · Graph cut · Fuzzy entropy · Iterative scheme

1 Introduction

The human iris has emerged as an effective biometric modality due to its uniqueness, stability and secure nature [1]. Automated person identification and verification systems based on the iris biometric have become increasingly popular over the past few years due to the availability of efficient and accurate iris recognition algorithm. It has been utilized or considered in financial field. For example, ATMS are a major area where iris recognition is being trailed [2]. The use of this technology with ATMS means that customers can discard their plastic cards and PINS thus eliminating the possibility of having cards and PINS stolen or lost. The banking industry is also involved in looking at implementing the technology in over the counter transactions with customers [3]. This would result in faster transaction times that leave the bank teller with more time to concentrate on the level of service provided to the customer.

Iris segmentation is a crucial step in every iris recognition system. It consists of extracting the set of pixels contained in the iris. However, it is hard to get an ideal iris images for accurate segmentation. Since the input images require a significant amount

© Springer International Publishing Switzerland 2016
H. Cao et al. (Eds.): PAKDD 2016 Workshops, LNAI 9794, pp. 238–247, 2016.
DOI: 10.1007/978-3-319-42996-0_20

of user cooperation during image acquisition, thereby these constraints limit the application of iris recognition system in ATMS.

Multilevel image thresholding as a segmentation approach has recently emerged as a powerful technique. One classic example is the fuzzy c-partition entropy segmentation proposed by Cheng et al. [4]. Though the performance of fuzzy c-partition entropy segmentation is encouraging, a few limitations still remain. Firstly, the spatial correlation among adjacent pixels is ignored because the labeling decision is independently made for each pixel using only its intensity information. Secondly, the running time increases exponentially as the number of thresholds increases. This makes such an approach less adopted for iris segmentation. As a result, how to perform fuzzy entropy segmentation for non-ideal images in an unsupervised manner is yet to be explored.

In this perspective, this paper proposes an iris segmentation approach based on the use of a multilevel thresholding step and Graph Cut (GC). The one considerably reduces running time sharply and delimits the iris region in the eye image so well. The major contributions are summarized as follows:

- The iterative scheme for accelerating the fuzzy 4-partition entropy calculation is proposed. This approach can not only cache all the entropy function values for subsequent calculation, but is also independent to the partition number.
- We combine the fuzzy 4-partition entropy segmentation with GC to intensify the spatial correlation of fuzzy 4-partition by using the probabilities of fuzzy events to define the costs of different label for each region in GC, so that the globally optimal partitioning threshold and the local spatial coherence are respected.
- The presented algorithm is quantitatively evaluated using the West Virginia University (WVU) Non-Ideal iris database and achieves highly competitive results compared with the state-of-the-art methods.

The remainder of the paper is organized as follows: Sect. 2 presents the related work. Section 3 discusses how to propose an iterative scheme for calculating the fuzzy 4-partition entropy efficiently. Section 4 explains how to applying GC over the regions and implementing the segmentation. Experiments on 20 test images are carried out in Sect. 5, where comparisons with existing multilevel thresholding method and GC algorithms are made. Finally, Sect. 6 concludes the paper.

2   Related Work

Being the most critical step in any iris biometric system, iris segmentation can be defined as the isolation of the iris from the captured eye image. Many approaches have been proposed in this respect. Daugman proposed the integro-differential Operator (IDO), which is a process that behaves as a circular edge detector that searches iteratively for approximating the iris boundaries as perfect circles [5]. The main drawback of this approach is that it does not work properly in the presence of noise, in the case of images generated under non-ideal conditions.

Another widely used segmentation algorithm is that of Wildes who suggested a histogram-based model-fitting approach accomplished by the implementation of hough transform for iris boundaries localization [1]. This approach suffers the fact that it requires large storage spaces and so costs high computation time.

Recent fuzzy c-partition entropy is also widely used in the iris segmentation, which consider the fuzziness of the iris image and utilize the fuzzy entropy to delimit the iris image into several different fuzzy classes [6]. But this method only use intensity information to partition the image while the spatial correlation among adjacent pixels is ignored, leading in noisy segmentation results. And the running time for searching the optimal thresholds increases exponentially with the number of partition increasing.

Another interesting approach for iris image segmentation is that of Pundlik who present a GC based algorithm for iris segmentation [7]. With this approach, the eye is modeled as a Markov Random Field and GC are used to minimize an energy function that enforces spatial continuity in the region labels found. However it is hard to set the likelihood item of the energy function, dying to fuzziness of the non-ideal iris image.

Motivated by the above observations, we here propose a novel iterative computation scheme for fuzzy c-partition entropy with $c = 4$ which combines with the EA can search optimal thresholds efficiently. Then, the GC algorithm has been conducted on the segmentation images, for enforcing the smoothness of the segmentation results.

3 Efficient Fuzzy 4-Partition Entropy Calculation Using an Iterative Scheme

It was mentioning that only the red channel of the color iris image is employed to implement the segmentation. The fuzzy 4-partition entropy is used for multilevel thresholding segmentation in order to partition the iris image into 4 fuzzy sets which are belongs to iris, pupil, eyelashes and background. Based on this idea, S membership functions are selected to divide the image into 4 suitable fuzzy sets, which is defined as:

$$S(x, u, v, w) = \begin{cases} 1 & x \leq u \\ 1 - \frac{(x-u)^2}{(w-u)(v-u)} & u < x \leq v \\ \frac{(x-w)^2}{(w-u)(w-v)} & v < x \leq w \\ 0 & x > w \end{cases}. \tag{1}$$

Then the opposite Z-function can be written as $Z(x, u, v, w) = 1 - S(x, u, v, w)$.

Three pairs of S-functions and Z-functions, which classify the pixels into four fuzzy sets, referred as dark set E_d, middle set E_{md}, bright set E_{mb} and most bright set E_b. The related membership functions are defined as below:

$$M_d(k) = S(k, u_1, v_1, w_1); \tag{2}$$

$$M_{md}(k) = \begin{cases} Z(k, u_1, v_1, w_1) & k \leq w_1 \\ S(k, u_2, v_2, w_2) & w_1 < k \leq w_2 \end{cases}; \tag{3}$$

$$M_{mb}(k) = \begin{cases} Z(k, u_2, v_2, w_2) & w_1 < k \leq w_2 \\ S(k, u_3, v_3, w_3) & k > w_2 \end{cases} ; \tag{4}$$

$$M_b(k) = S(k, u_3, v_3, w_3); \tag{5}$$

where k is the gray level of a pixel in the image, so we have $0 \leq k \leq 255$; $0 \leq u_1 < v_1 < w_1 < u_2 < v_2 < w_2 < u_3 < v_3 < w_3 \leq 255$ are the parameters determining the shape of the above membership functions. E_d, E_{md}, E_{mb} and E_b are defined as:

$$p_d = \sum_{k=0}^{255} h(k)M_d(k); \quad p_{md} = \sum_{k=0}^{255} h(k)M_{md}(k);$$

$$p_{mb} = \sum_{k=0}^{255} h(k)M_{mb}(k); \quad p_b = \sum_{k=0}^{255} h(k)M_b(k), \tag{6}$$

where $h(\cdot)$ is the normalized histogram function, which gives the occurrence probability of a given gray level. The entropy of the fuzzy 4-partition is given by

$$H(u_1, v_1, w_1, u_2, v_2, w_2, u_3, v_3, w_3)$$
$$= -p_d \log(p_d) - p_{md} \log(p_{md}) - p_{mb} \log(p_{mb}) - p_b \log(p_b). \tag{7}$$

Finding the maximum value of H requires calculating all combinations $(u_1, v_1, w_1, u_2, v_2, w_2, u_3, v_3, w_3)$. Straightforward implementation of the above process involves redundant calculations. To address this problem, iterative schemes are proposed [8]. But, their methods are designed solely for the fuzzy 2-partition entropy. So, a novel iterative approach is presented for fuzzy 4-partition entropy. Let p_d in the Eq. (5) expand as Eq. (8). P_{md}, P_{mb} and P_d can be rewritten in the same way.

$$p_d = \frac{1}{(w_1 - u_1)(w_1 - v_1)} \sum_{k=v_1+1}^{w_1} (k - w_1)^2 h(k) -$$
$$\frac{1}{(w_1 - u_1)(v_1 - u_1)} \sum_{k=u_1+1}^{v_1} (k - u_1)^2 h(k) + \sum_{k=0}^{v_1} h(k), \tag{8}$$

Those expanded equations all contain three similar sum terms. Hence conducting iterative computation and saving iterative values for the shared sum terms can reduce redundant computation. Now let $E(a, b) = \sum_{k=a+1}^{b} (k - a)^2 h(k)$, $F(a, b) = \sum_{k=a+1}^{b} (k - b)^2 h(k)$, $G(a, b) = \sum_{k=a}^{b} h(k)$. First let $E(a, b)$ varies along with b, and it can be rewritten as

$$E(a,b) = \sum_{k=a+1}^{b} (k-a)^2 h(k)$$

$$= \sum_{k=a+1}^{b-1} (k-a)^2 h(k) + (b-a)^2 h(b) \qquad (9)$$

$$= E(a,b-1) + (b-a)^2 h(b).$$

So the iterative calculation of $E(a,b)$ becomes:

$$\begin{cases} E(a,b) = E(a,b-1) + (b-a)^2 h(b), & b = a+2, \cdots, 255 \\ E(a,a+1) = h(a+1) \end{cases} \qquad (10)$$

For $F(a,b)$, when b is fixed, $F(a,b)$ varies along with a. And the iterative calculation of $F(a,b)$ becomes:

$$\begin{cases} F(a,b) = F(a+1,b) + (a-b+1)^2 h(a+1) & a = 0, \cdots, b-2 \\ F(b-1,b) = 0 \end{cases} \qquad (11)$$

Finally, the iterative process of the $G(a,b)$ is denoted as follow:

$$G(a,b) = \sum_{k=a}^{b} h(k) = G(a,b-1) + h(b). \qquad (12)$$

All the iterative values of $E(a,b)$, $F(a,b)$ and $G(a,b)$ can be stored for the subsequent exhaustive algorithms, where $0 \leq a < b \leq 255$, resulting in the computational cost of the fuzzy entropy H calculation being greatly reduced.

4   Enforcing Spatial Coherence Using Graph Cut

The optimization procedure discussed in the previous section computes the optimal combination of $(u_1, v_1, w_1, u_2, v_2, w_2, u_3, v_3, w_3)$ that yields the maximum entropy. Images can be segmented by computing the optimal threshold values. However, such a pixel-based approach leads in noisy results [9]. In order to address this problem, GC algorithm is applied to enforce the smoothness of the segmentation [10].

Firstly, a Gaussian filter and a median filter are applied to the localized eye image I in order to mitigate the noise level which is commonly affect observed for the image acquired in the unconstrained conditions. Then, a standard watershed algorithm is conducted using the gradient image to oversegment the input image into regions. All pixels belonging to the same watershed region are assigned to the same label. This allows us to perform GC over these regions, instead of individual pixels, which speeds up the GC optimization process. The data costs for assigning four labels (background, pupil, iris and eyelashes) corresponds to most bright set E_b, dark set E_d, bright set E_{mb} and middle set E_{md}. So a given region R is calculated using Eq. (13).

$$E_{\text{data}}(l_R = \text{``dark''}) = -\log \sum_{k=0}^{255} h_R(k)M_d(k);$$

$$E_{\text{data}}(l_R = \text{``middle''}) = -\log \sum_{k=0}^{255} h_R(k)M_{md}(k);$$

$$E_{\text{data}}(l_R = \text{``middle bright''}) = -\log \sum_{k=0}^{255} h_R(k)M_{mb}(k);$$

$$E_{\text{data}}(l_R = \text{``bright''}) = -\log \sum_{k=0}^{255} h_R(k)M_b(k);$$

(13)

where l_R is the label of region R, $h_R(k)$ is the normalized histogram of pixels inside region R.

To enforce the labeling coherence among adjacent regions, the smooth term E_{smooth} in GC is defined based on the one proposed by Boykov et al. [11]:

$$E_{smooth} = \exp(-\frac{(I_P - I_q)^2}{2\sigma^2}) \cdot \frac{1}{dist(p,q)},$$

(14)

where I_P and I_q are the average intensities of regions p and q. $dist(p,q)$ is the average distance between the regions p and q. Parameter σ is related to the level of variation between neighboring regions within the image. The value of σ shall stay in the range of $[0, 1]$; and we default it to 0.9 in our experiments. With the graph constructed for all the regions, the optimal label assignment for different regions is computed using the $\alpha-\beta$ swap operator [12].

5   Experimental Results

In this section, we evaluate the performance of the proposed iris segmentation algorithm from different aspects. In the Sects. 5.1 and 5.2, the segmentation results of the proposed method are compared with existing per-pixel threshold-based methods and the GC based method respectively. At last, discussions about algorithm complexity are given in Sect. 5.3.

All of the algorithms presented in this paper are implemented in Matlab 7.0 on a PC with 2.4 GHz CPU, 2G RAM, running Windows XP. Quantitative evaluations are conducted using 20 classical test images from West Virginia University (WVU) iris database. However, due to space limits, the segmentation results for 3 representative and challenging images are shown in the paper.

5.1   Comparison with Existing Threshold-Based Methods

We compare our results with the ones produced by existing algorithms, including the multi-thresholding segmentation method proposed by Otsu [13] and the histogram-based algorithm [14].

Since these approaches do not enforces spatial coherence, our per-pixel thresholding results obtained without GC are used for comparison. The uniformity measure (U) [15] is used to evaluate the quality of segmentation results.

$$U = 1 - 2(f - 1)\frac{\sum_{j=0}^{f-1} \sum_{i \in R_j} (k_i - u_j)^2}{N(k_{\max} - k_{\min})^2},$$ (15)

where f is the partition number; R_j is the segmented region j; k_i is the gray level of the pixel i; u_j is the mean of the gray levels of those pixels in the segmented region j; N is the number of total pixels in the given image; $k_{\max}$ and $k_{\min}$ are the maximum and minimum gray level of pixels in the given image. Higher value of U means the quality of the chosen thresholds is better.

The measured U values for all the 20 test images are showed in the Fig. 1. From the figure we can observe that our results have the highest U values under most settings.

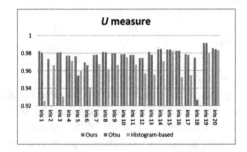

Fig. 1. Comparison of different segmentation methods for 20 iris images using U measurement. (Color figure online)

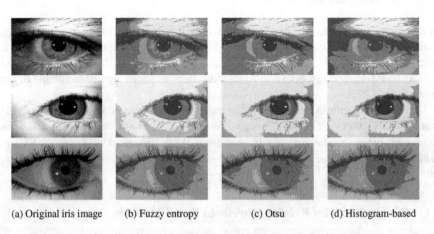

(a) Original iris image   (b) Fuzzy entropy   (c) Otsu   (d) Histogram-based

Fig. 2. Visual comparison of different segmentation methods on iris images.

Figure 2 provides visual comparisons among the segmentation results of different approaches. They confirm that the proposed approach generates the most visually pleasing results, whereas the existing approaches output subpar results in many cases.

5.2   Comparison with an Existing Graph Cut Based Methods

In order to demonstrate the effective of proposed segmentation approach, our segmentation results are compared with the publicly available implementation of Pundlik's algorithm [7]. The segmentation results on 3 non-ideal iris images from the databases are shown in Fig. 3. From that we can see, our extracted iris mask is more completed and can be used to iris recognition later. While Pundlik's result lost more detailed information.

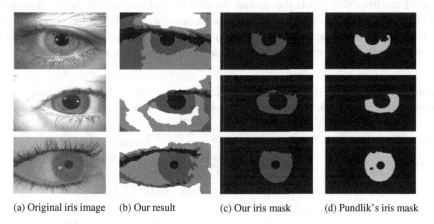

(a) Original iris image   (b) Our result   (c) Our iris mask   (d) Pundlik's iris mask

Fig. 3. Compared results of our algorithm and Pundlik's algorithm on 3 non-ideal iris images from the WVU database.

Besides that the evaluation function F proposed by Liu and Yang [16] is used to measure the quality of segmentation. This measure is widely adopted, with variants being proposed for evaluating image segmentation when the ground truth is unavailable. The F measure is defined as:

$$F = \sqrt{c} \sum_{i=1}^{c} \frac{e_i^2}{\sqrt{A_i}}, \tag{16}$$

where c is the partition number in the segmented image; A_i is the area or the number of pixels of the cth regions; and e_i is intensity error of region i. e_i is defined as the sum of the Euclidean distance of the intensity vectors between the original image and segmented image of each pixel in the region. In this paper, the F is normalized by the size of the image and is scaled down by the factor 0.0001. Figure 4 plots the F values of our and Pundlik's results. As expected, Our results get smaller F scores than Pundlik's results, suggesting our method can provide better segmentation quality.

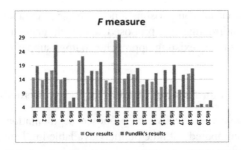

Fig. 4. Comparison with our algorithm and Pundlik's GC based method on 20 test images (Color figure online)

The proposed algorithm is further validated by considering the ground truth segmented results. Table 1 lists the various parameters of the extracted ground truth data on 20 test iris images. We measured both the percentage of mislabeled iris pixel as well as the error in the parameters of the estimated pupil and iris. Our algorithm clearly outperforms Pundlik's results, achieving a average segmentation error of 3 %.

Table 1. Characteristics of the 20 manually labeled images from the WVU database. And comparison of our algorithm and Pundlik's algorithm using the ground truth data.

Parameter	20 non-ideal iris images				Average error/standard deviation (pixels)	
	Average	Max	Min	Std	Ours	Pundlik's
Iris area (pixels)	24692	38315	14000	5693	2.3/2.8	4.5/10.2
Pupil area (pixels)	4244	14175	1231	2520	2.1/2.5	3.6/3.3
Iris occlusion (%)	27	54	3	13	3.0/2.8	3.7/4.5

5.3   Analyses on Algorithm Complexity and Running Time

The total time of the proposed method is mainly composed of 2 parts: the first part is spent on the iterative calculation scheme discussed in Sect. 3. The complexity of this iterative calculation is $O(n^2)$. Then GC optimization is also computationally efficient since it is conducted over a small number of regions, instead of all the pixels which can save lots of time. Generally speaking, the runtime for performing algorithm on the whole image of 256 × 256 resolution is around 3 s.

6   Conclusion

This paper presented an efficient iris segmentation for ATM based approach which is developed based on the fuzzy 4-partition entropy and GC algorithm. The main contributions of this paper include: (1) an iterative scheme for accelerating the fuzzy 4-partition entropy calculation is proposed, so the maximum entropy search time can be greatly reduced. (2) The probabilities of fuzzy events in the fuzzy 4-partition is used to define the costs of different label for each region in GC, so that the results are robust against isolated noise. Our experiment results have illustrated significant improvement in segmentation precision, especially for the images acquired under visible illumination. Hence, it can be used in the ATMS for accurate personal identification.

Acknowledgements. This work is supported by the Major Project of National Natural Science Foundation (No. 91218301), the Fundamental Research Funds for Central Universities-Innovation Team Project (No. JBK150503) and the Central Universities-Yong Scholar Development Project (No. JBK150134), the Youth Fund Project of National Natural Science Foundation (No. 61502396). Besides that, this work is also supported by the Internet Financial Innovation and Regulatory Collaborative Innovation Center.

References

1. Wildes, R.P.: Iris recognition: an emerging biometric technology. J. Proc. IEEE **85**(9), 1348–1363 (1997)
2. Sowjanya, J., Srivani, S.: Iris recognition for ATM based approach. J. IJCER **2**(4), 583–585 (2013)
3. Bechelli, L., Bistarelli, S., Vaccarelli, A.: Biometrics authentication with smartcard. J. Istituto di Informamatica e Teleomatica (ITT) **12**, 1–12 (2002)
4. Cheng, H., Chen, J.R., Li, J.: Threshold selection based on fuzzy c-partition entropy approach. J. Pattern Recogn. **31**(7), 857–870 (1998)
5. Daugman, J.G.: High confidence visual recognition of persons by a test of statistical independence. J. IEEE Trans. Pattern Anal. Mach. Intell. **15**(11), 1148–1161 (1993)
6. Tsai, C.C., Lin, H.Y., Taur, J., et al.: Iris recognition using possibilistic fuzzy matching on local features. J. IEEE Trans. Syst. Man Cybern. Part B: Cybern. **42**(1), 150–162 (2012)
7. Pundlik, S.J., Woodard, D.L., Birchfield, S.T.: Non-ideal iris segmentation using graph cuts. In: IEEE Computer Society Conference on Computer Vision and Pattern Recognition Workshops, CVPRW 2008, pp. 1–6 (2008)
8. Tang, Y., Mu, W., Zhang, Y., et al.: A fast recursive algorithm based on fuzzy 2-partition entropy approach for threshold selection. J. Neurocomput. **74**(17), 3072–3078 (2011)
9. Tang, Y., Zhang, X., Li, X., et al.: Application of a new image segmentation method to detection of defects in castings. J. Int. J. Adv. Manuf. Technol. **43**(5–6), 431–439 (2009)
10. Peng, B., Zhang, L., Zhang, D., et al.: Image segmentation by iterated region merging with localized graph cuts. J. Pattern Recogn. **44**(10), 2527–2538 (2011)
11. Boykov, Y., Veksler, O., Zabih, R.: Fast approximate energy minimization via graph cuts. J. IEEE Trans. Pattern Anal. Mach. Intell. **23**(11), 1222–1239 (2001)
12. Gu, Y., Kumar, V., Hall, L.O., et al.: Automated delineation of lung tumors from CT images using a single click ensemble segmentation approach. J. Pattern Recogn. **46**(3), 692–702 (2013)
13. Otsu, N.: A threshold selection method from gray-level histograms. J. Autom. **11**(285–296), 23–27 (1975)
14. Papamarkos, N., Gatos, B.: A new approach for multilevel threshold selection. J. CVGIP: Graph. Models Image Process. **56**(5), 357–370 (1994)
15. Kullback, S.: Information Theory and Statistics. Courier Corporation, New York (1968)
16. Liu, J., Yang, Y.-H.: Multiresolution color image segmentation. J. IEEE Trans. Pattern Anal. Mach. Intell. **16**(7), 689–700 (1994)

Matching Product Offers of E-Shops

Andrea Horch$^{(\boxtimes)}$, Holger Kett, and Anette Weisbecker

Fraunhofer Institute for Industrial Engineering IAO, 70569 Stuttgart, Germany
andrea.horch@iao.fraunhofer.de
http://www.iao.fraunhofer.de

Abstract. E-commerce is a continuously growing and competitive market. There are several motivations for e-shoppers, sellers and manufacturers to require an automated approach for matching product offers from various online sources referring to the same or a similar real-world product. Currently, there are several approaches for the assignment of identical and similar product offers. These existing approaches are not sufficient for performing a precise comparison as they only return a similarity value for two compared products but do not give any information for further calculations and analyses. The contribution of this paper is a novel approach and an algorithm for matching identical and very similar product offers based on the pairwise comparison of the product names. For this purpose the approach uses different similarity values which are based on an existing string similarity measure. The approach is independent from a specific product domain or data source.

Keywords: Web mining · Product resolution · E-commerce

1 Introduction

E-commerce is a constantly growing market. In 2014 the European turnover has been raised by 16.3 % to 363.1 billion Euros. The 264 million e-shoppers in Europe could choose from an estimated set of 645,000 online retailers for making their purchases [1]. As it is very important for e-shoppers to find the lowest price online [2], it is essential for online retailers to be aware of the prices and product range of their competitors in order to remain competitive. Considering the huge number of European online retailers offering numerous products within their e-shops as well as the message of [3], which implies that online prices are updated daily or even more often comparing the products and prices manually would be a hard and time consuming job. Thus, online merchants need software support to automatically compare products and prices.

To be able to compare products or product prices there is a need for an approach which identifies and matches product offers presenting identical or similar products. In [4–6] we propose approaches for (1) automatically identifying and extracting product records from e-shop websites and for (2) detecting and collecting different product attributes within product records. The approach presented in this paper uses the extracted product names to compare different product

© Springer International Publishing Switzerland 2016
H. Cao et al. (Eds.): PAKDD 2016 Workshops, LNAI 9794, pp. 248–259, 2016.
DOI: 10.1007/978-3-319-42996-0_21

offers in order to determine different product descriptions referring to the same or a very similar real-world product. While existing approaches depend on a specific product domain or data source the proposed approach is independent from both.

2 Related Work

The term *entity resolution* describes the problem of identifying, extracting and matching entities within structured and unstructured data from same or different sources [10]. Over the years many approaches for entity resolution have been published as the work presented in [11,12] or [13]. The matching of product offers (*product resolution*), which is a special variation of entity resolution has been profoundly investigated foremost over the last decade. Matching product offers describes the identification of product descriptions within the same or different structured or unstructured data sources which represent the same real-world product [14]. An early work on product resolution can be found in [7] where a weighted-tree similarity algorithm is described in order to match product or service requests and offers advertised by buyers and sellers on common e-marketplaces. The authors of [14] use an adaptive string similarity measure for matching product offers. In [8] the similarity of products within the domains *electronics* and *toys* is determined by measuring the similarity of defined attributes of the products. A system for mapping unstructured product offers to structured product descriptions is designed in [15]. The system acts as a prototype of a commercial search engine which matches the product offers returned by Bing Shopping[1] to structured product records from the Bing product catalog stored in the database of the system. A learning-based approach for matching product offers based on the extraction and comparison of product attributes is proposed in [16]. The authors of [9] present an algorithm for matching product titles from different data feeds. The approach introduced in [17] extends the product titles of product data from Web sources with tokens from a Web search to match different product offers for the same real world product entity similar to the algorithm proposed in [9]. A novel mining metric called *product identity-clustering* is presented in [18]. Additionally, the authors introduce innovative similarity metrics to improve the product identity-clustering as well as novel performance metrics to measure the performance of the proposed algorithms.

The existing approaches have investigated, extended and improved diverse current similarity measures and clustering methods for matching product offers from different Web sources. For some approaches even new metrics were created to compute the product similarity of product title pairs or a pair of complete product descriptions. However, the existing approaches depend on specific product categories (domains) or are created for product data of particular data sources as e.g. specific market places or search engine result pages whereas the approach proposed in this paper is independent from a product domain or data source.

---

[1] Bing Shopping had been discontinued in 2013.

3   Creation of the Approach

The approach was created to identify identical or very similar products of different e-shops based on the pairwise comparison of the product names. Additionally, the approach shall provide a hint regarding unit differences of the products in order to be able to automatically compare the product prices, as the prices of 200 mg of a product will be lower than of 400 mg of the same product. To create an adequate method to automatically compare the product names the following steps need to be performed:

1. Determine an appropriate similarity/distance measure to identify identical and similar product names.
2. Define suitable similarity values in order to compare the product names.
3. Determine an adequate combination of the defined similarity values in order to identify correct product matches.

The steps were implemented by performing different measurements on real online product offer data. The dataset was automatically collected from six different e-shops of three different product domains. The details of the used data and the further processing are described in detail in the following paragraphs.

3.1   Data

The data analysed to build the approach was collected from three e-shops of different countries selling products of the most popular product categories as presented in [2]. To be able to develop and verify a matching approach for each of the three e-shops, a competitor e-shop was needed. The first three e-shops were selected by performing the following Google searches:

1. `home electronics shop .uk`
2. `cosmetics,skincare,haircare shop .de`
3. `food shop .gr`

We picked out the first e-shop of the expected country and product domain from the result list of the search engine and included it into our result list of e-shops for the extraction of the product dataset. As an adequate competitor was required for each e-shop to build the matching approach for each selected e-shop, we ran another Google search in order to find a competitor. For this purpose we randomly chose a product within each e-shop and created the following search queries by stringing the name of the selected product together with the keyword "shop" and the top-level-domain of another country:

1. `CANON EOS 5D Mark III shop .gr`
2. `Aveda Be Curly Shampoo shop .uk`
3. `Dr Pepper 330ml shop .de`

Table 1. E-shops for dataset extraction

No.	Domain	E-shop	Records	Competitor	Records	Total records
1	Electronics	pixmania.co.uk	782	adorama.gr	926	1, 708
2	Haircare	myhaarzauber.de	380	thehairshop.co.uk	599	979
3	Food	brfoods.gr	850	usa-drinks.de	4, 773	5, 623

The result list of e-shops and the corresponding competitors are shown in Table 1. The identification and extraction of the product records of the e-shops was performed by our approach described in [5]. The product attribute extraction was done by our methods presented in [4,6].

The resulting data set contained a total of 8,310 product records extracted from the e-shops shown in Table 1. The dataset includes 1,708 data records of the product domain *home electronics*, 979 data records of the domain *cosmetics, skincare and haircare* and 5,623 data records of the domain *food*. A data record contains the following information about a product: (1) e-shop ID, (2) product name, (3) product manufacturer, (4) product units, (5) actual product price, (6) regular product price and (7) currency of prices. The collected data set is used to determine an appropriate measure and adequate similarity values in order to develop an optimal matching approach to find identical or very similar product offers within a data set of product offers.

3.2 Determination of the Similarity/Distance Measure

The similarity values to compare the product names were developed based on an existing string similarity/distance measure. To find the most suitable measure for our purposes we searched for the measure out of a defined set of measures returning the best precision and recall values for a certain threshold value when comparing the product names of the e-shops and their corresponding competitors given in Table 1. The considered set of similarity/distance measures was the following: $M = \{$*Levenshtein Distance, difflib.SequenceMatcher, Sorensen Distance, Jaccard Distance*$\}$.

Levenshtein Distance. The Levenshtein Distance calculates the minimum count of edit operations, which are necessary to amend a string into another string. The edit distance can be calculated as shown in Eq. 1.

$$d_{i,j} = min(d_{i,j-1} + d_g, d_{i-1,j} + d_g, d_{i-i,j-1} + d_{m(x_i,y_i)}) \tag{1}$$

$d_g = 1$
$d_{m(x_i,y_i)} = 1 \quad if \ x_i \neq y_j, otherwise : d_{m(x_i,y_i)} = 0$

Using the Levenshtein Distance the similarity of the compared strings is calculated by the following equation:

$$sim(string_1, string_2) = 1 - \frac{d(string_1, string_2)}{max(|string_1|, |string_2|)}) \tag{2}$$

Python Class difflib.SequenceMatcher. The class *SequenceMatcher* of the Python library *difflib* is based on the *Ratcliff-Obershelp similarity algorithm* shown in Eq. 3.

$$d_{ro} = \frac{2c_m}{|s_1| + |s_2|} \tag{3}$$

c_m : *number of matching characters*
$|s_1|$ *and* $|s_2|$: *lengths of strings* s_1 *and* s_2

The similarity of strings is calculated by using the ratio method of the class *difflib.SequenceMatcher.*

Sorensen Distance. The Sorensen Distance determines the distance of strings by calculating the ratio between their common species (intersecting set of species) and their combined length as given in Eq. 4.

$$d_{so} = \frac{2c}{a + b} \tag{4}$$

a : *number of species in set A*
b : *number of species in set B*
c : *number of common species of set A and set B (intersecting set)*

Jaccard Distance. The Jaccard Distance is very similar to the Sorensen Distance. It calculates the ratio between their common species (intersecting set of species) and their combined length of the compared strings in order to determine the distance of two given strings as Sorensen, but in contrast to Sorensen for the Jaccard Distance the common species are not double-weighted.

$$d_{jac} = \frac{c}{a + b - c} \tag{5}$$

a : *number of species in set A*
b : *number of species in set B*
c : *number of common species of set A and set B (intersecting set)*

Selection of an Adequate Similarity/Distance Measure. To find the best measure out of the defined set of measures $M = \{$*Levenshtein Distance, difflib.SequenceMatcher, Sorensen Distance, Jaccard Distance*$\}$ we calculated the string similarities by using each of the measures of M for every product name of the original e-shops and each product name of the corresponding competitor's e-shop of the data set of Table 1. For each resulting product domain data set we searched for the threshold values where (1) recall = 1, that means for all True Positives and no False Negatives, and (2) max(precision), that means for a maximum of True Negatives and a minimum of False Positives. Precision and recall are defined as given in Eqs. 6 and 7.

$$Precision = \frac{TP}{TP + FP} \tag{6}$$

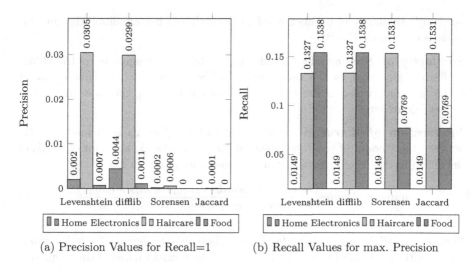

(a) Precision Values for Recall=1   (b) Recall Values for max. Precision

Fig. 1. Results for max. precision and max. recall (Color figure online)

$$Recall = \frac{TP}{TP + FN} \tag{7}$$

TP : *True Positives*; *identified correct matches*
FP : *False Positives*; *identified incorrect matches*
FN : *False Negatives*; *not identified correct matches*

The results for (1) the precision when the recall is 1 are shown in Fig. 1a and (2) the recall when max(precision) are presented in Fig. 1b. As expected, the resulting precision and recall values for the used measures are not really good since in the most cases the product names of different e-shops are differ in several aspects: Some e-shops only use the raw product name from manufacturer, some add specific features and in some cases there are some additional words as "on sale" or "new" added to the line including the product name. In other cases the product names are very close to each other although the products are even not the same product type since the products belong to the same product line, as a shampoo and a conditioner belonging to a product line called "Fruit Love".

To overcome this issues novel similarity values need to be created which are based on the measure having the best results. Looking at the results shown in Fig. 1a and b the similarity calculated by using SequenceMatcher is the most promising basis measure for all domains. Thus, the new similarity values to match product names were created based on it.

3.3 Definition of Similarity Values

After a deep manual analysis of all product names of all domains we created five different kinds of similarity values: (1) similarity of strings, (2) intersection of words, (3) similarity of number words, (4) maximum n-gram similarity and (5) average n-gram similarity.

Similarity of Strings. The *similarity of strings* corresponds to the difflib similarity calculated by the ratio method of SequenceMatcher. That means it is the raw comparison of the two product names by using the ratio method of SequenceMatcher.

Intersection of Words. The value *intersection of words* is defined as ratio between the amount of common words of both strings and the count of words of the string having the maximum count of words as shown in Eq. 8.

$$i(string_1, string_2) = \frac{common(words(string_1), words(string_2))}{max(words(string_1), words(string_2))} \qquad (8)$$

Similarity of Number Words. To calculate the *similarity of number words* the algorithm searches for the longest word of the product name of the original e-shop containing numbers and letters and calculates the similarity of the identified word and all words within the product name of the competitor by using the ratio method of difflib.SequenceMatcher. The maximum result value of all word comparisons is the *similarity of number words* for the compared product names.

Maximum N-Gram Similarity. The strings of the product names for comparison are disassembled into all possible consecutive fragments of a certain length. The fragments are words and the length is n. We have split the strings into 3-, 4- and 5-grams. All n-grams of a string were compared to those of the other string by using the ratio method of difflib.SequenceMatcher. The maximum value for that comparison was taken as *maximum n-gram similarity* of those strings.

Average N-Gram Similarity. Similar to *maximum n-gram similarity*, but here not the maximum but the average value of all n-gram similarities of the strings is taken to measure the similarity of the strings.

3.4   Determination of an Optimal Similarity Value Combination

To determine an optimal combination of the defined similarity values we calculated all similarity values for all combinations of product names of the original e-shops and the corresponding competitor's e-shops of the data set described in Sect. 3.1. For each domain and similarity value we determined the threshold to achieve the best possible precision and recall values. That means, instead of calculating the precision for a recall value of 1 we calculated the precision as well as the recall to get a maximum value of True Positives and a minimum value of False Positives, thus we did not aim to get a minimum of False Negatives or a maximum of True Negatives as we did in Sect. 3.2 in order to find the most adequate similarity/distance measure.

The average results over all three domains are shown in Fig. 2, but we also considered the results per domain in order to detect particular deviations within the different domains: The best precision values for the domain *Home Electronics* could be achieved by the similarity values *Intersection of Words* (0.28), *Average 5-gram Similarity* (0.28) and *Maximum 3-gram Similarity* (0.24), whereas the best results for recall were *Similarity of Number Words* (0.81), *Maximum 3-gram Similarity* (0.69) and *Maximum 4-gram Similarity* (0.63). For the domain *Haircare* the maximum precision values were obtained for the similarity values *Similarity of Strings* (0.93), *Maximum 5-gram Similarity* (0.89) and *Average 5-gram Similarity* (0.88), the highest recall values had the similarity values *Similarity of Strings* (0.83), *Maximum 3-gram Similarity* (0.75), *Intersection of Words* (0.65) and *Maximum 4-gram Similarity* (0.65). Best precision values for the domain *Food* were achieved by the similarity values *Average 3-gram Similarity* (0.18), *Intersection of Words* (0.14) and *Similarity of Strings* (0.11).

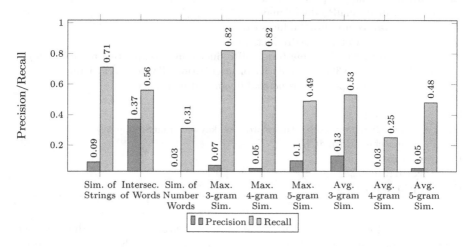

Fig. 2. Precision and recall for all domains and similarity values (Color figure online)

Considering the average results shown in Fig. 2 over all three domains the peaks for the recall were obtained by the similarity values *Maximum 3-gram Similarity* (0.82), *Maximum 4-gram Similarity* (0.82) and *Similarity of Strings* (0.71). The only sufficient value for precision was achieved by the similarity value *Intersection of Words* (0.37). Having regard to these results we except to obtain the best results for the matching of product names of arbitrary e-shops and product domains by combining the similarity value returning the best results for precision (*Intersection of Words*) and the similarity value providing the best recall ((*Maximum 3-gram Similarity*) and (*Maximum 4-gram Similarity*)). Therefore, we combine the similarity values *Intersection of Words* and *Maximum 3-gram Similarity* to filter the best matches. As the *Maximum 3-gram Similarity* is used the *Maximum 4-gram Similarity* is redundant.

A threshold (θ) needs to be found in order to separate the matches (True Positives) of a dataset from the non-matches (True Negatives). The threshold defines the smallest value which one of the identified similarity values (*Intersection of Words* or *Maximum 3-gram Similarity*) must have to be considered as a match (True Positive). Inspecting the identified matches (True Positives) of the three datasets the threshold (θ) for the domain *Home Electronics* is 0.33, the threshold for the domain *Haircare* is 0.36 and that one of the domain *Food* is 0.5. As the thresholds of the domains *Home Electronics* and *Food* are not very close a specific threshold for each domain needs to be found by using a small subset of the dataset of each domain. The observations and the resulting findings concerning the similarity values and thresholds result in Algorithm 1.

Algorithm 1. Matching Algorithm

```
 1: procedure MATCH(datasetA, datasetB, θ)
 2:     for all originalShopProducts do
 3:         cleanOriginalProductName
 4:         for all competitorProducts do
 5:             cleanCompetitorProductName
 6:             calculateSimValues(originalProductName, competitorProductName)
 7:             if ((max3GramSimilarity or intersectionOfWords) > θ) then
 8:                 competitorPorducts.add(competitorProduct)
 9:             end if
10:         end for
11:         match = max(competitorPorducts, key=averageSimilarity)
12:         matches.add(match)
13:     end for
14:     return matches
15: end procedure
```

The input for the algorithm is the dataset containing the products of the original e-shop and those of its competitor. Additionally, a threshold to separate the matches and non-matches need to be specified based on their calculated values for their *Intersection of Words* and their *Maximum 3-gram Similarity*. The threshold can be determined by analysing the similarity values of matches of a subset of the dataset to process. The algorithm runs though all products of the original e-shop (see line 2) and compares them to all products of the competitor (see line 4). Before the similarity values of the products are calculated the product names of the original shop and those of the competitor need to be preprocessed. That means hyphens and non-word characters are removed by Regular Expressions and the strings are converted to lower case. In addition to the *Intersection of Words* and the *Maximum 3-gram Similarity* of the strings the average similarity of those similarity values is calculated in line 6 of the algorithm. All competitor products with a similarity value greater than or equal the defined threshold (θ) are stored to a list of probable matching competitor products (see lines 7 and 8). The competitor product having the highest average similarity value is considered as match (see line 11). Products of the original e-shop where no competitor product with a similarity value greater than or equal θ could be found do not have any matching competitor product.

4   Experiment

The adequacy of our proposed approach was verified by an experiment on real-world data. The experiment and its results are described in the following.

4.1   Experimental Set-up

In order to demonstrate the adequacy of our approach we tested the algorithms introduced in Sect. 3.4 on real-world data collected from e-shops of further categories presented in [2]. The dataset was selected and collected as the dataset for the creation of the approach as described in Sect. 3.1. Detailed information about the experimental dataset is given in Table 2.

Table 2. Experimental dataset

No.	Domain	E-shop	Records	Competitor	Records	Total records
1	Clothing	weare.de	355	shop.microxtreme.gr	563	918
2	Books	whsmith.co.uk	284	globalbooks.de	178	463

We determined the threshold (*theta*) for each domain by pre-processing a small subset of the datasets and by selecting the smallest value for one of the defined similarity values (*Intersection of Words* or *Maximum 3-gram Similarity*) providing the best matching results as described in Sect. 3.4. The resulting thresholds were the following: $\theta_{Clothing} = 0.68$, $\theta_{Books} = 0.73$. Having identified adequate thresholds we executed the matching algorithm (Algorithm 1).

4.2   Experimental Results

The results of the experiment are shown in Fig. 3. For the domain *Clothing* we could achieve a precision of 0.89 and a recall of 0.86. For the domain *Books* the precision was 0.69 and the recall was 0.96.

The results of the experiment are sufficient. The precision for the domain *Books* is not as good as that of the domain *Clothing* what is caused by the small string distance of the product names of that domain (e.g. *Harry Potter and the Half-Blood Prince* and *Harry Potter and the Deathly Hallows*) which may increase the amount of False Positives. But as the recall value is 0.96 we expect that within such kinds of domains, where the strings of non-matches can be very close, almost all true matches can be found. On a Windows 8 machine with 2×2.53 GHz CPU and 32 GB RAM the algorithm needs 0.0028 s to compare two products, thus to compare a very large set of products the comparison needs to be parallelized and distributed over several machines.

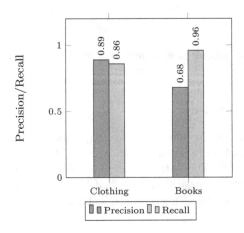

Fig. 3. Experimental results (Color figure online)

5   Conclusions

The paper proposes a novel approach to match products of different e-shops based on their product names. The approach is independent from the product domain and data source. That means products of arbitrary e-shop websites can be compared as long as the e-shops belong to the same product domain. The approach is based on the Python class *difflib.SequenceMatcher*. The paper describes the creation and identification of similarity measures which are suitable to match products by a pairwise comparison of their product names. The most adequate similarity values are used to build a matching algorithm. The developed algorithm and included similarity values are verified by an experiment on real-world data collected from two e-shops of the domains *Clothing* and *Books*. The experiment demonstrates the adequacy of the approach.

The matching of product descriptions based on product names is a first step to compare the product offers of e-shops. An extension of the approach by further research should refine the matching results by using additional product attributes as colour or weight to obtain even more precise matching results.

References

1. Nagelvoort, B., van Welie, R., van den Brink, P., Weening, A., Abraham, J.: Europe B2C E-commerce LIGHT Report 2014 (2014). https://www.ecommerce-europe. eu/website/facts-figures/light-version/download
2. PostNord: E-Commerce in Europe 2014 (2014). http://www.postnord.com/en/ media/publications/e-commerce-archive/
3. Civic Consulting: Consumer market study on the functioning of e-commerce and Internet marketing and selling techniques in the retail of goods (2011). http:// www.civic-consulting.de/reports/study_ecommerce_goods_en.pdf

4. Horch, A., Kett, H., Weisbecker, A.: Mining e-commerce data from e-shop websites. In: Proceedings of the 2015 IEEE Trustcom/BigDataSE/ISPA, pp. 153–160 (2015)

5. Horch, A., Kett, H., Weisbecker, A.: A lightweight approach for extracting product records from the web. In: Proceedings of the 11th International Conference on Web Information Systems and Technologies, pp. 420–430 (2015)

6. Horch, A., Kett, H., Weisbecker, A.: Extracting product unit attributes from product offers by using an ontology. In: Proceedings of the Second International Conference on Computer Science, Computer Engineering, and Social Media, pp. 67–71 (2015)

7. Yang, L., Sarker, B.K., Bhavsar, V.C., Boley, H.: A weighted-tree simplicity algorithm for similarity matching of partial product descriptions. In: IASSE, pp. 55–60 (2005)

8. Balog, K.: On the investigation of similarity measures for product resolution. In: Proceedings of the Workshop on Discovering Meaning on the Go in Large Heterogeneous Data 2011, pp. 49–54 (2011)

9. Gopalakrishnan, V., Iyengar, S.P., Madaan, A., Rastogi, R., Sengamedu, S.: Matching product titles using web-based enrichment. In: Proceedings of the 21st ACM International Conference on Information and Knowledge Management, pp. 605–614 (2012)

10. Getoor, L., Machanavajjhala, A.: Entity resolution: theory, practice & open challenges. In: International Conference on Very Large Data Bases (2012)

11. Wang, J., Kraska, T., Franklin, M.J., Feng, J.: CrowdER: crowdsourcing entity resolution. Proc. VLDB Endow. **5**, 1483–1494 (2012)

12. Kolb, L., Rahm, E.: Parallel entity resolution with Dedoop. Datenbank-Spektrum **1**, 23–32 (2013)

13. Passos, A., Kumar, V., McCallum, A.: Lexicon infused phrase embeddings for named entity resolution. In: Proceedings of the Eighteenth Conference on Computational Natural Language Learning, pp. 78–86 (2014)

14. Thor, A.: Toward an adaptive string similarity measure for matching product offers. Informatik 2010: Service Science - Neue Perspektiven für die Informatik, Beiträge der 40. Jahrestagung der Gesellschaft für Informatik e.V. (GI) **1**, 702–710 (2010)

15. Kannan, A., Givoni, I.E., Agrawal, R., Fuxman, A.: Matching unstructured product offers to structured product specifications. In: Proceedings of the 17th ACM SIGKDD International Conference on Knowledge Discovery and Data Mining, pp. 404–412 (2011)

16. Köpcke, H., Thor, A., Thomas, S., Rahm, E.: Tailoring entity resolution for matching product offers. In: Proceedings of the 15th International Conference on Extending Database Technology, pp. 545–550 (2012)

17. Londhe, N., Gopalakrishnan, V., Zhang, A., Ngo, H.Q., Srihari, R.: Matching titles with cross title web-search enrichment and community detection. Proc. VLDB Endow. **7**, 1167–1178 (2014)

18. Yetgin, Z., Gözükara, F.: New metrics for clustering of identical products over imperfect data. Turk. J. Electr. Eng. Comput. Sci. **23**, 1–14 (2014)

Keystroke Biometric Recognition on Chinese Long Text Input

Xiaodong Li and Jiafen Liu[✉]

School of Economic Information Engineering,
Southwestern University of Finance and Economics,
Chengdu, People's Republic of China
jfliu@swufe.edu.cn

Abstract. Keystroke Biometric is useful in distinguishing legal users from perpetrators in online activities. Most previous keystroke studies focus on short text, however short text keystroke can only be used in limited scenarios such as user name and password input and provide one-time authentication. In this paper, we concentrate on how to detect whether current user is the legal one during the whole activity, such as writing an E-mail and chat online. We developed a JAVA applet to collect raw data, and then extracted features and constructed 4 classifiers. In the experiment, we required 30 users to choose a topic randomly and then type in a text about 400 Chinese characters on it. This experiment repeated 9 times in different days under the same typing environment. The accuracy of different methods shifts from 94.07 % to 98.15 %, the FAR reaches to 0.74 % and FRR to 1.15 %. In summary, Chinese free long text keystroke biometric recognition can be used to authenticate users during the whole online activity with satisfactory precision.

Keywords: Biometric features · Chinese free-text · Keystroke dynamics · Authentication

1 Introduction

With the rapid development of information technology in China, Internet has penetrated into all sides of our life and work. Communication between peoples has been extended. We can talk to someone on the other side of the earth in a chat room or via email, no matter whether we have met before. Hence the information security is facing greater challenges than before. Many imposters leverage the Internet to steal others' property, which could seriously challenge the fairness and justice of the society. Imagine that your account and password got into the wrong hands, and then the attacker may impersonate you, chat with your contacts and deceive them. This happens often in reports. If the imposter's tone sounds like you, it is hard to perceive. We need a reminder to help us to recognize whether the user is our friend or just an imposter, though we can't see the one who is using the account. Identification of legal users becomes vitally important for all online applications, especially those about money.

To avoid the fraudulent attack, considerable efforts have been taken in this field by predecessors. The biometric recognition technology is one of the most promising. Each

H. Cao et al. (Eds.): PAKDD 2016 Workshops, LNAI 9794, pp. 260–271, 2016.
DOI: 10.1007/978-3-319-42996-0_22

person has his (her) inherent biometric features, unique, rarely change and difficult to copy or imitate. Generally, biometrics can be classified to physiological characteristics and behavior characteristics. The former contains fingerprint, DNA, iris, body smell, vein, etc. The latter contains signature, walk behaviors, cellphone-use behaviors or other operation behaviors. Nowadays biometric recognition technology has got more attention for its higher security, reliability and effectiveness. However, recognition based on physiological features needs specialist equipment to collect data, and it will hinder its further application. Moreover, many users felt that they were monitored and invaded and refused to cooperate unless necessary. Keystroke biometric recognition may therefore be a better option for most online applications. Only a keyboard is needed, and keystrokes can be collected unobtrusively without additional training or supervision. Therefore, its born advantages, low-cost, not invasive, simple, easy to use attract much more researchers to research on keystroke biometric recognition for identifying different users [1].

In 1895, a research paper on the radio operators shows that every operator has his own unique typing pattern while sending the same radio message, which opens the door to the keystroke dynamics research [2]. At the beginning of the 20th century, psychologists had confirmed that the people's behavior feature can be predicted when people do some repetitive works [3]. Keystroke dynamics has been used as an effective feature for many years, dating back to the Second World War, the allied forces leveraged the Morse Code typing rhythms to recognize whether the sender was ally or not [4].

In the early researches, the majority of works focus on the short text input, mainly in the field of passwords recognition during the log-in phase. Forsen et al. [3] is the first to introduce the idea that whether keystroke dynamics can be identify users by typing their own names. And then variety of methods have been adopted and innovated to improve the recognition accuracy. Gain et al. [5] acted as a pioneer to propose that the keystroke time could be effective to enhance the identification accuracy, their experiment reported false alarm rate of 5.5 % and imposter pass rate of 5.0 %. Umphress and Williams [6] refined the keystroke time and introduced statistic in 1985 to gain time feature, such as mean and standard. Candler et al. [7] improved the recognition system by using classical logistic methods to innovate it, their experiment based on the Bayes classifier reports FRR of 8.1 % and FAR of 2.8 % for 26 subjects, while FRR reduced to 3.1 % and FAR reduced to 0.5 % for 32 subjects. Legett et al. [8] proposed the static identification and dynamic identification, though their result seems unsatisfactory, the significance lies in the inspiration for later researches. Napierl et al. [9] improved Legett's model by adopting the statistic methods innovatively, and reduced FAR and FRR a little. Neural Networks had also been used in this area by Brown and Rogers [10]. Obaidat and Balqies [11] added keystroke transition time and hold time to the feature vector, and got a really high accuracy of 100 % by running Artificial Neural Networks algorithm for classification. In the author's opinion, though the classifier is thought to be effective, it consumes too much time in training phase. DE RU, Tapiador et al. [12] applied another popular algorithm, fuzzy logic to classification in 1990s. Robinson et al. [13] designed a model by combining inductive learning classifiers and statistical methods, and the model performs well with error rate about 9 %. Other short-text input algorithms and feature choosing algorithms report high performance, such as K-means, KNN, SVM, HMM, the R method, A method, R+A or RA method etc., in which the R+A or RA method is a combination of R and A method [14, 15]. As more researchers join in this field, short text keystroke recognition performs better, and many corporations launch applications and products on keystroke biometric recognition, such as American Net Nanny with its BioPassord, Australian National University with its TRUST, etc.

However, the short text contains limited information and is not enough to express the users' complete typing pattern, thus affects the performance of the recognition systems [16]. Long text keystroke recognition gradually came to people's view. In 1999, Monrose [17] proposed to expand the identification to the whole computer-use period involving free text input. Euclidean distance, Non-weight probability, and Bayes were adopted in the experiment with the recognition rate from 85 % to 92.4 %. Researchers in Pace University like Curtin et al. [16] published a paper to elaborate on his long text keystroke study, in which a Nearest Neighbor classifier using Euclidean distance was applied, reaching a recognition rate of 94.7 %. Patrick and Hafez [18] designed a new algorithm to achieve continuous recognition throughout the whole typing period. New distance method and Reward and Punishment Mechanism enable the system to continuously identify the user as long as he types.

Most studies in keystroke recognition focused on English input due to wide usage of English in the world, and a few scholars have done some exploratory research on other languages. Gunetti et al. [19] designed an experiment crossing two different languages, Italy and English. Subjects was required to use these two languages, and the result shows that identification rate in Italy is 93.3 % and reduced to 90 % in English. This experiment demonstrates that users' invisible typing pattern can be identified by keystroke dynamics no matter which language the user types. A door to research different languages has been opened. Many domestic scholars have also done a great deal of researches on Chinese keystroke recognition. For example, Dexu and Xiaoqin [20] chose common-used digraphs in Chinese phonetic alphabet, like ai, an, ao, in, ng, ni, on, ou, sh, wo, zh, used distance measure to improve the model and achieved an identification rate of 95 %. Based on these keystroke thoughts, free Chinese text keystroke dynamics has been pushed forward in domestic studies.

There is still a long way to go in keystroke recognition on Chinese long text input. The case will be more complicated when it comes to Chinese input than that in English, due to the linguistic features and input characteristics of Chinese. For example, we may need to click more than one key to input a Chinese letter. Keystroke on Chinese long text may contain massive biometric information and need to be mined further. Insufficient samples on Chinese long text make the results unconvincing. Arbitrary feature selection simply copied from that in English may not reflect the real typing pattern well. In this paper, a special system is designed to improve effectiveness of keystroke recognition based on Chinese long text.

The remainder of the paper is organized as follows. Section 2 presents the detail of our keystroke biometric system, including all stages from original raw data collection to establishment of the system. Section 3 presents the experimental design and Sect. 4

shows the experimental results and our analysis. We conclude with possible applications of our system in Sect. 5.

2   Keystroke Biometric System

Keystroke biometric system, just as its name implies, identifies and authenticates a user by his inherent typing pattern with keyboard. Typing pattern can be characterized by feature vector series extracted from raw data containing only key codes, key press time and key release time. The main function of our system is collecting user's Chinese long input and analyzing the typing pattern to identify the user. Our keystroke biometric system mainly consists of three modules: raw data collection, feature extraction, and pattern classification. The following are the details.

2.1   Data Collection

Different from English input, input of Chinese characters depends on third-party input softwares or plugins, such as popular Sougou Pinyin from domestic company or Microsoft Pinyin from Microsoft Company. It's hard to capture the complete key messages when user types using any Chinese input software, because the input software will intercept keyboard messages from the Windows kernel. To solve this problem, we applied HOOK to our data collection module. HOOK monitors all kinds of events, including keyboard messages, in applications or processes from the underlying operating system with efficiency. We developed a Java applet based on HOOK to collect Chinese input keystroke data. All 30 subjects are required to fill in some information firstly: name, and the number of input times. And then each user should choose a topic from 20 topics predefined in our system. After clicking the start button, they can write a short passage of 400 characters in Chinese according to the topic, and click the finish button to end input. Why we need a topic when user types in the experiment? It is similar to our input environment in real life. We think about what we want to express on the topic, choose words and build sentences, then type via keyboard. Besides, a specific topic helps to gain high quality data by avoiding meaningless casual keystrokes.

Our applet captures key events while user inputs, transforms and stores as raw data. The raw data file contains these 4 items: press time, release time, virtual key and character. Table 1 shows a segment of raw data collected in our experiment.

2.2   Feature Extraction

Everyone has a different typing pattern, so everyone's feature vector should be different from the others. In fact, massive raw data can not be directly used to characterize users' typing pattern. Our system will extract a feature vector to describe user's typing pattern from the raw data. Based on mathematic knowledge, the features are specially designed. Key information in raw data is key-press time and release time of each key in the input series. The details of keystroke are presented below.

Table 1. The fragment of raw data from a free text

Press time	Release time	Virtual key	Character
...	...	...	...
2962593	2962703	83	S
2962703	2962796	72	H
2962812	2962906	69	E
2962937	2963015	78	N
2963078	2963109	68	D
2964640	2964765	8	BackSpace
2965312	2965406	77	M
2965406	2965500	69	E
2965562	2965625	72	H
2965750	2965828	85	U
2965812	2965921	73	I
2965984	2966109	74	J
2966078	2966218	73	I
2966296	2966453	78	N
2966515	2966625	160	Shift_left
2966625	2966703	72	H
2966765	2966812	20	Caps Lock
2966765	2966812	65	A
2966812	2966906	78	N
2967046	2967109	71	G
...	...	...	...

Suppose that there are arbitrary two keys: key A (first key) and key B (second key). A is pressed first, then B. There are 3 different situations according to the key event sequence: Type 1, Type 2, and Type 3. The former two types were described by Villani et al. in literature [21] and Type 3 is another case we found by observing the process of keystroke.

Type 1: this is the most common situation. Key A is pressed and then released, and then key B is pressed and released. There is no overlapping time between two keys.

Type 2: key A is pressed, then key B is pressed before A is released, and then key B is released after A is released. There exists a short overlapping time.

Type 3: In this situation, key B's key-press time and release time is contained within the interval of key A's press and release time. Overlapping time definitely exists, and more than one key may be included in the interval. For example, if we want to type a word 'EXAMPLE' in capital letter, we may press down 'Shift' first, and will not release it until we have typed all 7 letters in the word, hence 7 keys are pressed and released in the duration of 'Shift' key.

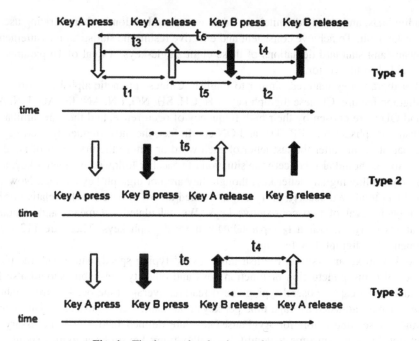

Fig. 1. The keystroke sketch map for three types

Symbols used in Fig. 1 are explained as follows.

t_1: duration time of key A, equals to the difference of the release time and the key-press time.

t_2: duration time of key B.

t_3: the transition time from the key-press time of A to the key-press time of B.

t_4: the transition time from the time when A is released to the time when key B is released. In Type 3 we mentioned above, value of t4 may be negative, because the release time of key B may be earlier than that of key A.

t_5: the transition time from the time when key A is released to the time when key B is pressed. And in Type 2 and Type 3, the value may also be negative, because the key-press time of key B may be earlier than the release time of key A.

t_6: the transition time from the key-press time of A to the release time of B.

In the process of constructing feature vectors, we expected to maximize the utilization of the raw data as sufficient as possible. There is no doubt that the duration time and the transition time should be used to construct feature vector. Besides that, we took more considerations on characterizing individual's typing pattern on Chinese long text input. Feature vector of our recognition system consisted of three aspects: single key features, digraph features and statistic features.

For single key features, scholars noticed that in Chinese phonetic alphabets, I, N, A, U, E and H had the highest frequency according to the statistical results [22]. Moreover, the key 'spacebar' and 'shift' are also typed frequently. So users' behavior of clicking these eight keys contains essential information to reveal the invisible custom of individuals, and should definitely be taken into consideration in characterizing user's keystroke habit. To achieve consistent and effective result, the statistical measurements of means and standard deviations of these eight single-keys, a total of 16 parameters were added to the vector.

For digraph key features, similar to English, Chinese phonetic alphabets also have the digraph feature. Chinese digraph keys ZH, CH, SH, NG, EN, AN, IN, AO, UN, AI, EI and OU were chosen by their high frequency of occurrence, and they are similar to English digraphs such as ER, TH, and ON etc. In fact, the most frequently used key is spacebar, it occurs after the last letter of each word or before the first letter of another word. So we should also concern the situation of spacebar followed by a letter key, and a spacebar following any letter key, though they are not digraph keys in fact. Now we have 14 in total. We used t_3, t_4, t_5 and t_6 defined above to describe the relative order and time interval of two consecutive keys. We calculated the means and standard deviations of t_3, t_4, t_5 and t_6 separately for these digraph keys. There are 112 measurements for digraph key features.

As keystroke analysis on English input, users' typing speed, pause rate, the preferences of using punctuation or function keys and other typing habits should also be considered. To capture users' typing speed feature, average time per keystroke (short for AvgTime), adjusted average time per keystroke (short for AdjustedAvgTime), and average pause time (short for AvgPauseTime) are defined below. It is necessary to point out that duration time beyond 0.5 s without any keystroke activities should be regarded as pause time [1].

$$\text{AvgTime} = \frac{the\ whole\ typing\ time}{the\ number\ of\ whole\ keystrokes} \tag{1}$$

$$\text{AdjustedAvgTime} = \frac{the\ whole\ typing\ time\ -\ the\ whole\ pause\ time}{the\ number\ of\ whole\ keystrokes} \tag{2}$$

$$\text{AvgPauseTime} = \frac{the\ whole\ typing\ time}{the\ number\ of\ pause} \tag{3}$$

To capture users' typing feature when editing text, We counted the pause rate, the usage rate of backspace, spacebar, punctuation and function keys, and other preferences. When a user think about a topic, the interval of thinking may affect the whole time and number of pause, and it reflects the users' thinking habits in keystroke way. The preferences of the users vary from person to person. Some of them are inclined to use more commas, or use more function keys in place of mouse operations, and input a series of Chinese characters after typing a series of letters, and even prefer the left-handed 'shift' or the right-handed one, etc.

$$\text{PauseRate} = \frac{total\ pauses}{total\ keystrokes} \tag{4}$$

$$\text{BackspaceRate} = \frac{total\ backspaces}{total\ keystrokes} \tag{5}$$

$$\text{SpacebarRate} = \frac{total\ spacebars}{total\ keystrokes} \tag{6}$$

$$\text{PunctuationRate} = \frac{total\ punctuations}{total\ keystrokes} \tag{7}$$

$$\text{FunctionRate} = \frac{total\ function\ keys}{total\ keystrokes} \tag{8}$$

In Formula 8, the function keys mainly contain End, Home, ESC, four Arrows, Ctrl, Shift, Page UP, Page Down, Alt, TAB, and Enter.

As we can see on the standard keyboard, some special function keys including Shift, Ctrl and Alt lie on both the left and right sides, and number keys from '0' to '9' can be found on the top of main board and on the NumPad section. We use a formula based on sigmoid function to quantify user's preference for left-handed or right-handed inputting some special keys that exists on both sides.

$$F(N_1, N_2) = \begin{cases} 0, & if\ N_1 \neq 0, N_2 = 0 \\ \frac{1}{1+e^{\left(\frac{N_2}{N_1}\right)}}, & if\ N_1 > N_2 \\ 0.5, & if\ N_1 = N_2 \\ \frac{1}{1+e^{-\left(\frac{N_1}{N_2}\right)}}, & if\ N_1 < N_2 \\ 1, & if\ N_1 = 0, N_2 \neq 0 \end{cases} \tag{9}$$

In Formula 9, N1 and N_2 indicate the number of left keystrokes and right keystrokes separately. According to the ratio of N_1 and N_2, the formula falls into 5 parts.

If $N_1 = 0$, $N_2 \neq 0$, then $F(N_1, N_2) = 1$, it means that the user extremely prefers right keys. If $N_1 \neq 0$, $N_2 = 0$, then $F(N_1, N_2) = 0$, the user extremely prefers left keys. In case of $N_1 = N_2$, we thought that the user had no obvious tendency on both sides. These three situations occur largely due to insufficient raw data, and the following two cases are more common. If $0 < N_1 < N_2$, we compute the value of N_1/N_2, then introduce sigmoid function. The other case is $N_1 > N_2$, we compute reciprocal and negative value of N_1/N_2, and then use sigmoid function to get a value. It is closer to 1, the user prefers to use the right-hand keys more, and vice versa.

Now we have 16 single-key features, 112 digraph key features and 10 statistic features. 138 measurements in total. The next process is outlier removal. Those measurements far from the mean measurements will be removed. And then make features standardized by Formula 10. Standardization will convert all measurements with outlier removal into the interval from 0 to 1.

$$x = \frac{x - x_{min}}{x_{max} - x_{min}} \tag{10}$$

2.3   Pattern Classification

The system armed with different algorithms will automatically learn from the samples (so called training set), once the pattern classifier has been trained well, new test data can be identified. At the same time, we used four classifiers in our system, Naïve Bayes (NB), Support Vector Machine (SVM), Decision Tree classifier J48 (DT-J48), and Random Forest (RF). Naïve Bayes is a simple technique for categorization based on applying Bayes' theorem, it requires strong or naïve independence assumption between the features and runs quickly. Support Vector Machine is an advanced classifier, it belongs to supervised learning models, and supports linear classification and non-liner classification. Decision Tree J48 is a popular algorithm used to generate a decision tree and classify the test samples, and it is often considered as a statistical classifier. Random Forest is a classifier containing multiple decision trees. It can handle a mass of variables input and construct classifier with high prediction accuracy.

3   Experimental Design

3.1   Subjects and Data Collection

Since the model has been created, the effect of model needs to be measured in a general metric. The most commonly adopted metrics to evaluate the recognition system are False Accept Rate (FAR) and False Refuse Rate (FRR) [5], they represent respectively specificity and sensitivity of the system. As mentioned earlier, input of Chinese characters needs third-party software, and Sougou Pinyin application is adopted based on an overall consideration for its easy-to-use, popularity. The most important to us, its personal lexicon enables users to construct his own conventional words set and thus reduce the times of keyboard clicking. Using personal lexicon will reinforce user's input habit further.

Meanwhile, there are total 30 subjects to be invited to type a paragraph of text under the same software and hardware condition. For every subject, he/she will choose a topic from the given topics and input a text about 400 Chinese characters on the topic so as to provide representative information, it will be repeated for 9 times. That is to say, everyone will type 9 free texts about 400 Chinese characters corresponding to 9 topics.

3.2   Experimental Design

Considering that a sample of 400 Chinese characters contains about $1400 \sim 2200$ keystrokes, we could split each sample into several subsamples to increase sample size. Our study consisted of two experiments to enhance the persuasiveness of the results. We divided each sample into 3 subsamples in Experiment 1, and divided each sample into 4 subsamples in Experiment 2. In Experiment 1, there are 27 samples for each user, and 810 in total. There are 36 samples for each user, and 1080 samples altogether in Experiment 2. In both experiments, 66 percent of the data was put under training set and the rest 34 % was used to validate our models. In compliance with other researcher's work, we also adopted recognition accuracy, False Accept Rate, False Reject Rate, Area under Curve, and F1-measure to evaluate the performance of our models.

4 Experimental Results

We run Naïve Bayes, Support Vector Machine, decision tree classifier J48, and Random Forest on different data set in Experiment 1 and Experiment 2 independently. And we observed outcome under different settings and adjusted parameters to make our model work well and get better feedback. Table 2 shows the performance of 4 classifiers on different data set.

Table 2. Performance of 4 classifiers on different data set

No.	Classifiers	Accuracy	FAR	FRR	AUC	F1-Measure
Exp. 1	NB	98.15 %	1.11 %	0.76 %	0.901	0.662
	SVM	94.07 %	4.44 %	1.53 %	0.5	0.383
	DT-J48	97.78 %	1.11 %	1.15 %	0.868	0.666
	RF	98.15 %	0.74 %	1.15 %	0.943	0.749
Exp. 2	NB	97.22 %	1.39 %	1.14 %	0.851	0.583
	SVM	94.72 %	3.61 %	1.72 %	0.5	0.387
	DT-J48	96.94 %	1.94 %	1.15 %	0.729	0.593
	RF	97.50 %	1.11 %	1.43 %	0.937	0.608

In Experiment 1, SVM shows 94.07 % accuracy, and the AUC is 0.5, the classification effect seems not satisfactory. In fact, negative samples is much more than positive samples. Though the SVM classifier reject many positive samples, the accuracy keeps high. ROC curve is irrelative to number of positive and negative samples, so AUC can fairly reflect the performance of the models. And SVM shows low AUC. And other three classifiers get similar results, up to 98.15 % accuracy with AUC close to 1. The FAR of Naïve Bayes is higher than the Random Forest, but the FRR of Naïve Bayes is lower than the Random Forest. To some degree, we prefer lower FAR to assure the account security. And the F1-Measure of Random Forest is the highest. Taken together, both Naïve Bayes and Random Forest perform well but Random Forest is better.

In Experiment 2, recognition accuracy of Naïve Bayes reaches 97.22 %, but its F1-Measure of 0.583 is too low. Obviously the SVM doesn't performance well. Random Forest's accuracy of 97.50 % and F1-Mesure of 0.608 are higher than other classifiers, and its 1.11 % FAR is the lowest of all. Among these classifiers, the Random Forest shows better performance.

Compared to experiment 1, the accuracy, AUC and F1-Measure of the experiment 2 are lower. We thought that probably because we split a text into four samples, and each sample could not supply enough information to the feature vector, many measurements of features might be missing.

5   Conclusions and Future Work

In this paper, we presented our methods for Chinese long text keystroke dynamics and did some experiments on keystroke data on 30 subjects. The experimental result shows that our Chinese keystroke recognition system can obtain satisfactory results, the accuracy reaches to 98.15 %, FAR to 0.74 % and FRR to 1.15 %. At the same time, the high performance indicates that our selected features of keystroke on long Chinese input are effective to reflect characteristics of individual typing habit. Finally, the comparison between Experiment 1 and Experiment 2 indicates that when we construct a feature vector, enough keystroke data of a sample is necessary. Better expression of a feature vector is also helpful to perform better.

In our future study, much work needs to be done. We will expand our experiment by increasing samples of more users, and enhance the process of feature extraction and classification. Keystroke recognition under different conditions, such as different keyboards, contents and application environment etc., is worthy to study in our future work.

Acknowledgment. This work was supported by National Natural Science Foundation of China [60903201, 91218301]; and the Fundamental Research Funds for the Central Universities [JBK120505, JBK140129].

References

1. Lisa, M.V., Lina, Z., Andrew, S.: Automated stress detection using keystroke and linguistic features: an exploratory study. Int. J. Hum Comput Stud. 10(67), 870–886 (2009)
2. Bryan, W.L., Harter, N.: Studies in the physiology and psychology of telegraphic language. Psychol. Rev. 1(4), 27–53 (1970)
3. Forsen, G.E., Nelson M.R., et al.: Personal attributes authentication techniques. Personal Attributes Authentication Techniques (1977)
4. Salima, D., Jan, R.M.: The reliability of user authentication through keystroke dynamics. Stat. Neerl. 4(63), 432–449 (2009)
5. Gaines, R.S., Lisowski, W., et al.: Authentication by keystroke timing: some preliminary results. Authentication by Keystroke Timing Some Preliminary Results (1980)
6. Umphress, D., Williams, G.: Identity verification through keyboard characteristics. Int. J. Man Mach. Stud. 3(23), 263–273 (1985)
7. Candler, S., Johnson, R.S.: Computer-access security systems using keystroke dynamics. IEEE Trans. Pattern Anal. Mach. Intell. 12(12), 1217–1222 (1990)
8. Leggett, J., Williams, G., et al.: Dynamic identity verification via keystroke characteristics. Int. J. Man Mach. Stud. 6(35), 859–870 (1991)
9. Napier, R., Laverty, W., et al.: Keyboard user verification: toward an accurate, efficient, and ecologically valid algorithm. Int. J. Hum Comput Stud. 2(43), 213–222 (1995)
10. Brown, M., Rogers, S.J.: User identification via keystroke characteristics of typed names using neural networks. Int. J. Man Mach. Stud. 6(39), 999–1014 (1993)
11. Obaidat, M.S., Sadoun, B.: Verification of computer users using keystroke dynamics. IEEE Trans. Syst. Man Cybern. B Cybern. 2(27), 261–269 (1997)

12. Tapiador, M., Sigenza, J.A., et al.: Fuzzy keystroke biometrics on web security. In: Automatic Identification Advanced Technologies (2000)
13. Robinson, J.A., Liang, V.W., et al.: Computer user verification using login string keystroke dynamics. IEEE Trans. Syst. Man Cybern. Part A Syst. Hum. 2(28), 236–241 (1998)
14. Gunetti, D., Picardi, C.: Keystroke analysis of free text. ACM Trans. Inf. Syst. Secur. 3(8), 312–347 (2005)
15. Pilsung, K., Sungzoon, C.: Keystroke dynamics-based user authentication using long and free text strings from various input devices. Inf. Sci. 308, 72–93 (2015)
16. Curtin, M., Tappert, C., Villani, M., et al.: Keystroke biometric recognition on long-text input: a feasibility study. In: Proceedings of International Workshop SCI Comp/Comp Stat (IWSCCS), Hong Kong (2006)
17. Monrose, F., Rubin, A.D.: Keystroke dynamics as a biometric for authentication. Future Gener. Comput. Syst. 4(16), 351–359 (2000)
18. Patrick, B., Hafez, B.: Continuous authentication using biometric keystroke dynamics. In: The Norwegian Information Security Conference (NISK), pp. 1–12 (2009)
19. Gunetti, D., Picardi, C., Ruffo, G.: Dealing with different languages and old profiles in keystroke analysis of free text. In: Bandini, S., Manzoni, S. (eds.) AI*IA 2005. LNCS (LNAI), vol. 3673, pp. 347–358. Springer, Heidelberg (2005)
20. Dexu, Z., Xiaoqin, H.: Dynamic free text keystroke continuous identification based on the rewards and punishments algorithm with frequency. J. Netw. New Media 2, 41–49 (2015). (in Chinese)
21. Villani, M., Tappert, C., Giang, N., et al.: Keystroke biometric recognition studies on long-text input under ideal and application-oriented conditions. In: Computer Vision and Pattern Recognition Workshop, pp. 39–39 (2006)
22. Cheng, Y., Yunkai, W., Ruilong, H.: Behavior research of internet user passwords based on pinyin analysis. Comput. Eng. 09, 174–177 (2014). (in Chinese)

Recommendation Algorithm Design in a Land Exchange Platform

Xubin Luo[✉] and Jiang Duan

555 Liutai Avenue, Wenjiang District,
Chengdu 610041, China
xluo@swufe.edu.cn

Abstract. In China the majority of the farmlands are small pieces, which should be circulated and aggregated to a larger scale and pave the way for modern farms. A Platform needs to be built to connect the small landowners and the potential new farmers or investors. This paper proposes an efficient recommendation algorithm that takes both the space attributes and other properties of farmland pieces into consideration and produce best selection for the intended potential new farmers or investors with customized object functions.

1 Introduction

In China the property rights of rural lands are collectively owned by all the families in a village. In late 1970s, the lands are divided into pieces and contracted by different families. Each family is responsible for cultivating the lands and for the output of the lands. In order to make it fair to all the families, each family should get same share of lands different class of lands. Therefore the lands were divided into very small pieces. The typical size of each lands ranges from dozens to hundreds of square meters. Each family has quite a few pieces of small lands, which in most cases, are distributed at difference locations. It was indeed a great move forward for the agriculture and countryside in early 1980s. However, this situation of lands distribution facing more and more problem after more than 30 years of fast growth of Chinese economy. When the growth of the Chinese economy keeps growing the agriculture is facing a very tough question: the payoff the old farming is too low that, not the young generation, but anyone who could get a job in the factory, has left the countryside [1]. The scattered small land pieces causes difficulties in utilizing the lands more efficiently—it is too small for large agriculture machine and automatic farming. Obviously a new way of farming and agriculture industry must be established to replace the old and outdated ones. However, no modern agriculture can be built on those small and scattered pieces of farmlands. The scattered farmlands must be aggregated to form bigger farms with moderate size. Otherwise it is economically infeasible.

This work was funded by *MOE (Ministry of Education of China) Youth Project of Humanities and Social Sciences* (Project No. 10YJC870024).

© Springer International Publishing Switzerland 2016
H. Cao et al. (Eds.): PAKDD 2016 Workshops, LNAI 9794, pp. 272–279, 2016.
DOI: 10.1007/978-3-319-42996-0_23

In recent years the transfer of lands (or land exchange) is getting more and more popular. Farmlands are aggregated in some area and big and modern farms are hence established. However, a serious problem is hindering the process. There is no systematic land registration system for farmlands, although the farmlands were already recognized as property right in the *Property Law of the People's Republic of China*, which was adopted at the 5th session of the Tenth National People's Congress in 2007. Without land titling and accurate registration data, the land transfers and exchanges are facing big uncertainty [2], which hinders the progress and quality of the land aggregation. Most of the big farms established in this environment usually have strong local connection so that they have the ability to deal with those uncertainties. Thus the farmlands exchange market is more localized and new farms in most cases are not so efficient as expected [3].

In viewing of this situation, China started a huge land-titling project in early 2013 to pave the way for a more efficient and market oriented land exchange market, to facilitate the formation of land aggregation. The project aims to register all the farmlands, which totals around 2.2 billion *mu*, or *Chinese acres*, and give all the farmers the land property rights, so that the farmlands could be transferred to others in a more efficient way. The information registered for each piece of farmland includes location, boundary, size, ownership and its aerial picture. The project make the information regarding the land ownership transparent and authentic for the land exchange market, eliminating the difficulties that previously raises the cost of the land exchange transactions or sometimes, make the transaction even not feasible. Once the lands are registered, land exchange could aggregate the small pieces together and form big and modern farms [4], which can bring economic benefits to the previous landowners and the new farmer or investor on both sides.

With the authentic land registration data, we can expect that the land exchange platform would play a more important role in connecting the old landowners and the new farmers or investors. With the authentic data available, the land exchange could happen more globally to maximize the benefits of the transactions. Therefore the party exchange platform is in great need. We have built a land exchange platform that could serve this purpose and it has attracted much attention in this field.

However, for the new farmer or investor of the modern farms, it is costly as well as frustrating to search for and compare vast number of small lands. If you need to look at a combination problem of thousands of small pieces of farmlands to get a farm of two hundred *mu*, it is too much. For example, if the land pieces are not aggregated but scattered around vast area, the cost to cultivate and manage would be much higher than the those ones which are close to each other. Besides locations, we also need to consider the price of the lands, the soil type and other properties associated with the lands. With proper databases, we could provide a recommended set of lands to optimize the utility for the potential buyer or investor.

Since detailed information regarding the farmlands were not until the land titling project, most of existing work are on the connecting of general information and to the best of our knowledge there are no existing work addressing the problem considered in this paper.

2 Problem Modeling

In this paper, the problem that we consider is how to select and recommend a set of lands that benefit the one who is going to acquire a set of lands and start a modern farm—who we assume as the acquirer. We assume the utility function of the acquirer as *Total_Profit*. The set of available land pieces are B: $\{b_1, b_2, b_3, \ldots\ldots, b_n\}$. For each of the blocks, they have a set of attributes, i.e., $a_i^1, a_i^2, \ldots, a_i^m$ are m attributes for the land block b_i. The attributes for each block could be the cost, location and other attributes. The cost and profit of each block can both be associated with the all the attributes. That means, $cost(b_i) = f^c(a_i^1, a_i^2, \ldots, a_i^m)$ *and* $profit(b_i) = f^p(a_i^1, a_i^2, \ldots, a_i^m)$. Meanwhile, the cost and profit as a whole are also associated the connections between the land blocks. If two blocks b_i and b_j, the cost to cultivate them is determined by the function $cost(b_i, b_j)$.

The objective of this problem is to recommend a set of lands E as the subset of B so that the utility function of E is maximized.

3 ILP Formulation

For the new farmers or the investors, land selection is a complex process, and sometimes even the factors to be considered has nothing to do with the land, which could be culture, emotional, or even political factors. To simplify the model, this article only consider land and agriculture related considerations. Therefore, we put forward the floof this problem:

- s: an input value that denotes the minimum size of the farm project as required by the land acquirer. Usually the acquirer may want to set a minimum scale of the farm project with other consideration even though the optimal point may be at less scale. s can be set to zero if no such minimum requirement is needed.
- $cost(b_i)$: an input value that represents the annual cost to rent the land block b_i. This variable is input value as set by the given information. In most cases the $cost(b_i)$ would be proportional to the size of the land block but also varies with the land condition and the intention of the land owners.
- $size(b_i)$: an input value that denotes the size of the land block b_i;
- $cost(b_i, b_j)$: an input value that represents the cost connection land blocks b_i and b_j, which is determined by their locations. If they are bordering with each other, then the cost is zero. Otherwise the cost is proportional to the distance between the two blocks. For simplicity, we do not consider the more complicated cases in which the cost includes transportation or the road conditions, since those situation does not affected the real consideration of this problem.
- $profit(b_i)$: an variable that denotes the output profit of the land block b_i;

Therefore, in this recommendation algorithm design, our objective is to maximum the object function:

$$U = \sum_{i=1}^{n} profit(e_i)b_i \qquad (1)$$

where $b_i = 1$ if e_i is selected, 0 otherwise.
which subject to the following constraints:

$$profit(e_i) = property\_profit(e_i) + relation\_profit(e_i) \qquad (2)$$

where *property_profit* represents the profit obtained from the output of the land block which is derived from Eq. 3 and the *relation_profit* denotes the relation between the land block in consideration and all the other neighboring land blocks which could be derived from Eq. 4.

$$property\_profit(e_i) = \sum_{j=1}^{k} f_j(e_{ij}) \qquad (3)$$

$$j \in [1, k]$$

$$relation\_profit(e_i) = \sum_{m=1, m \neq i}^{n} g(e_i, e_m) \qquad (4)$$

In some cases, it may require the total area be below a certain number, as well as the total purchase cost must not exceed a certain amount, these requirements would become constraint:

$$\max total\_profit = \sum_{i=1}^{n} \left(\sum_{j=1}^{k} f_j(e_{ij}) + \sum_{m=i+1}^{n} g(e_i, e_m) \right) b_i \qquad (5)$$

In crop investment projects, investors are primarily concerned with land pH, illumination time, rainfall and other attributes, because these attributes will affect the growth of crops, thus affecting the output. Furthermore for different types of farms, the same set of attributes my produce different impacts. Usually the profit and cost function by land attributes will not be strictly a fixed value, usually a value interval, so the impact of land property value gains on investment projects, can be transformed into investment needs and the extent of land property fit impact on investment income $f_j(x_{ij}) = a_j demand_j(x_{ij}) s_i,$

then

$$property\_profit(e_i) = \sum_{j=1}^{k} f_j(e_{ij}) = \sum_{j=1}^{k} a_j demand_j(e_{ij}) s_i \qquad (6)$$

$$j \in [1, k]$$

$$relation\_profit(e_i) = \sum_{m=1,m\neq i}^{n} g(e_i, e_m) = \omega * relation(b, e) \tag{7}$$

Investment projects are also affected by the relationship between the lands for investment income, which primarily reflect the impact of the distance between the lands. It generally requires the distance between plots as small as possible to minimize the cost of transportation, management and operations. Based on the above assumption, the relationship between land blocks are formulated as follow:

$$relation(b, e) = \sum_{i=1}^{n} b_i \sqrt{\left(x_i - \frac{\sum_{i=1}^{n} s_i x_i b_i}{\sum_{i=1}^{n} s_i b_i}\right)^2 + \left(y_i - \frac{\sum_{i=1}^{n} s_i y_i b_i}{\sum_{i=1}^{n} s_i b_i}\right)^2} \tag{8}$$

Then the final solution:

$$\max total\_profit = \sum_{i=1}^{n} \sum_{j=1}^{k} a_j demand_j(e_{ij}) s_i b_i + \sum_{i=1}^{n} b_i \omega \sqrt{\left(x_i - \frac{\sum_{i=1}^{n} s_i x_i b_i}{\sum_{i=1}^{n} s_i b_i}\right)^2 + \left(y_i - \frac{\sum_{i=1}^{n} s_i y_i b_i}{\sum_{i=1}^{n} s_i b_i}\right)^2}$$

$$where \begin{cases} \sum_{i=1}^{n} e_{ij} b_i \leq c_j \\ j \in [1, k] \\ b_i = 0, 1 \\ \dots \end{cases} \tag{9}$$

4 Heuristic Algorithm

While the formulation in previous section obtains the optimal set of land pieces, it is infeasible when the scale of this problem grows due to the exponential complexity. This is especially true when the total number of land pieces is very large. Therefore, we propose in addition to the previous formulation a effective heuristic algorithm that are not only close to the optimal solution but the time it consumes grows polynonimally with the scale of the problem. The algorithm is shown as follows.

In this algorithm, we start from selecting the blocks with the highest profit as the seed blocks and expand from those blocks. The reason behind it is that the blocks with the highest profit are either the largest blocks or the one with the highest the profit rate, and typically the area where they are located exhibit the same features. Thus it would be good seeds for our selections. For each high profit block selected we select the one from all the neighboring blocks with the longest shared bordering line. In this way the connection cost for each neighboring block is minimized. Once the right neighboring block is selected we merge the two block into a single block and put it back in to the

1.   Set T, O as null, bo as zero;
2.   For each b in B, if b satisfy the basic requirements, put b into T.
3.   Calculate the direct profit from each block in T.
4.   Repeat: select the one with biggest profit b_i in T
5.   Repeat: select the one b_j from T with largest shared border with b_i
6.   If profit b_i and b_j combined are not below bo
7.   if $bo ==$ zero, set bo as $profit(b_i+b_j)$
8.   otherwise, set bo as $bo/2 + profit(b_i+b_j)/2$
9.   remove b_i and b_j from T
10.   insert b_i+b_j as a new block into T
11.   end if
12.   end repeat
13. end repeat
14. Sort all the element in T in descending order of the proft
15. Repeat: select from b from T
16.   If $O+b$ satisfy the requirements
17.   insert b into O
18. end repeat
19. end

pool of land blocks and wait to be selected again. The loop for merging with the neighboring blocks will not end until no more neighbors could be found. When the repeat loop ends, we can expect that the pool of lands would have different land blocks that were produced from the merging. The lands will be merged to form a cluster of islands, which are not connected to each other. Then the task left is to select the right islands to form the output, which is done by the loop from line 15 to line 18.

5   Simulation

In the simulation, a kiwi planting farming project is set as an example to simulate the above algorithms. We assume an investor need to set up a farm focus on cultivation of kiwi for the purpose of selling kiwifruit as it main source of income. In this case, investors are primarily concerned with the impact of kiwifruit growing and production of land property, including plots pH, potassium content, exposure time, of course, land area and land prices are all the key attributes that should be taken into consideration in the decision making process of land acquiring. In the simulation, the set of lands available for selection is randomly generated. We compare the profit as obtained by the integer linear programming (ILP) formulation and the heuristic algorithm.

Figures 1 and 2 show the comparison between the ILP and the heuristic algorithm by the results obtained and the time consumption. As we can see from Fig. 1, the profit obtained by the heuristics algorithm is by average less than 10 % below the optimal solution. However, as shown in Fig. 2, although ILP global optimal solution is obtained, as the solution scale increases, the time consumption grows exponentially. As the scale after solving reach 50, the time required to solve more than 50 h, which hard to accept. The heuristic algorithm's time complexity is O (n3).

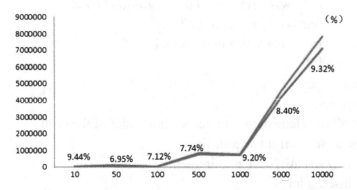

Fig. 1. Comparison between ILP and heuristic algorithm (profit)

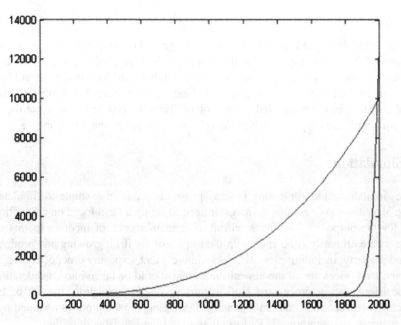

Fig. 2. Comparison between ILP and heuristic algorithm (time)

6 Conclusion

This paper proposes an efficient recommendation algorithm that takes both the space attributes and other properties of farmland pieces into consideration and produce best selection for the intended potential new farmers or investors with customized object functions. The problem is formulated with integer linear programming equations and an effective heuristic algorithm is also proposed. The simulation shows that the proposed heuristic algorithm obtained results close to the optimal solution while significantly reduce the time consumption. The heuristic is especially important considering the huge amount of available lands in practice.

References

1. Mu, R., Giles, J.: Village political economy, land tenure insecurity, and the rural to urban migration decision: evidence from China. World Bank Policy Research Working Paper 7080 (2014)
2. Li, L.: Land titling in China: Chengdu experiment and its consequences. Chin. Econ. J. **5**(1), 47–64 (2012)
3. Ellickson, R.C.: Costs of complex land titles: two examples from China. Brigham-Kanner Prop. Rights Conf. J. **1**, 1–281 (2012)
4. Hsing, Y.: The Great Urban Transformation: Politics of Land and Property in China. Oxford University Press Catalogue, Oxford (2012)

Erratum to: Normalized Cross-Match: Pattern Discovery Algorithm from Biofeedback Signals

Xueyuan Gong[1]([⊠]), Simon Fong[1], Yain-Whar Si[1],
Robert P. Biuk-Aghai[1], Raymond K. Wong[2],
and Athanasios V. Vasilakos[3]

[1] Department of Computer and Information Science,
University of Macau, Macau, China
{yb47453, ccfong, fstasp, robertb}@umac.mo
[2] School of Computer Science and Engineering,
University of New South Wales, Sydney, Australia
wong@cse.unsw.edu.au
[3] Department of Computer Science, Electrical and Space Engineering,
Lulea University of Technology, Lulea, Sweden
athanasios.vasilakos@ltu.se

Erratum to:
Chapter 14 in: H. Cao et al. (Eds.):
Trends and Applications in Knowledge Discovery and Data Mining, LNAI 9794, DOI: 10.1007/978-3-319-42996-0_14

The spelling of the fourth author's name was incorrect. Instead of "Robert P. Biuk-Agha" it should be read as "Robert P. Biuk-Aghai". The original chapter was corrected.

The updated original online version for this chapter can be found at
DOI: 10.1007/978-3-319-42996-0_14

Author Index